WISCHNITZER'S RESIDENCY MANUAL

Residency is a defining period in a physician's life because it is the decisive stage for personal growth, intellectual challenge, and emotional stress. It is a major transitional period transforming a medical student into a practice-ready physician. This role change for the physician-in-training usually takes place in a new setting and necessitates coping with conflicting demands, heavy responsibilities, and long work hours. Adding to the resident's burden is the ongoing need to manage financial, social, and work demands.

This manual was designed to help medical students in this final critical segment of their journey to becoming practicing physicians. It will enhance the students' awareness of the potential obstacles along the way and provide them with guidance on how to avoid them. The book includes selecting an appropriate specialty, maximizing the chances of being chosen, surviving residency, and beginning practice.

Dr. Saul Wischnitzer, a former Chairman and Professor of Anatomy, has written 10 books in the field of biomedicine and published about 50 scientific papers. He taught at, among various institutions, New York Medical College and the Hadassah Medical School in Jerusalem. He also served for nearly two decades as a Premedical Advisor.

Dr. Wischnitzer has been a major contributor to medical education. His *Guide to Medical and Dental Schools*, which recently appeared in an 11th edition, is the most popular guidance manual for premeds. A second edition of his *Survival Guide for Medical Students* is in preparation. *Wischnitzer's Residency Manual* will serve to assist medical students completing the final, lengthy, postgraduate training interlude facing prospective physicians.

Edith Wischnitzer, Research Associate for this project, has been actively involved in the publication of many of the senior author's books.

Wischnitzer's Residency Manual

Selecting, Securing, Surviving, Succeeding

Saul Wischnitzer

Edith Wischnitzer

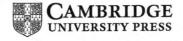

CAMBRIDGE
UNIVERSITY PRESS

CAMBRIDGE
UNIVERSITY PRESS

32 Avenue of the Americas, New York NY 10013-2473, USA

Cambridge University Press is part of the University of Cambridge.

It furthers the University's mission by disseminating knowledge in the pursuit of education, learning and research at the highest international levels of excellence.

www.cambridge.org
Information on this title: www.cambridge.org/9780521675161

First published 2006

A catalogue record for this publication is available from the British Library

Library of Congress Cataloguing in Publication data

Wischnitzer, Saul.
Wischnitzer's residency manual : selecting, securing, surviving, succeeding / Saul Wischnitzer, Edith Wischnitzer.
      p. ; cm.
Includes bibliographical references and index.
ISBN-13: 978-0-521-67516-1 (pbk.)
ISBN-10: 0-521-67516-2 (pbk.)
1. Residents (Medicine) – Handbooks, manuals, etc.   I. Wischnitzer, Edith.   II. Title.
III. Title: Residency manual.
[DNLM: 1. Internship and Residency.   2. Vocational Guidance.   W20W811w   2006]
RA972.W57   2006
610'.92 – dc22   2006002831

ISBN 978-0-521-67516-1 Paperback

This book is dedicated
to our
children and grandchildren,
who have brought us
genuine joy.
May they be blessed with good health
and much happiness.

ACKNOWLEDGMENTS

We are very pleased to acknowledge the invaluable computer assistance of our son, Judiah M. Wischnitzer, and the encouragement of our friends, Melvin N. Zalefsky, M.D., and Michael S. Frank, M.D., both of the Albert Einstein College of Medicine.

Contents

Tables and Forms

Tables

Forms

Preface

Residency is the defining period in a physician's life. This is because it is the decisive stage for personal maturation and professional growth, as well as a time of intellectual challenge and emotional stress. It represents the major transitional interlude during which the graduated medical student is transformed into a practice-ready physician. This role change for the physician-in-training usually takes place in a new setting. Moreover, it necessitates coping with conflicting demands, heavy responsibilities, and long work hours. Adding to the resident's burden is the simultaneous need to manage acquired medical school debt, retain interpersonal relationships with family and friends, and build new ties to colleagues and supervisors. Consequently, the success of a resident, working under such demanding circumstances, depends to a very large extent on choosing the most appropriate specialty and training at a desirable facility. Both of these decisive factors are to a large extent under the resident's control.

In view of the very limited free time available to medical students, the ability to focus their attention on concerns relative to residency is quite restricted. Thus, it is important to provide prospective residents, *in a single volume*, with this wide-ranging residency guidance manual. This book is designed to facilitate their successful journey through a very demanding process that critically affects their professional future. It is especially written to meet the goal of providing invaluable advice and information that will impact very favorably on residents, by facilitating their journey both professionally and personally.

To ensure adequate coverage of the subject, the book considers all four major elements of residency. Postgraduate medical training initially involves *selecting* the most appropriate specialty compatible with your interests and abilities. The book next aims to maximize your chances of *securing* a residency appointment at an appropriate program. It then offers you concrete advice on *surviving* the rigors of a residency. Finally, the book considers the issues to be faced after your residency ends, so as to initiate your *succeeding* in practice.

Given the time constraints of medical students, the information provided is highly organized and concisely presented. This book will enhance your awareness of the many potential obstacles along the way and provide you with advice on how to avoid them. It is also designed to make your life as a resident more manageable and thus fulfilling, thereby contributing to professional growth and career satisfaction.

The career path you have undertaken is very challenging, highly responsible, and potentially deeply rewarding. After finishing the premedical and medical school phases, you have completed about two-thirds of the long journey toward becoming a practicing physician. This book is designed to be your road map for the final, critical segment toward this goal. We wish you much success.

Saul Wischnitzer, Ph.D.
Edith Wischnitzer

Message to the Reader

The challenge that you face as a medical student is enormous. You will be forced to make critical decisions as to your future professional life. These will impact very significantly on you and your family's personal life for years to come. This book is designed to assist you significantly in the decision-making process. To be successful, it is essential to be strongly motivated to take the issue of postgraduate training seriously early on, even if committing yourself to any specific specialty is not imminent. It is especially important that you proceed with residency planning in an organized and timely manner. To achieve this goal, a timetable is presented below for your guidance and to facilitate this vital process.

Residency attainment timetable while in medical school

FIRST YEAR

■ Establish a diary to begin to record *briefly* any exceptional experiences, impressions, and feelings you have as you proceed through each year of medical school.

■ Seek to establish friendly relationships with faculty, residents, and upper-level students who can provide you with useful information regarding postgraduate training planning.

■ If possible, find a suitable advisor/mentor, even at this early stage.

■ When time permits, such as during holidays and weekends, seek to gain some exposure to specialties by joining a hospital treatment team or a physician making rounds.

■ If possible, try to participate in a medically oriented extracurricular activity, such as a free health clinic in your vicinity.

■ Focus your efforts not only on mastering the material being taught, but also on securing attractive grades. For the latter, obtaining proficiency in test taking can be especially helpful.

■ Focus on acquiring good study habits (if you have not done so already) to facilitate your efforts to excel in your performance.

POST-FIRST-YEAR SUMMER

■ Although having a relaxing vacation is useful, securing research experience will be especially valuable when applying for a residency appointment, especially in certain specialties.

■ Make a self-assessment as to your performance thus far, noting your strengths and weaknesses. Determine any areas where improvement can be made (e.g., time management, study, or test-taking skills).

■ Seek to become informed about current events in health care by reading appropriate medical journals and relevant newspaper articles. Discuss the issue of the provision of health care with your family physician and others that you know to gauge how it may impact you in the future.

SECOND YEAR

■ If you haven't as yet selected an advisor/mentor you should to do so now. The help you get may prove invaluable for both your professional and personal life.

■ Continue to update your diary with relevant impressions of important experiences, especially those related to clinical medicine.

■ Continue to focus on excelling in your studies as the academic year proceeds.

■ Seek information on specialty options from upper-class students and Internet sources, supplementing that found in this book.

■ Develop a study plan for Step 1 of the USMLE, whose results may prove critical to your chances for success in securing a residency, of choice.

■ Review your diary notes and see if there are any preliminary conclusions you can draw concerning your interests and abilities.

THIRD YEAR

■ Make a serious effort to briefly record your reactions, both emotional and intellectual, to your clerkship experiences. The information can prove decisive in the residency selection process.

■ Identify clerkships that are especially appealing and those that are clearly not so.

■ When you achieve a favorable performance grade and evaluations in a clerkship, secure a letter of recommendation from the supervising attending for your file in the dean of students' office. It will prove valuable when a composite dean's letter has to be prepared on your behalf during your senior year, for submission to residency programs.

■ Start to develop a resume for use when you apply later in the year for your residency appointment.

◼ Participate in specialty identification programs such as the Glaxo approach and complete the specialty selection protocol presented in this book (see Chapter 2).

◼ Start planning your senior year curriculum in consultation with your advisor/mentor, which permits flexibility in choosing electives of special interest. Choose electives that will be of value relative to your specialty selection process.

◼ Secure and complete the student agreement for the NRMP.

◼ In *May* you should initiate contacts with prospective residency programs to secure relevant information from them.

FOURTH YEAR

◼ In *June* or *July* prepare a preliminary list of residency programs that are of interest to you and then meet with your advisor/mentor to discuss the appropriateness of your choices.

◼ During *July* arrange that all letters of recommendation from faculty members are dispatched to the dean of students' office. Be sure that you have submitted a request that the dean of students prepare his/her letter in support of your residency applications.

◼ Secure a letter of recommendation from the chairperson of the department in which you seek a specialty. He/she should also be provided with a copy of your resume at the time that you make your request.

◼ Develop a system to accurately keep track of your residency application activities.

◼ In *September* prepare and review your resume and personal statement with your advisor/mentor.

◼ Make sure that the NRMP receives your agreement materials by *mid-November*.

◼ Arrange for residency interviews at suitable dates during the interview season, which usually extends from *November* to *January*.

◼ Your Rank Order List should be prepared and reviewed with your advisor/mentor by the end of *January*. This list should be submitted by *mid-February*.

◼ Match Day is in *mid-March*.

◼ Letters of appointment or a contract are sent out by residency program directors within a month after Match Day.

Bear in mind that although the above timetable is a useful guideline, you should seek to meet all deadlines as early as possible. This will minimize any difficulties that may arise from unforeseen events that interfere with your scheduled residency planning activities.

Abbreviations

Note: Many of the terms listed here are defined in the glossary.

AAMC	Association of American Medical Colleges
AHA	American Hospital Association
AMA	American Medical Association
AMWA	American Medical Women's Association
AOA	American Osteopathic Association
CaRMS	Canadian Resident Matching Service
COTH	The Council of Teaching Hospitals
C. V.	Curriculum vitae – a resume
ECFMG	Educational Commission for Foreign Medical Graduates
ERAS	Electronic Residency Application Service
EVMG	Exchange-visitor international medical graduate
FLEX	Federation Licensing Examination
FMG	Foreign national physicians who are IMGs
FMGEMS	Foreign Medical Graduate Examination
FNIMG	Foreign national international medical graduates
FREIDA	AMA Fellowship and Residency Electronic Interactive Database Access
FSMB	Federation of State Medical Boards of the United States
HMO	Health maintenance organization
HPSP	Health Professions Scholarship Program
IAP-66	Visa document issued to a J-1 visa holder
IMG	International medical graduate
IPA	Individual provider association
LCME	Liaison Committee on Medical Education
MCO	Managed care organization
NBME	National Board of Medical Examiners

NBOE	National Board of Osteopathic Examiners
NBOME	National Board of Osteopathic Medical Examiners
NRMP	National Residency Matching Program
OSCE	Objective structured clinical examination
PC	Professional Corporation
PGY-1	Postgraduate year-1 of a residency program
PPO	Preferred provider organization
ROL	Rank Order List of residency appointment preferences of the applicant
ROLIC	Rank Order List input code
SPEX	Special purpose examination
TOEFL	Test of English as a Foreign Language
USIMG	A U.S. citizen whose medical degree was not approved by the LCME
USMLE	United States Medical Licensing Examination

PART ONE

SELECTING A SPECIALITY

I F YOU ASK COLLEGE STUDENTS TAKING THE REQUIRED PREMEDICAL SCIENCE courses and studying for the MCAT exam why they are doing so, the obvious answer that they will give is, "I want to become a physician." The focus of these students' efforts, justifiably, is on getting into medical school, preferably the one of their choice. They quite naturally must defer the issue of what specialty they wish to work in as physicians for an appropriate later time. Once they are enrolled in medical school, this major issue comes to the foreground all too soon.

Making the selection of an area for postgraduate training is a key life decision that requires very careful consideration. It is a complex task, for it involves (a) candid self-assessment of your interests, abilities, and lifestyle needs; (b) becoming knowledgeable as to the many specialty options available; and (c) careful execution of the varied components of the timetable relative to securing a residency. (See front matter, *Message To the Reader* section.)

Professional activities associated with the practice of medicine are extremely diverse, medicine being a composite of many areas of specialization. Also, there is a wide disparity between specialty activities of, for example, an allergist and a urologist in their approach, skills, and practice (although though they have had a common educational core of knowledge and experience). Complicating the choosing of a specialty is the fact that the exposure of students to specialties and subspecialties during medical school is very brief and limited in scope. Moreover, it takes place essentially in the context of hospital and clinic settings. Although anesthesiologists and pathologists have hospital-based practices, most specialties are primarily office-based or are combined office-based and hospital-based practices. Thus career decisions are commonly made by medical students based on inadequate knowledge of the overall realities of medical practice. This limitation goes as far as not considering some areas for specialization because the prospective resident may not even be aware of their existence.

It therefore behooves medical students, first of all, to acquaint themselves with the very wide spectrum of specialty opportunities available. If you assess yourself and compare your personal abilities and interests with those that the specialty calls for, making a choice becomes much easier and more realistic. The six chapters of Part One that follow will facilitate becoming knowledgeable as to possible career choices and familiarizing yourself with how best to make a determination as to what area is most suitable for you.

1 | Considering Your Options

Overview

For the greater part of the first half of the 20th century, graduates of U.S. medical schools would automatically complete one of several types of internships. Most of these doctors would then directly enter practice. This was possible because there was a limited amount of medical knowledge available, and physicians could therefore treat patients with a wide variety of illnesses. Specialization was an uncommon path for the bulk of medical school graduates. If undertaken, it frequently involved overseas postgraduate training. This obviously had limited appeal for most graduates.

The situation changed dramatically in the second half of the century. The internship period was transformed into postgraduate year one (PGY-1). Major and remarkable advances in medical knowledge and technology mandated that graduating physicians secure postgraduate training to acquire the background and skills needed to serve as generalists or specialists. This situation usually requires medical students to make challenging and decisive career choices at some point during their undergraduate medical education. The choice that has to be made is among three fundamental options. Each choice will have its own advantages and liabilities. Furthermore, each path will require subsequent difficult decisions as you narrow your focus. Your basic options are selecting a

■ Generalist track or

■ Specialist track or

■ Transitional year.

Each of these will be discussed separately.

Choosing a generalist track

Over the past several decades, with the onset of radical changes in health care management, the position of the generalist physician has assumed much greater significance in the provision of patient services. This came about because the long-standing, very costly health care system had strongly emphasized specialty and subspecialty treatment. To improve the situation, an ongoing effort exists to establish a more equitable balance between the number of generalists and specialists entering the profession.

Generalists are viewed as those engaged in primary care specialties, namely, family practice, internal medicine, and general pediatrics. These areas are characterized by

■ Treating a wide range of illnesses affecting different body systems.

■ Providing ample opportunity to offer continuity of care.

■ Commonly providing services in an ambulatory setting.

■ Usually treating readily curable illnesses of children or adults.

■ Facing simple technological demands in the course of one's practice.

■ Having to treat patients with both medical and psychological problems.

■ Serving as community-based practitioners, with local hospital affiliations.

■ Responding to the needs of patients with multiple illnesses.

One can decide between the three primary care options noted earlier by a process of elimination. Thus those strongly interested in children will obviously choose pediatrics. Those wishing a wider scope of activity, such as working with adults, will elect internal medicine as a specialty. On the other hand, for those seeking to serve the widest segment of the patient population, entering family practice is the appropriate choice. It should be noted that the three aforementioned specialty areas are discussed in detail in Chapter 3, whereas the basic subject of choosing a specialty is covered in Chapter 2.

One should be aware that diagnosing problems in primary care specialties is not necessarily straightforward, because a decisive answer is not always readily and clearly available. Thus a tolerance for practicing, at times, in a state of ambiguity is highly desirable for those serving as generalists.

Choosing a specialist track

Specialists are considered experts in their fields. In this book, areas of clinical practice are categorized into (a) major specialties (Chapter 3) and (b) three groups of subspecialties. The latter comprise of medical, surgical, and other subspecialties (Chapters 4, 5, and 6, respectively). It should be recognized that there are also physicians devoting themselves full time to administrative and research activities.

An alternative, but less clearly defined, classification scheme involves characterizing specialists as secondary, tertiary, and support professionals. In addition to these three areas, the other group is obviously primary care specialists or generalists. In this categorization, both specialists and subspecialists are placed in either secondary or tertiary care categories.

Secondary care specialists are exemplified by general surgeons and pediatric subspecialists. They secure patients by referral and provide services in treatment or consultation modes, and their practices are largely hospital-based. They usually have an association with their patients for a limited period of time.

Tertiary care specialists can be exemplified by ophthalmologists who treat only patients with retina problems or orthopedic surgeons who are involved exclusively with joint replacement procedures. These specialists usually have a practice that is restricted to a single structural entity in a limited area of the body. The medical problems they face may be quite challenging, and patients usually are seen by referral for both consultation and treatment. Such practices frequently require a high degree of specific technical expertise.

Clinically supportive specialists are pathologists, radiologists, and anesthesiologists. They facilitate other physicians in carrying out their diagnostic and treatment responsibilities. Work in these fields may have no or merely short-term patient contact. They work primarily in hospitals, medical centers, or private facilities. Technology usually plays a vital role in their activities.

Choosing a transitional year

A transitional year is a broad-based training period, comparable to the third year of medical school, except that a PGY-1 resident's level of responsibility is obviously more meaningful than that of a clerkship.

A little less than one-fourth of medical students make their specialty choices when they are in their preclinical years. Almost half of them do so when they are in their third year of medical school and nearly another fourth do so during their fourth year. Less then 10% defer making a specialty choice until some time after graduation. Uncertainty as to the appropriate selection or a sense of insecurity that an inappropriate decision may result in career failure inhibits some students from making a selection regarding postgraduate training.

It should also be recognized that for several specialties, one can apply *only* during PGY-1 for admission to residency programs. In such a case an internship-type year is needed as a prerequisite. This is the situation for such specialties as anesthesiology, ophthalmology, and radiology. In such cases, deferring a decision in order to undertake a transitional year of postgraduate training may be advisable. Moreover, the clinical experience gained during an interlude when one is genuinely uncertain about future plans can for some prove especially valuable. Thus, a transitional year can provide a suitable alternative under specific circumstances. Should these exist, this option then merits careful consideration.

There is, however, a negative side to the transitional year. To use this year simply because of a desire to procrastinate in making a career decision can be self-defeating. This is because for most PGY-2 (advanced matches) you need to obtain an appointment before the end of the senior year of medical school. Moreover, many specialties (internal medicine, pediatrics, etc.) do not accept the transitional year as counting toward completion of a PGY-1 residency requirement. Thus, even after gaining enhanced clinical competence during a transitional year, you might be forced to repeat it to gain entrance into a desired residency program. To be forced to serve a second internship year is obviously a very unappealing prospect. Another reason against electing to take a transitional year is that your career goals remain unfocused and your future plans are in a state of limbo, which is psychologically challenging.

An alternative approach that obviates these difficulties is to seek a preliminary rather than a categorical residency in medicine or surgery. Such programs can meet the PGY-1 requirements in these two areas as well as their many subspecialties. Preliminary residencies are not excessively difficult to secure.

You should be aware that there is a risk that the intense demands and burdens of a transitional internship can be so excessive as to motivate an individual to accept a residency appointment even in a field of secondary interest. This is done merely because it serves to resolve a burdensome career dilemma, albeit in a far less than ideal way. This approach should be avoided, because the consequences of the wrong choice can very negatively impact an individual's professional life in terms of work-related satisfaction.

An additional negative consequence of the transitional year may be induced by trying to resolve the residency problem by seeking to apply to two specialties simultaneously. This has its own inherent risk, namely that your ploy will be uncovered. You may then find that no attractive program in either field seeks your services as a resident and it may therefore prove difficult to secure adequate training.

2 | Selecting Your Specialty

Overview

Medicine as a profession is going through turbulent times. Medical education and patient reimbursement are among issues in a state of flux. Nevertheless, as a medical student, you can exercise considerable control over your personal career. This is because your choice of a specialty will determine (1) how long a training period you will have, (2) how many programs will be accessible to you, and (3) the geographic area of your training site. To achieve a favorable outcome of the specialty selection process, careful planning is essential.

Medical students, being intensively involved in demanding educational activities, may find themselves pressured into choosing a specialty with undue haste, not giving it the thought that this very important decision deserves. Some elect to choose the specialty of a physician they admire, or of their medical school mentor, trying merely to imitate a person looked upon as a role model. These motivating factors present serious risks, due to the inherent differences that usually exist between individuals, and the sought-after results may not materialize.

The specifics of choosing a specialty will be discussed later in this chapter, but some generalizations are in order at this point. In seeking to establish a *tentative* choice of specialty, try to determine what approach to medicine appeals to you most.

- Do you prefer to focus on wellness or on sickness?
- Are you interested in treating adults of varying ages?
- Do you prefer short- or long-term patient relationships?
- Do you favor contact with peers in your profession or with patients?
- Do you prefer a contemplative or decisive approach to solving problems?
- Do you require a professional and personal lifestyle that is organized and orderly?
- Do you prefer the challenges of professional activities that are unpredictable?

Your responses to such basic questions can help you focus on the type of specialty that you will find most satisfying. Some preliminary guidelines that will assist you in your selection process are noted below:

- If the concept of maintaining wellness is appealing, then investigate such fields as family medicine, pediatrics, internal medicine, and obstetrics/gynecology. In these areas long-term patient relationships are a common feature. There is also a special need for being empathetic and providing counseling in such fields.
- Should you prefer long-term patient relationships in the context of holistic treatment and desire a stable lifestyle, then fields such as physical medicine/rehabilitation, psychiatry, or rheumatology can prove satisfying.
- If you seek a well-organized practice with regular hours but also want relatively short-term patient contact, then consider dermatology carefully.
- Some physicians are interested in the concept of wellness, but are not committed to close personal patient relationships. Rather they are more interested in maintaining the health of society as a whole. For these groups, public health, general preventive medicine, and infectious diseases offer an appealing outlet for their interests. In these areas one can work with groups of individuals to help resolve significant medical problems.
- Those who feel they would like the satisfaction provided by the dual aspects of medicine and surgery can benefit from a career in ophthalmology, otolaryngology, or obstetrics/gynecology.
- There are individuals who seek to have a major impact on people without a long-term relationship. For them, such fields as emergency medicine and surgery (including its many subspecialties) will be especially appealing.
- For those who prefer interacting with their peers rather than with patients, specialties such as pathology and radiology are particularly attractive. However, these fields do not have much prestige or power in the medical hierarchy.
- For those who seek intellectual challenge, a field such as neurology is an attractive option.

■ For individuals with good manual dexterity for whom creativity is important, plastic surgery can offer personal fulfillment.

■ For those who favor procedures and data analysis, gastroenterology will be especially appealing.

Specialties and subspecialties

There are numerous specialties and subspecialties, as will be seen in Table 2.1. New areas are still emerging and some of these are described briefly at the end of Chapter 6. To receive recognized status, a specialty needs to gain recognition by the American Board of Medical Specialties (ABMS). This is the nationally recognized organization that can confer official status allowing certification of MDs who have satisfactorily demonstrated the level of competency established for the field.

The ABMS is a not-for-profit organization, consisting of 24 distinct medical specialty boards, which is concerned with overseeing certification in the United States. Its mission, for well over half a century, has been to improve the quality of medical care in this country. It does so by assisting member boards in developing and implementing educational standards to evaluate and certify physician specialists. Consequently, the ABMS is recognized by accreditation organizations as the source of board certified specialists for accreditation purposes.

The 24 specialty boards recognized by the AMBS are identified in Table 2.1 and their associated subspecialties are shown in the adjacent column. These specialties and many of their subspecialties will be discussed in detail in four groupings. These are major specialties, (Chapter 3), medical subspecialties (Chapter 4), surgical subspecialties (Chapter 5), and other specialties (Chapter 6).

General considerations

Five general considerations associated with selecting a specialty need to be considered. Each of these will be briefly discussed.

1. Be realistic. Many medical students set their specialty goals in their youth. For some this desire, after a while, can become a firm inner conviction. It may have been brought on by the favorable contact with a specialist or in response to a serious family illness. In any case, such early plans need to be carefully reevaluated at your current, more mature stage of life, when you are more familiar with your personal assets and limitations. Thus, if you are determined to become, for example, an ophthalmologist and find that your fine motor skills involving hand–eye coordination or your color vision is somewhat impaired, you need to seriously reconsider your plans for entering this field. It behooves medical students to assess their career goals bearing in mind any personal permanent limitations that they currently have.

Table 2.1 Specialties and subspecialties

Specialty	Subspecialty
Allergy & immunology	Clinical & laboratory immunology
Anesthesiology	Critical care medicine Pain
Colon & rectal surgery	———
Dermatology	Dermatologicpathology Clinical laboratory dermatological immunology Dermatological pathology
Emergency medicine	Medical toxicology Pediatric emergency medicine Sports medicine
Family practice	Geriatric medicine Sports medicine
Internal medicine	Cardiovascular disease Critical care medicine Endocrinology, diabetes, and metabolism Gastroenterology Geriatric medicine Hematology Infectious diseases Medical oncology Nephrology Pulmonary medicine Rheumatology
Medical genetics	Molecular genetic pathology
Neurological surgery	———
Neurology	Child neurology
Nuclear medicine	———
Obstetrics & gynecology	Critical care medicine Gynecologic oncology Maternal & fetal medicine Reproductive endocrinology
Ophthalmology	Retina-vitreous Glaucoma Pediatric ophthalmology Neuro-ophthalmology
Orthopedic surgery	Hand surgery
Otolaryngology	Otology Pediatric otolaryngology Plastic surgery within the head & neck
Pathology	Blood bank/transfusion medicine Chemical pathology Cytopathology Dermatologic pathology Forensic pathology

Specialty	Subspecialty
	Immunopathology
	Medical microbiology
	Medical genetic pathology
	Neuropathology
	Pediatric pathology
Pediatrics	Adolescent medicine
	Clinical & laboratory immunology
	Development-behavioral pediatrics
	Neonatal–perinatal medicine
	Neurodevelopmental disabilities
	Pediatric cardiology
	Pediatric critical care
	Pediatric emergency medicine
	Pediatric endocrinology
	Pediatric gastroenterology
	Pediatric hematology–oncology
	Pediatric nephrology
	Pediatric pulmonology
	Pediatric rheumatology
	Sports medicine
Physical medicine & rehabilitation	Pain management
	Pediatric rehabilitation medicine
	Spinal cord injury medicine
Plastic surgery	Hand surgery
	Plastic surgery within the head & neck
Public health and preventive medicine	Occupational medicine
Psychiatry	Addiction psychiatry
	Child & adolescent psychiatry
	Forensic psychiatry
	Geriatric psychiatry
	Clnical neuropsychiatry
	Pain management
Radiology	Musculo-skeletal radiology
	Neuroradiology
	Nuclear radiology
	Pediatric radiology
	Vascular interventional radiology
Surgery	Pediatric surgery
	Surgical critical care
	Vascular surgery
Thoracic surgery	———
Urology	———

It is essential to evaluate to what extent any significant handicap would limit you in a specific field. What counts is not only the type of work you would like to do, but your capacity for doing such work well.

2. Determine your interests. Students have many novel and diversified experiences during their initial two years in medical school. This is especially true because exposure to patients, clinical issues, and some electives commonly takes place during this interval, if to a limited extent. To benefit from such experiences, keep a brief, accurate log of the meaningful ones. Jot down their nature, your impressions, and how they impacted your thinking. A collection of such comments can be a useful starting point for serious consideration of specialty options. As you proceed through clinical rotations, briefly note important impressions in your log as they occur: what experiences provide you with special satisfaction, fit your innate interests, and allow you to demonstrate your unique skills. These can significantly influence the choice of a specialty and reinforce or negate your initial thoughts as to possible residency fields. Such a diary may require an investment of time, but ultimately it may pay large dividends when it comes to selecting a specialty.

3. Seek a mentor's advice. After having selected a compatible mentor early on (see Chapter 7), see him/her periodically so that they can really get to know you. Because mentors usually are faculty members, they can provide an insight as to what demands and responsibilities different specialties entail or put you in contact with someone knowledgeable who can do so. Your mentor should be able to give an objective insight into your own personality, abilities, and interests, which should help steer you in an appropriate direction. You should welcome their suggestions on selecting a specialty or on modifying your own choice based on their perception of your innate talents (e.g., changing from adult to pediatric cardiology). The final decision, however, should ultimately be your own.

4. Maximize your grades and USMLE score. These two elements will strongly impact your choice of specialty options. They are used by program directors to assess your potential. The higher they are, the more favorable are your residency appointment chances. Thus, when you are considering the most competitive appointments, low grades in relevant courses or clerkships or a low score on Step I of the USMLE will be a serious impediment to being placed. You should not rely on the prestige of the medical school you are attending to make up for deficiencies in these areas.

5. Get exposure. Be adventurous enough to gain experience in a variety of electives that offer the possibility of broadening your specialty selection choices. Gaining exposure also means getting to know attendings and their daily professional routines, as well as the extent of their career satisfaction. Becoming acquainted with residents and their activities and the motivation for their specialty choices can also help to provide a realistic perspective on a specialty's characteristics.

Timing your specialty choice

There is no set time during medical school when you need to decide on your specialty choice. Obviously, the earlier you arrive at your choice, the less pressure you will find yourself under. However, should you make a premature selection and you may be forced to reconsider if you find another area more appealing.

Starting to think about a specialty early on, even during the second year of medical school, is not premature, but the most serious consideration and decision-making should take place in the third and fourth years.

In spite of their most genuine efforts, some students will not have made their choice even as late as when graduation rolls around. Such individuals have a number of options:

- Completing a transitional year (see Chapter 1).
- Securing a preliminary (rather than categorical) residency.
- Obtaining a Master's in Public Health.
- Devoting a year to research.

Relevant specialty criteria

Selecting a specialty involves taking a wide variety of factors into consideration. Each student will naturally have their own personal priorities as to the importance of the factors discussed below for their situation.

For the present generation of medical students, patient contact is now commonly initiated quite early in the curriculum. Often some clinical exposure takes place even during the first semester of the freshman year. It is most intense during the third, clerkship year, where it is the dominant educational activity. This intimate contact obviously can significantly influence specialty choice. Aside from professional contacts, medical students are influenced by their response to interacting with patients, their evaluation of their ability to assist people, the intellectual challenge of the medical issues they encounter, and the manner in which they respond to them.

In an age where health care management is in a state of flux, it is now more important than ever to take into consideration factors other than the influence of a period of very limited patient contact (viz., clerkships or electives) or the strong positive impression made by a physician role model in the choice of a specialty.

A wide variety of factors deserve attention in considering this issue. Five of these are discussed below.

1. Income prospects. Substantial debt accumulated by almost all medical students is an accepted consequence of undergraduate medical education. Students quite naturally hope to be able to repay their loans from the income they anticipate earning after they start practicing. Moreover, it is a reasonable assumption that a well-established physician's net annual income is, on average, quite substantial (ca. $175,000). For different specialties annual income varies considerably and may also depend on the specific nature of the practice. For procedure-oriented areas such as surgery and anesthesiology, income is significantly higher than average (ca. $215,000). On the other hand, those who are involved in cognitive or thinking specialties such as psychiatry or pediatrics have a significantly lower level of remuneration (ca. $150,000).

Although there may be a linkage between specialty choice and the extent of a student's debt, the evidence in support of this premise is quite inconclusive. Nevertheless, the idea of eliminating debt by selecting a highly remunerative specialty is simplistic. This is because securing a residency appointment in a high-income specialty is problematic, because such residencies are highly competitive. Nevertheless, it needs to be recognized that (a) with interest accruing on loans, there can be a significant increase in a student's total debt over time, (b) it takes usually about 10 years to reach peak earning capacity from the start of a practice, and (c) a lower-income specialty can prolong repayment of a substantial loan. Consequently, it is clear that the issues of specialty choice, income prospects, and debt repayment are quite complex.

2. Challenge of securing a residency. It is readily possible to determine the extent of competition and thus the overall difficulty of securing an appointment in a specific specialty. This can be done by comparing the number of openings with the number of applicants in the past year or two. However, to identify your chances as an individual is far more difficult. This is because they depend on (a) how many interviews you have had, (b) at which institutions they took place, and (c) how confident you are in your judgment when you prepare your Rank Order List for the Match.

By objectively assessing your residency interview performance at each specific site and making a realistic judgment of what the programs seek in a candidate on the basis of the interview, you can prepare a potentially more successful Rank Order List. Consequently you stand a better chance of making the right match and hence being selected for a residency opening at an institution you favor. All of this assumes that your academic record, recommendations, and USMLE Step I scores make you a competitive candidate to start with.

3. Length of training. Length of training factor has the most influence on students considering generalist or support specialist careers. The impact of assuming greater debt because of the demands of extended postgraduate training is one of the considerations in avoiding medical or surgical specialties or subspecialties. It should also be noted that investing more time to attain specialist status does not necessarily correlate with greater income.

4. Lifestyle. The intense work demands on all residents are certainly higher than the standard layman's 35-hour workweek. But there are significant work-time differences among practitioners in various specialties. Thus a recent estimate showed that the overall weekly work schedule in emergency medicine stood at a relatively low 48 hours, whereas that for obstetrics/gynecology was as high as 61 hours. This does not reflect the breakdown between day and night activities, which obviously varies in different specialties.

The variation in work hours between specialties is significant, because there is reason to believe that the residency schedule mimics the work schedule in actual practice. Specialties are available for those who have a desire for intensely paced work, on one hand, and those who prefer a slower-paced regime, on the other.

5. Career prospects. There has been considerable speculation as to future demands for physicians as a whole as well as for personnel needs in varying specialties. Predictions of physician shortages in the past have failed to materialize. Currently a strong case even can be made that a shortage of physicians may even be in the offing.

As to the need for physicians in various specialties, although some trends as to future prospects can be hypothesized, scientific and technological advances in medicine preclude making definitive judgments in this regard. Thus, for example, angioplasty, the opening of clogged coronary arteries by passing a catheter through them, has generated a need for more cardiologists trained in invasive procedures. As a consequence, this development has lowered the need for the services of thoracic surgeons, who are skilled in operative bypass procedures. Speculation along similar lines is applicable to other specialties. Thus demographic changes, which may bring with them a lower birth rate, may generate a need for fewer obstetricians and pediatricians. It becomes apparent from such considerations that future needs for specialists are unpredictable. This is because need is subject to uncontrollable events such as major medical breakthroughs, unexpected newly diagnosed diseases, and changes in demographics or in public attitudes toward health care practitioners and their services. Consequently, it is probably advisable that you place less emphasis on future specialty needs when formulating your career plans.

Specialty selection methods

Selecting a specialty as a future area of practice needs to be viewed from a long-term perspective. The key issue to be faced is whether you will enjoy your professional activities over the long haul, which should last for more than 30 years. Making the proper choice requires becoming familiar with various methods associated with deciding on a specialty and utilizing those that best meet your needs.

Medical students use varying approaches to assess their future career interests. These include the following:

Clinical exposure. Medical students have an opportunity, albeit relatively briefly during their clerkships, to evaluate the nature of the *major* specialties. They can gain some exposure to subspecialties during various stages of medical school by taking electives. The long-established requirement of direct personal participation in clinical care during the course of successive rotations, commonly in the third year, has built-in weaknesses. This is due to the unrealistic nature of the clinical exposure, given that it takes place essentially in an academic setting. The response to a rotation is entirely dependent on the nature of one's clinical experience. This in turn is determined by (a) a student's interaction with their supervising attending physician, (b) the nature of the collaboration with their treatment team of residents, (c) the type of cases being treated, and (d) the extent of responsibility delegated to the student. These four factors can prove exhilarating or disappointing, in whole or in part, depending on unforeseeable circumstances of the specialty in question and the established protocol at the institution as to the content of student responsibilities.

Many successful physicians have obviously made the proper choice by the hit or miss method of relying exclusively on their undergraduate clinical exposure. Unfortunately, others have not fared so well. Thus, although clinical exposure is an approach of considerable value, it is preferable that it not be used as the exclusive criterion for formulating your career decision. It is desirable that it be supplemented by clinic or office practice experience and also enhanced by utilizing one or more of the other approaches described below. This approach can maximize one's chances for making the most appropriate decision.

Interest assessment tests. Many high schools and colleges offer their students interest assessment protocols to ascertain potential career pathways. This approach can also be used to point people in the direction that may be the most appropriate medical specialty.

■ *Strong Vocational Interest Inventory*. This protocol matches student interests with those of practitioners in seven specialties. The results of such tests have been validated by their longstanding use and they have been found to be valuable when taken in the upper years of your medical school studies. Such tests are administered by dean of students' offices at most medical schools. This approach merits your exploration to determine what guidance it can provide you.

■ *Glaxo Wellcome Medical Specialty Profiles*. This book is a key component of this pharmaceutical company's program designed to assist medical students in selecting a specialty. This program seeks to determine a student's decision-making style and provides insights into the essential factors involved in this issue. Almost all medical schools offer this program, which consists of group lectures, videotapes, and decision-making exercises. This program is usually taken during the first half of the third year. Although time-consuming, it is a very worthwhile endeavor and has proven beneficial to many students who have completed it.

■ *Self-Assessment Protocol.* A method for specialty selection is presented below. It can supplement either of the aforementioned approaches in meeting the challenging problem of specialty choice.

A specialty selection protocol

Three approaches to specialty selection, namely, obtaining clinical exposure, completing an interest assessment test, and enrolling in the Glaxo Wellcome Program, were discussed above. A supplementary approach that can prove quite valuable in helping you arrive at a choice of a specialty is the following *self-assessment* protocol, which will be discussed in detail. It should be utilized after employing the other aforementioned specialty selection processes. Because specialty selection is such a critical issue, the protocol has been designed in a logical, structured, and self-validating manner to ensure maximal dependability.

This self-assessment protocol involves the use of two sets of parameters that, when matched, provide guidelines to selecting an appropriate specialty. These parameters are (a) your *professional interests* relative to practicing medicine, surgery, or both and (b) your *personal attributes* relative to those mandated by specific specialties and subspecialties. By matching these two sets of characteristics, using the five-step protocol outlined below, you should be able to identify and then establish the career direction that may be most suited for you.

At this point, it is desirable to understand more fully the rationale behind this protocol before going into its details. Step 1 involves your making a preliminary determination as to which of three major physician career pathways, namely medicine, surgery, or both, you best fit into (or if none of these, see options in Chapter 6). Next you need to establish *a personal reference framework*, based on your interests and abilities (Steps 2 and 3). This is then followed in Step 4 by your identifying the *specific practice areas* that you find to be most appropriate, from one or two categories. These categories are (a) major specialties (Chapter 3, containing medical or medical–surgical areas) and/or medical subspecialties (Chapter 4) and/or surgical subspecialties (Chapter 5). Should it be necessary to validate the suitability of a practice area's attributes to your own, you can use the personal framework as a support tool. Finally, you will need to formulate a prioritized list of the three most suitable practice areas, by coordination with input from other sources (Step 5). A definitive decision as to a specialty can be arrived at after completing a *specialty reality check* (Chapter 8).

The multistep specialty selection protocol consists of:

Step 1. Identifying your major professional pathway: medicine, surgery, or both.

Step 2. Determining an in-depth inventory of your professional interests.

Step 3. Determining a professionally relevant inventory of your personal attributes.

Step 4. Identifying prospective practice areas that best meet your professional needs.

Step 5. Coordinating and validating your specialty choices using multiple sources.

Details regarding each of these five steps are given below.

Step 1. Preliminary identification of medicine, surgery, or both as your career pathway. The practices of medicine and surgery have much in common, which is not surprising, because they are interdependent. They differ, however, in a general way in a number of significant respects. These are obvious from a comparison of major characteristics of both areas, as is shown below:

Characteristics	Medicine	Surgery	Medicine/Surgery
Involves high-risk procedures	no	yes	yes
Requires superior manual dexterity	no	yes	yes
Emphasizes preventive health care	yes	no	yes
Provides intimate personal services	yes	yes	yes
Involves long-term relationships	yes	no	yes
Practice is largely office-based	yes	no	yes

Make your choice by circling the appropriate response for each item and drawing your conclusion from the column that has the predominant number of circles. This should tell you if your interests fit better with medicine, surgery, or a combination of both fields (as is the case for such areas as ophthalmology, otolaryngology, obstetrics/gynecology, and urology).

Step 2. Determine an inventory of your professional interests by self-assessment. It is important to thoughtfully record your professional interests and the intensity of your feelings about them. This will serve as a frame of reference for relating these interests to each of the three major activities of training: medicine, surgery, or both (Step 1), and for better judging your specific practice areas of interest within these three categories.

Proceed to identify and define the extent of your professional interests in the varied activities of practicing physicians, using Form 2.1. These are clustered into five groups. Indicate the extent of your interest by noting *A*—appealing, *T*—tolerable, or *U*—unappealing next to each function.

Form 2.1 Professional interests

Group I: Type of patient treated

_____ Children and adolescents

_____ Adults of varying ages

_____ Senior citizens

_____ Critically ill patients

Group II: Type of professional activity

_____ Providing preventive care

_____ Providing comprehensive care

_____ Providing extensive workups

_____ Providing office care

_____ Securing referrals and providing consultations

_____ Ordering laboratory tests

_____ Utilizing one's manual dexterity

_____ Performing repetitive standard procedures

_____ Working as a consultant for other physicians

_____ Working with technological equipment

_____ Being involved in long-term relationships

Group III: Type of patient illness

_____ Treating complex problems

_____ Treating major diseases

_____ Treating acute illnesses and injuries

_____ Treating incurable diseases

_____ Treating life-threatening illnesses

_____ Treating infectious diseases

_____ Treating terminally ill patients

Group IV: Type of services provided to patients

_____ Providing medical services

_____ Providing surgical services

_____ Providing psychological services

_____ Providing medical and surgical services

_____ Providing rehabilitation services

Group V: Preferred area of body system to be treated

_____ Dealing with the musculoskeletal system

_____ Dealing with the digestive system

_____ Dealing with the respiratory system

(continued)

Form 2.1 (continued)

_____ Dealing with the circulatory system

_____ Dealing with the urinary system

_____ Dealing with skin problems

_____ Dealing with the nervous system

_____ Dealing with the reproductive system

Step 3. Determining an inventory of your personal attributes. Associated with each specialty or subspecialty are personal attributes that make an individual especially suited for a particular field. Thus, for example, superior manual dexterity is an asset for all surgical practices, but of no value for psychiatry. For the latter, however, being a good listener is essential.

Form 2.2 contains a list of desirable personal attributes that you should identify as being: *A*—genuinely applicable, *I*—decidedly inapplicable, *U*—uncertain.

Note: Your response can serve as a reference source when identifying relevant attributes associated with each specific practice area that are discussed in Chapters 3 to 6.

Form 2.2 Desirable personal attributes

_____ Prefers directly providing patient services

_____ Desires to utilize one's superior manual dexterity

_____ Has a long attention span

_____ Anxious to secure prompt results

_____ Desires scheduled professional activities

_____ Works well under intense stress

_____ Responds rapidly when circumstances necessitate

_____ Detail-oriented

_____ Very patient and "laid back" personality

_____ Seeks to have extensive expertise in a limited area

_____ Willing to do repetitive procedures

_____ Has superior observational ability

_____ Likes challenging situations

_____ Has good communication skills

_____ Likes to assume a leadership position

_____ Likes working with a health care team

_____ Likes working with other physicians

_____ Likes long-term patient relationships

_____ Seeks variability in patient care

_____ Satisfied with breadth rather than depth of knowledge

_____ Prefers doing rather than thinking

_____ Prefers working primarily in an office practice

_____ Prepared for unscheduled interruptions

_____ Seeks to offer comprehensive care

_____ Prepared to work long hours

_____ Prepared to accept an erratic work schedule

_____ Likes to use sophisticated technological equipment

_____ Has abundant self-confidence

_____ Seeks the challenge of complex problem-solving

_____ Prefers helping patients with treatable diseases

_____ Likes to focus on details

Step 4. Identifying possible specific practice areas. Having ascertained which category of medicine, surgery, or a combination of both merits being pursued (Step 1), you can now move on to be more specific as to determining your potential career choices. This can be done by proceeding to read the appropriate career descriptions of major specialties (Chapter 3) or subspecialties of medicine (Chapter 4) or surgery (Chapter 5) that are of special interest to you. If necessary, you also can look into subspecialties that are outside of the traditional ones, as well as emerging subspecialties (Chapter 6).

When investigating practice areas, first get an overview of the field from the description provided, and then focus your attention especially on the section within each individual career description presented in Chapters 3–6 that is entitled "Desirable Personal Attributes and Interests." Identify those relevant to you by placing an X in the appropriate boxes. Where you have checked off *at least* 7 out of 10 attributes you should investigate the area further. If in doubt as to a specific attribute's relevance, check your reference framework, namely, Form 2.1 or 2.2 of your completed personal inventory. The total number of attributes for each should be noted in the summary sections at the ends of Chapters 3–6.

When you have identified the major specialties and/or subspecialties that merit further consideration, note them in the appropriate section(s) of Form 2.3. Bear in mind that some areas combine medical and surgical components (e.g., ophthalmology, a otolaryngology, obstetrics/gynecology, and urology).

Form 2.3 Possible specialties and subspecialties meriting serious consideration

A. Major Specialties   B. Medical Subspecialties

1._____   1._____

2._____   2._____

3._____   3._____

C. Surgical Subspecialties   D. Other Subspecialties

1._____   1._____

2._____   2._____

3._____   3._____

Step 5. Coordinate and validate findings. Completion of the previous steps allows you to arrive at some *tentative* conclusions as to your most appropriate potential areas for specialization. These should be correlated with the data secured by the use of other approaches to specialty determination that were noted previously, namely, clinical exposure, interest assessment testing, and the Glaxo method. In addition, completing the third-year clerkships and possibly some relevant electives will enable you to better judge how relevant some of the practice areas are for you.

Conclusions. This self-assessment protocol should guide you in selecting areas that merit further possibilities. These may be subspecialty electives that are direct off-shoots of internal medicine or surgery. They may also be unrelated subspecialties. Completing electives will allow you to determine how genuine your interest in and suitability for a specific career are. Conversations with attendings and visits to the offices of practitioners will serve to round out your picture and allow you to make a sound decision on this vital issue. The more comprehensive a picture you have of a practice area, the more likely will be the soundness of your ultimate choice.

Once you have achieved a sense of confidence in the possible choices of a career, you should note up to three most suitable choices in a prioritized fashion on Form 2.4.

Form 2.4 Prioritized list of prospective specialties

1._____

2._____

3._____

Before proceeding further, however, it is *essential* to perform a *reality check* on each of your prospective choices (see p. 116). This should be done preferably before taking an elective to see if you are a viable candidate for an appointment. This depends on your level of competitiveness in relation to the competitiveness for securing a residency appointment in the specific specialty. Carrying out a reality check is outlined in Chapter 8. Completing a reality check as well as an elective and getting additional input from other specialty selection approaches as well as from your advisor/mentor should help you narrow down your choice of a specialty to the most realistic one, thus helping ensure your potential for success. Once your choice is made, guidance to facilitate achieving your goal of obtaining a residency appointment in the specialty of your choice is provided in Part Two of the book.

Advice from the pros

An overall approach to specialty selection having been presented, it can prove profitable at this point to gain insights from some physicians who were faced with the challenge of choosing a specialty. Given that hindsight should be a profitable teacher meaningful advice from professionals is presented below for your consideration:

■ Medical students should not feel pressured to make early and self-imposed irrevocable career decisions.

■ My advice to students who are trying to decide what to do in medicine is keep your options open. Let your interests and experiences define what you do.

■ Medical students should keep an open mind even after they think they have made a firm commitment.

■ With rotating internships gone, if you are vacillating about what area to enter, start with straight medicine, because it offers the best foundation for whatever specialty is ultimately chosen.

■ A year spent reviewing your decision, if you compare that with a lifetime in practice, is a small investment in formulating long-term goals.

■ I recommend that medical students try to find an interesting project that provides a taste of what being a doctor is like.

■ In mapping a medical career, you should continue to maintain broad interests and test a number of areas through your academic clinical experiences.

■ Spend more time than average on clerkships of special interest and get to know some of the residents. Choose one who could be most beneficial in teaching you and let him serve as a role model for a while.

■ I do not believe that the choices you make in medical school and early residency have to be irrevocable. Nor should they generate excessive anxiety. If you are comfortable with yourself, you'll be happy in a variety of areas, once you've made the larger selection of surgery versus medicine.

■ The choice between generalist and specialist is mostly by happenstance. For the generalist, the family or child is the focus of professional life, since diseases come and go, but the patient stays. For the specialist, the disease stays and the patients come and go.

■ Time, place, and people have a lot to do with the decision of what field to enter.

■ Most students look on selecting a specialty as an analytic process that involves balancing assets against liabilities. In the end, it is a good to make a decision by balancing positives and negatives, but remember that feelings count a great deal.

■ There is no absolutely correct decision, since a person can be happy in many fields. Without doubt, there are similar personalities in the various specialties and for whatever reason they tend to group. That fields have their defined personality types may be a valid generalization, but for individuals there can be great variation.

■ If you reach the end of medical school and are still not sure of your generalist or specialist orientation, pediatrics affords you an opportunity to continue to keep your options open.

■ One should not look upon specialists as less caring, since this is confusing breadth of interest with depth of commitment.

■ Specialty care frequently involves a team of professions including nurse practitioners, social workers, and therapists of various kinds.

■ Some discover that they like a more surgical or a more instrumental kind of work such as anesthesiology, where personal interactions are less intense and easier to cope with. Others, albeit a smaller number, go into such fields as pathology and radiology to move away from direct patient contact. There are some who are so caught up in emotional problems of children, but they do not wish to deal with medical illness. Yet liking children, they move into child psychiatry.

Finally, perhaps your personal physician can shed light for you on this important issue, in view of his/her own personal experience.

3 | Major Specialties

Overview

The 20th century was a period of momentous change in both physician education and advances in patient care. Early on during this interval, medical education was placed on a sound scientific footing as a result of publication of the famous Flexner Report in 1910. The consequence of this report was the closing of many institutions claiming to train physicians, in conjunction with a coexisting apprenticeship system. All surviving and newly established medical schools were mandated to offer a structured curriculum for the training of medical students, utilizing distinct basic and clinical science departments. During the course of the last few decades of the 20th century, there occurred several major innovations in the medical school curriculum design. Consequently, each school now has its own unique program specifically designed to fulfill its mission.

Physicians during the first half of the century were trained to serve as general practitioners. For those seeking specialty training prior to World War II, a residency at a European medical center, especially in Germany and Austria, was a common occurrence. As the quality of our medical education establishments gradually improved, attractive postgraduate training opportunities in this country rapidly multiplied. In addition, subspecialty areas emerged as offshoots, for the most part, from the fields of internal medicine and general surgery. New subspecialties have come into being in recent years (e.g., emergency medicine and geriatrics) and more can be anticipated (e.g., trauma surgery and sports medicine). It can be envisioned that future dramatic innovations (e.g., gene therapy) and advances in technology will generate as yet unforeseen subspecialties.

Descriptions of fields of specialization and subspecialization can be presented in alphabetical order. However, it is probably more useful if they are classified into four groupings, namely, the major specialties and three groups of subspecialties. The former will be described below; the medical, surgical, and other subspecialties are considered in the next three chapters.

Table 3.1 summarizes the characteristics of the major specialties. A detailed discussion of each of them follows.

Definitions

The following definitions apply to the *capsule headings* that are used in this chapter, as well as in Chapters 4, 5, and 6.

Status: A classification identifying the nature of the specialty.

Projected need: The anticipated future needs for specialists in this field.

Securing a residency: How challenging it is to obtain an appointment in this field. This estimate is based on current projections and trends and thus is subject to change. Five levels of competitiveness are used.

Training programs: Approximate number of postgraduate training programs in this specialty including, where appropriate, both first- and second-year openings.

Positions open: The number of all entry-level residency appointments available annually. Where relevant, combined first- and second-year figures are given. The number of women residents in the area is also noted.

Training period: The number of years needed to become eligible for meeting basic certification requirements as a board certified specialist in this field.

Weekly patient contact hours: This refers to the amount of direct exposure you will have to patient care, but it does not include other professional responsibilities, such as conferences and lectures (which can be estimated as taking up an additonal five hours).

Patient contact hours are defined as follows:

Above average: 55 and above

Average: 45–55

Below average: 40–45

Attaining patients: The manner in which a specialist obtains patients is identified.

Remuneration: Monetary level of compensation when starting a practice and median income, in relation to the average of physicians in general.

Table 3.1 The major specialties

Specialty	Nature of work	Prereq. year(s)	Training area	Training period min.	max.
Anesthesiology	Inducing loss of pain sensation by drugs or gases	One	Clinical base	Three	Four
Dermatology	Treatment of skin diseases	One	Medicine	Three	Three
Family practice	Provide general preventive of acute medical care for the family	–	–	Three	Three
Internal medicine	Diagnosis and medical treatment of the diseases of adults	–	–	Three	Three
Neurology	Diagnosis and medical treatment of diseases of the nervous system	One	Clinical base	Three	Four
Obstetrics/ gynecology	Care during pregnancy and labor; treatment of diseases of female reproductive system	One	Clinical base	Three	Four
Ophthalmology	Diagnosis and treatment of eye diseases medically or surgically	One	Optional	Three	Four
Otolaryngology	Diagnosis and treatment of ear, nose, and throat diseases	One	General surgery	Three	Four
Pathology	Analysis of changes in the body tissues due to disease processes	One	Optional	Four	Four
Pediatrics	Care of infants and children and treatment of their diseases	–	–	Three	Four

Table 3.1 *(continued)*

Specialty	Nature of work	Prereq. year(s)	Training area	Training period min.	max.
Physical medicine and rehabilitation	Treatment by various means for restoration of function	One	Medicine and surgery	Three	Three
Psychiatry	Diagnosis and treatment of emotional mental diseases	One	Clinical base	Four	Four
Radiology	Diagnosis of disease by x-ray and other energy sources	One	Clinical base	Four	Four
Surgery	Treatment of diseases by surgical intervention	One	–	Four	Seven
Urology	Treatment of kidney, prostate, and bladder diseases	Three	General surgery		

Starting

Well above average	> $200,000
Above average	> $165,000–200,000
Average	> $125,000–165,000
Below average	< $125,000

Median

Well above average	> $275,000
Above average	> $225,000–275,000
Average	> $175,000–225,000
Below average	< $175,000

Night and emergency calls: The extent to which one can expect unscheduled disruptions to meet patients' needs.

The following definitions apply to text headings. Note that these apply to headings used in this chapter as well as in Chapters 4, 5 and 6.

Scope: A very brief summary of the specialty's area of coverage.

Activities: A description of the principal work-related responsibilities in the specialty.

Professional satisfaction: A summary of the major attractive features that motivate individuals to choose the specialty as the focus of their future careers.

Negative attributes: Elements of dissatisfaction with the specialty.

Desirable prerequisites: A summary of background educational experiences that will facilitate judging one's interest and abilities as well as enhancing the chances for securing a residency appointment.

Desirable personal attributes and interests: A checklist of personal characteristics that one should have when considering a residency in this specialty. This facilitates determining the suitability of a career as a specialist in this field by validating specialty selection choices.

Residency or specialty selection factors:

Postgraduate training/certification: The essential components of the residency training program and requirements to secure certification are presented.

Subspecialty options: A description of fellowship area opportunities within the specialty are provided. Some fellowships may result in certification of special competency.

For further information: The principal organization associated with the specialty is given at the end of each description, along with its Web site. Addresses also are provided in the organizations appendix at the end of the book.

The choices

Each of 15 major specialties will be discussed below.

Anesthesiology

Status: Supports surgical specialties

Projected need: Above average

Securing a residency: Extremely competitive

Training programs: Ca. 130

Positions open: Ca. 1000 (women residents ca. 300)

Training period: Four years (which includes a clinical base year)

Weekly patient contact hours: Average

Attaining patients: Assigned by the hospital or office practitioners

Remuneration: Starting, high: median, high

Night and emergency calls: Common

SCOPE. Anesthesiologists are involved in providing medical services that render patients insensitive to pain. Anesthesia is administered during surgical, obstetric, therapeutic, and diagnostic procedures. Exposure to critical care patients is a part of training in this specialty.

ACTIVITIES. Anesthesiologists, in addition to their routine clinical services, are trained to serve as critical care physicians. As such they are qualified to manage cases requiring cardiac and respiratory resuscitation and to treat unconscious patients and those with metabolic or electrolytic imbalances. Specialized anesthesiologists are also involved in treating cases involving pain management. Thus there is a spectrum of activities in which anesthesiologists can participate.

PROFESSIONAL SATISFACTION. Beyond attractive monetary remuneration, gratification comes from being in a position to allay the natural anxiety and fears of patients prior to surgical procedures. The major aspect of the work involves devising a personalized patient anesthesia protocol, administering it, and following its application to its conclusion in the recovery room, all within a time span.

NEGATIVE ATTRIBUTES. Schedule uncertainties, difficulties in working with some surgeons, and inadequate recognition are the principal complaints of some.

DESIRABLE PREREQUISITES. In addition to a solid internal medicine background, completing at least a one-month elective in this field, as well as electives in cardiology and pulmonary medicine, is recommended.

DESIRABLE PERSONAL ATTRIBUTES AND INTERESTS. Check off the desirable attributes and interests of anesthesiologists you know for certain that you have *in abundance.* Then indicate the total number of checks on the bottom of the list as well as on the summary page at the end of this chapter.

_____ Works well under intense stress
_____ Long attention span
_____ Detail-oriented work habits
_____ Quick thinking and fast acting
_____ Strong commitment to accuracy
_____ Superior manual dexterity
_____ Teamwork oriented
_____ Good interpersonal skills
_____ Desires an organized work schedule
_____ Prefers quick results for one's efforts
_____ Total

RESIDENCY SELECTION FACTORS. Having an impressive overall academic record is important, especially in physiology and pharmacology courses, as well as in one's internal medicine clerkship and anesthesiology elective. The residency interview is decisive. Demonstrating intellectual curiosity by means of research work is quite desirable.

POSTGRADUATE TRAINING/CERTIFICATION. Residency involves completion of a four-year training program, the first year of which can be a transitional, preliminary, or categorical internship in a clinical specialty. For some programs you may have to secure such an initial appointment on your own. The next three years are then devoted exclusively to clinical anesthesiology.

Certification requires completion of a three-year residency including two months of critical care experience. Passing written and oral examinations is essential to meet the requirements of the American Board of Anesthesiology.

SUBSPECIALTY OPTIONS. The one-year subspecialty options are as follows:

Critical care medicine (Ca. 100 positions) and *pain management* (Ca. 150 positions). Both require a prerequisite of three years of clinical anesthesia. Completion of subspecialty training results in a Certificate of Special Qualifications. There are also programs prior to eligibility for specialization, during PGY-4 of the residency program, in cardiothoracic, neurological, obstetric, and pediatric anesthesiology. These programs are distinct from routine anesthesiology and thus require a separate application for a residency appointment.

FOR FURTHER INFORMATION. American Society of Anesthesiologists, www. asahq.org.

Dermatology

Status: Major specialty

Projected need: Average to below average

Securing a residency: Strongly competitive

Training programs: Ca. 100

Positions open: Ca. 300 (women residents ca. 160)

Training period: Three years (after a year of internship)

Weekly patient contact hours: Below average

Attaining patients: Self or physician referral

Remuneration: Variable; starting, average; median, well above average

Night and emergency calls: Rare

SCOPE. Dermatologists are involved in the diagnosis and treatment of disorders and diseases of the skin, whether acute or chronic in nature.

ACTIVITIES. This is primarily an office-based specialty, with treatment being chemotherapeutic and/or surgical (including lasers). For those with chronic disorders, dermatologists also provide psychological support during prolonged treatment.

PROFESSIONAL SATISFACTION. The fact that for this specialty, most cases can receive therapeutic help and achieve a positive response and the outcome to measures taken promptly is especially gratifying. Being exposed to patients of varying age groups and using a variety of dermatological approaches is stimulating. There is also the challenge of correlating clinical observations and pathological findings.

NEGATIVE ATTRIBUTES. Few practitioners have complaints about the specialty except that its prestige is not as high as they would like.

DESIRABLE PREREQUISITES. An outstanding medical school record, including completing an elective in dermatology at a teaching clinic or service with a community dermatologist, is very desirable.

DESIRABLE PERSONAL ATTRIBUTES AND INTERESTS. Check off desirable attributes and interests of dermatologists you know for certain that you have *in abundance*. Then indicate the total number of checks on the bottom of the list as well as on the summary page at the end of this chapter.

_____ Acute vision

_____ Strong interpersonal skills

_____ Superior observational skills

_____ Strong manual dexterity

_____ Prefers an organized work schedule

_____ Favors precise diagnoses of problems

_____ Favors a prompt response to therapy

_____ Sensitive to patients' plight

_____ Receptive to patient complaints

_____ Desires independence as a practitioner

_____ Total

RESIDENCY SELECTION FACTORS. Securing strong supporting Dean of Students and Chairman letters, AOA membership, and attending a prominent medical school are important. Research work of good quality will enhance one's chances for securing a position.

POSTGRADUATE TRAINING/CERTIFICATION. Residency involves one year of a broad-based internship (e.g., family practice, internal medicine, surgery, pediatrics) followed by three years in dermatology. Applicants usually must secure their internship on their own. The interview for the residency appointment usually takes place at the end of the fourth year of medical school.

Certification requires completing a residency and passing a two-part exam, one written and the other involving visual aids and microscopic slides.

SUBSPECIALTY OPTIONS. There are two subspecialties in this field. They are as follows:

Dermatologic pathology. This involves a one-year fellowship after completion of a dermatology residency. Upon successful completion, one is awarded a Certificate of Special Competence. It is offered by ca. 40 programs with one fellowship each.

Clinical and laboratory dermatological immunology. This subspecialty also consists of a one-year fellowship program.

FOR FURTHER INFORMATION. American Academy of Dermatology, www.aad.org.

Family practice

Status: Major medical specialty

Projected need: Significant

Securing a residency: Not competitive

Training programs: Ca. 500

Positions open: Ca. 3,500 (women residents ca. 1,750)

Training period: Three years

Weekly patient contact hours: Average

Attaining patients: Self-referral

Remuneration: Starting, below average, median, below average

Night and emergency calls: Common

SCOPE. Family practice is a primary care specialty that covers a broad spectrum of individuals. It involves treating patients with acute or chronic common diseases.

ACTIVITIES. This specialty, which provides training in a wide variety of disciplines, has essentially absorbed the role formerly occupied by the general practitioner. Family practitioners spend most of their time in direct patient contact in an outpatient setting. The nature of their practice will depend on their training, interests, and location. They are also involved in dealing with behavioral and psychological issues their patients may present. Most practitioners are associated with some form of managed health care delivery system.

PROFESSIONAL SATISFACTION. Two elements that define this specialty are the sources of its attraction to practitioners. One involves providing broad-based medical care and serving many members of the same family. The other is the long-lasting relationships of trust that can be established between doctors and patient families. These prove to be very meaningful and gratifying elements.

NEGATIVE ATTRIBUTES. Friction with patients may occasionally arise, if they are overly dependent, excessively demanding, or terminally ill.

DESIRABLE PREREQUISITES. It is advisable to secure a preceptorship in this specialty in a community practice setting. You need to develop expertise in the diagnosis and management of common health problems (e.g., hypertension, diabetes, arthritis).

DESIRABLE PERSONAL ATTRIBUTES AND INTERESTS. Check off the desirable attributes and interests for family practice you know for certain that you have *in abundance*. Then indicate the total number of checks on the bottom of the list as well as on the summary page at the end of this chapter.

_____ Highly people-oriented

_____ Appreciates variety in challenges to problem solving

_____ Superior communication skills

_____ Satisfied with limited expertise in many areas of medicine

_____ Tolerant of uncertainty in formulating diagnoses

_____ Favors establishing long-lasting patient relationships

_____ Prefers an office-based practice

_____ Recognizes the need for schedule flexibility

_____ Not highly procedure-oriented

_____ Readily willing to refer patients to specialists when appropriate

_____ Total

RESIDENCY SELECTION FACTORS. These include a strong commitment to family practice, maturity, strong interpersonal skills, and a favorable Dean's letter. A large number of women are entering this specialty. An impressive personal statement will help secure an interview, which, in turn, is the key to securing an appointment to a residency.

POSTGRADUATE TRAINING/CERTIFICATION. The three-year residency program covers clinical training in a variety of relevant basic specialties. Clinical exposure is provided in a number of settings including family practice centers. Most residencies are sponsored by community hospitals rather than medical school/ university settings.

Certification requires completing a residency and passing a written examination. This specialty is unique, because it requires recertification by passing a written examination every seven years.

SUBSPECIALTY OPTIONS. One-year fellowships are available in *adolescent medicine, geriatric medicine*, and *sports medicine*, which result in being awarded a Certificate of Special Competence.

FOR FURTHER INFORMATION. American Academy of Family Physicians, www. aafp.org.

Internal medicine

Status: Major specialty

Projected need: Above average

Securing a residency: Somewhat competitive

Training programs: Ca. 400

Positions open: Ca. 6,500 (women residents ca. 1,800)

Training period: Three years

Weekly patient contact: Average

Attaining patients: Self-referral or by referral

Remuneration: Starting, average; median, below average

Night and emergency calls: Common

SCOPE. General internists provide primary health care to adults with acute and chronic medical conditions.

ACTIVITIES. Internists are generalists because they treat a broad range of medical conditions. Many of their older patients suffer from multiple chronic conditions. In rural areas, internists may act as consultants for complex cases. In urban areas, subspecialty internists provide the necessary expertise. Most of the practice of internists is office-based, but time may also have to be spent on hospital rounds, nursing home visits, and occasional house calls.

PROFESSIONAL SATISFACTION. The most attractive features of this specialty are the intellectual challenge in achieving accurate diagnoses and formulating appropriate treatment protocols and the gratitude of patients for services rendered. Satisfaction is also provided by the long-term relationships established with patients.

NEGATIVE ATTRIBUTES. The lengthy and frequently irregular office hours are the most common deficiency, because of their impact on one's personal life.

DESIRABLE PREREQUISITES. Exposure to many patients with medical problems during your internal medicine clerkship and related electives (e.g., cardiology, gastroenterology) will prepare you for a general internal medicine residency.

DESIRABLE PERSONAL ATTRIBUTES AND INTERESTS. Check off the desirable attributes and interests of internists you know for certain that you have *in abundance*. Then indicate the total number of checks on the bottom of the list as well as on the summary page at the end of this chapter.

_____ Prefers variety in the nature of medical problems being treated

_____ Enjoys long-term relationships with patients

_____ Favors diagnosing and prescribing rather than repetitive procedures

_____ Can patiently and empathetically listen to patients' concerns

_____ Prepared to treat patients with multiple chronic illnesses

_____ Willing to coordinate provision of health care services for seniors

_____ Can communicate well both orally and in writing with patients and physicians

_____ Desires primarily an office-based practice

_____ Willing to accept schedule interruptions with patient needs

_____ Tends to be accurate, thorough, and detail-oriented

_____ Total

RESIDENCY SELECTION FACTORS. The dean's letter and interpersonal skills, as well as one's internal medicine clerkship performance, are the important selection criteria for this specialty.

POSTGRADUATE TRAINING/CERTIFICATION. This specialty provides training along two tracts. The traditional one is an academic hospital-based tract, whereas a primary-medicine tract focuses more on training in ambulatory and continuity care clinics. The latter include electives in orthopedics, gynecology, and minor surgery. A variety of combined programs involve internal medicine and other specialties, the most common being internal medicine/pediatrics.

Completing a residency and passing a written examination are the requirements for certification.

SUBSPECIALTY OPTIONS. The wide variety of options are discussed in detail under medical subspecialties (see Chapter 4).

FOR FURTHER INFORMATION. American College of Physicians, American Society of Internal Medicine, www.acponline.org.

Neurology

Status: Major specialty

Projected need: Average

Securing a residency: Below average competition

Training programs: Ca. 129

Positions open: Ca. 500 (women residents ca. 45)

Training period: Three years (after a base internship)

Weekly patient contact hours: Average

Attaining patients: Referral

Remuneration: Starting, average; median, average

Night and emergency calls: Limited

SCOPE. Neurologists are concerned with the diagnosis and medical treatment of patients with diseases of the brain, spinal cord, and peripheral nerves, as well as neuromuscular disorders.

ACTIVITIES. Although this specialty is largely office-based, hospital service and consultations are an important part of professional activities in this field. Patients treated include those suffering from strokes, migraine headaches, vertigo, Parkinson's, Alzheimer's, and other neurological diseases.

PROFESSIONAL SATISFACTION. The field provides opportunities for those favoring very significant intellectual challenges, because it involves dealing with complex diagnostic problems. Neurology is especially attractive to those who find the intensely demanding procedural aspects of neurosurgery unappealing.

NEGATIVE ATTRIBUTES. Challenges faced in this specialty include the frustration of emergency calls and the unresponsiveness of some cases to treatment.

DESIRABLE PREREQUISITES. Securing meaningful exposure to neurology through an elective as well as gaining strong clerkship experience is important. A sound background in neuroanatomy as a medical student is strongly advised.

DESIRABLE PERSONAL ATTRIBUTES AND INTERESTS. Check off the desirable attributes and interests of neurologists you know for certain that you have *in abundance*. Then indicate the total number of checks on the bottom of the list as well as on the summary page at the end of this chapter.

_____ Enjoys intellectually challenging problems

_____ Favors scheduled patient care activities

_____ Desires variability in procedures and approach

_____ Has strong analytical skills in problem solving

_____ Desires patient contact for diagnostic and therapeutic reasons

_____ Seeks problems that are intellectually resolvable

_____ Desires independence as a practitioner

_____ Wishes for adequate remuneration for one's efforts

_____ Has patience to await long-term outcome from treatment

_____ Doesn't favor procedural activities as the approach of choice

_____ Total

RESIDENCY SELECTION FACTORS. These include medical school class rank and quality of recommendations. You should have a demonstrated interest in clinical neuroscience or in neurology and/or have taken a neurosurgical elective.

POSTGRADUATE TRAINING/CERTIFICATION. The program requires four years of training, with the first being an internship. Usually this is in internal medicine; however, an internship in family practice or pediatrics or in a transitional program is also acceptable. Most residencies are secured through the Neurology Matching Program, which provides fourth-year medical students with second-year residency appointments. Some first-year positions can be also secured through the NRMP. Programs that provide training in adult and child neurology and psychiatry.

Certification is obtained after completing a residency and passing a written and then an oral examination.

SUBSPECIALTY OPTIONS. Subspecialization in *child neurology* requires two years of pediatric training or one in pediatrics and one in internal medicine prior to starting the neurology program. Certification requirements are similar to those described above, but are focused more on child neurology.

FOR FURTHER INFORMATION. American Academy of Neurology, www.aan.com.

Obstetrics and gynecology

Status: Major medical–surgical specialty

Projected need: Greater than average

Securing a residency: Strongly competitive

Training programs: Ca. 250

Positions open: Ca. 1,100 (women residents ca. 800)

Training period: Four years

Weekly patient contact hours: Above average

Attaining patients: Usually self-referral

Remuneration: Starting, above average; median, above average

Night and emergency calls: Frequent

SCOPE. Obstetricians/gynecologists provide clinical care during pregnancy and delivery and also treat disorders of the female reproductive tract. These specialists tend to be involved in primary care of their female patients.

ACTIVITIES. Although primarily office-based, practitioners devote considerable time in hospital service for deliveries and surgery. Most specialists practice in both areas, but some restrict their activities to one or the other. Some specialists are concerned with problems of fertility. The high cost of malpractice insurance has resulted in some practitioners declining to clinically manage high-risk pregnancy cases; they may even restrict their practice to gynecology. Women are increasingly becoming attracted to practice in this field. Primary care especially involving women's health issues, has become an integral component of this specialty.

PROFESSIONAL SATISFACTION. Gratification comes from a variety of sources, including the multidisciplinary nature of the specialty, particularly its surgical component. Achieving successful outcomes with the delivery of normal, healthy children and the establishment of strong interpersonal relations with patients during the lengthy pregnancy are additional reasons for the satisfaction that this specialty provides.

NEGATIVE ATTRIBUTES. The unpredictability of the disruption of one's professional and personal life by women in labor is the standard unpleasant feature of this specialty.

DESIRABLE PREREQUISITES. Choose to improve your background by selecting electives from among such disciplines as general surgery, urology, internal medicine, and infectious diseases.

DESIRABLE PERSONAL ATTRIBUTES AND INTERESTS. Check off the desirable attributes and interests of obstetricians and gynecologists you know for certain that you have *in abundance*. Then indicate the total number of checks on the bottom of the list as well as on the summary page at the end of this chapter.

_____ Has superior manual dexterity

_____ Enjoys working with people

_____ Capable of working for long periods of time

_____ Willing to accept an unpredictable schedule graciously

_____ Has empathy for women in a special situation

_____ Is prepared to accept a varied work schedule

_____ Can establish good rapport with patients

_____ Can act decisively

_____ Can adjust as circumstances warrant

_____ Reacts calmly under intense pressure

_____ Total

RESIDENCY SELECTION FACTORS. Aside from securing good grades, a strong dean's letter, and an impressive USMLE Step I scores, you should also do well on your ob/gyn clerkship, seek some research experience in the field, and be concerned with women's health issues.

POSTGRADUATE TRAINING/CERTIFICATION. The four-year residency program provides clinical experience with both hospitalized and ambulatory patients, involving obstetric and gynecological patients. There is also a minimum six-month segment dealing with primary care, which is now a mandatory part of all residency programs.

Certification involves completing a residency and passing a written examination. After two years of practice an oral exam can be taken to complete the process.

SUBSPECIALTY OPTIONS. There are four different two-year fellowships available. These are *reproductive endocrinology* (fertility), *maternal–fetal medicine, gynecological oncology*, and *critical care medicine*. Completion of any of these programs results in a Certificate of Special Competence and enables the fellow to take the oral board examination after only six months of practice.

FOR FURTHER INFORMATION. American College of Obstetrics & Gynecologists, www.acog.org.

Ophthalmology

Status: Major medical–surgical specialty

Projected need: Limited

Securing a residency: Competitive

Training programs: Ca. 125

Positions open: Ca. 450 (women residents ca. 135)

Training period: Three years (after a clinical-based first year)

Weekly patient contact hours: Below average

Attaining patients: Usually self-referral

Remuneration: Starting, above average; median, above average

Night and emergency calls: Limited

SCOPE. Ophthalmology deals with the diagnosis and treatment of diseases of the eye.

ACTIVITIES. Largely office-based, an ophthalmology practice involves the use of sophisticated medical equipment for both diagnosis and treatment. Patients of all age ranges are seen and a wide variety of services are provided, ranging from fitting glasses and contact lenses to micro- and laser surgery of the eye.

PROFESSIONAL SATISFACTION. The major gratifying factor is being able to use one's skills to restore patients' vision to the maximum extent possible. A great deal of satisfaction is derived from carrying out surgical procedures (e.g., cataract surgery).

NEGATIVE ATTRIBUTES. The challenge is to avoid office routine generating a feeling of monotony that detracts from the interest of the specialty.

DESIRABLE PREREQUISITES. Taking an elective in this specialty is especially desirable to ensure your genuine interest in the field.

DESIRABLE PERSONAL ATTRIBUTES AND INTERESTS. Check off the desirable attributes and interests of ophthalmologists you know for certain that you have *in abundance.* Then indicate the total number of checks on the bottom of the list as well as on the summary page at the end of this chapter.

_____ Has superior manual dexterity

_____ Possesses impressive hand–eye coordination

_____ Very patient and exacting in decision-making

_____ Desires rapid tangible results for one's efforts

_____ Enjoys patient contact and developing long-term relations

_____ Willing to accept demanding working hours

_____ Prefers challenges that are both intellectual and manipulative

_____ Can take decisive action when called for

_____ Seeks variability in treatment modalities

_____ Prefers to be in an action-oriented specialty

_____ Total

RESIDENCY SELECTION FACTORS. The major considerations in securing an appointment in this specialty are high class standing in medical school, level of performance in the required clerkships, USMLE Step 1, board scores, and research experience.

POSTGRADUATE TRAINING/CERTIFICATION. Residency applications for the three-year program need to be submitted two years in advance through the

Ophthalmology Matching Program. There is a required one-year internship, obtainable through the NRMP, that is a prerequisite to undertaking the specialty training.

Certification involves completing a residency and taking a written exam and then an oral exam within the next two years.

SUBSPECIALTY OPTIONS. Fellowships are available in a variety of areas and are obtainable via the Ophthalmology Matching Program. The subspecialty areas are *retina–vitreous, glaucoma, cornea, pediatric ophthalmology, and neuro-ophthalmology*. There are, however, no board certified subspecialties.

FOR FURTHER INFORMATION. American Academy of Ophthalmology, www. aao.org.

Otolaryngology – head and neck surgery

Status: Major medical–surgical specialty

Projected need: Average

Securing a residency: Strongly competitive

Training programs: Ca. 100

Positions opens: Ca. 275 (women residents ca. 50)

Training period: Three or four years (after one or two years of a general surgery residency)

Weekly patient contact hours: Average

Attaining patients: Primarily referral

Remuneration: Starting, above average; median, average

Night and emergency calls: Limited

SCOPE. Work in this specialty may involve head and neck surgery, but the major emphasis is on the diagnosis and treatment of diseases of the ear, nose, and throat.

ACTIVITIES. This specialty has assumed a broader aspect than covering only diseases of the ear, nose, and throat. As noted, it now covers head and neck surgery, excluding the upper respiratory and GI tracts. It is a largely office-based specialty and much of the surgery is ambulatory.

PROFESSIONAL SATISFACTION. Practitioners find most gratification with working in this field, particularly in establishing diagnoses on the basis of a direct physical exam rather than via lab tests. Especially meaningful are the variety of patients seen and the ability of the specialist to resolve their medical problems effectively.

NEGATIVE ATTRIBUTES. Like others, these specialists dislike the paperwork associated with their work. They are also troubled that other specialists are not aware of the extent of head and neck surgery services that ENT people provide.

DESIRABLE PREREQUISITES. Seek to attain good grades, especially in your surgical clerkship. Be especially familiar with the anatomy of the head and neck, to be able to communicate well with patients and clarify for them their problems and treatment protocols developed to restore their health.

DESIRABLE PERSONAL ATTRIBUTES AND INTERESTS. Check off the desirable attributes and interests of otolaryngologists you know for certain that you have *in abundance*. Then indicate the total number of checks on the bottom of the list as well as on the summary page at the end of this chapter.

_____ Superior manual dexterity

_____ Desires to solve problems quickly and decisively

_____ Wants to observe treatment results relatively promptly

_____ Favors intellectual and technical challenges

_____ Desires an organized schedule

_____ Likes to work with their hands

_____ Enjoys patient contact and interpersonal interaction

_____ Enjoys being creative in their work

_____ Prefers an organized schedule

_____ Is an action-oriented individual

_____ Total

RESIDENCY SELECTION FACTORS. These include class rank, letters of recommendation, especially from an academic otolaryngologist, evidence demonstrating manual dexterity, an impressive performance in an ENT elective, and, if possible, significant research work.

POSTGRADUATE TRAINING/CERTIFICATION. This specialty requires one to two years of general surgery followed by four years of otolaryngology training. Selections for residency appointments are made by the Otolaryngology Matching Program. The prerequisite internships are arranged through the NRMP, through the matching program itself, or by applying for a preliminary surgical program directly. Training covers the seven subdivisions of the specialty: otology, laryngology, head and neck surgery, and allergy, as well as facial, plastic, and reconstructive surgery.

Certification requires at least five years of combined training in surgery and otolaryngology, as well as passing written and oral examinations.

SUBSPECIALTY OPTIONS. Fellowships are available in *pediatric otolaryngology and otology/neurology,* as well as in the above noted subdivisions of this specialty.

FOR FURTHER INFORMATION. American Academy of Otolaryngology – Head and Neck Surgery, www.aconns.org.

Pathology

Status: Major laboratory-based specialty

Projected need: Possibly above average

Securing a residency: Somewhat competitive

Training programs: Ca. 150

Positions open: Ca. 590 (women residents ca. 260)

Training period: Four or five years including a base internship

Weekly patient contact hours: Below average

Attaining patients: Hospital referral

Remuneration: Starting, above average; median, average

Night and emergency calls: Minimal

SCOPE. Pathology is involved in seeking to identify the presence of disease in body component specimens as well as to determine the diagnosis and manifestation of its character.

ACTIVITIES. These depend on subspecialty area, namely anatomic or clinical pathology. *Anatomic pathology* involves in carrying out autopsies to uncover causes of death and includes cytopathology and surgical pathology. *Clinical pathology* includes hematology, clinical chemistry, neurology, microbiology, and blood banking transfusion medicine. Training is also provided in medical informatics and management to prepare individuals for supervising large laboratories. Most pathologists are hospital-based. They may be involved also in academic medicine as teachers and researchers, in addition to their clinical responsibilities. Some clinical pathologists are responsible for the supervision of private laboratories.

PROFESSIONAL SATISFACTION. These include being consulted by a variety of specialists, the intellectual challenge of establishing diagnoses, having a fixed work schedule, and the ability to organize one's work activities to one's liking.

NEGATIVE ATTRIBUTES. The major frustrations in this specialty stem from bureaucratic impediments. These include governmental regulations and being held responsible for lost requisitions or lab work, which distract from the essence of the work.

DESIRABLE PREREQUISITES. Secure a solid scientific understanding of basic pathologic processes to serve as a foundation of postgraduate studies. Having a strong interest and abilities in gross and microscopic anatomy, especially histology, are important. Completing an elective in pathology and gaining research experience are strongly recommended.

DESIRABLE PERSONAL ATTRIBUTES AND INTERESTS. Check off the desirable attributes and interests of pathologists you know for certain that you have *in abundance*. Then indicate the total number of checks on the bottom of the list as well as on the summary page at the end of this chapter.

_____ Has well organized, methodical work habits

_____ Strong preference for working with peers rather than patients

_____ Diligent concern for scientific detail

_____ Strongly favors an organized and structured work schedule

_____ Prefers precise decisions on medical issues

_____ Partial to thinking rather than action-oriented approaches

_____ Focuses on accuracy in one's work habits

_____ Enjoys intellectual challenge

_____ Seeks variety in activities

_____ Satisfied with a salaried position

_____ Total

RESIDENCY SELECTION FACTORS. Performance in the relevant basic sciences and recommendations from relevant faculty are decisive factors in securing a residency.

POSTGRADUATE TRAINING/CERTIFICATION. Training involves a "credentialing year," consisting of a clinical internship or clinically related research. It is followed by three or four years of either anatomic pathology or clinical pathology. The residency can also be a combination of both areas, extending over four years.

Certification is offered after completion of a residency and passing of a written examination in anatomic or clinical pathology (or both).

SUBSPECIALTY OPTIONS. Special qualification certificates are offered after fellowship training in blood banking medicine, chemical pathology, cytopathology, dermatologic pathology, forensic pathology, immunopathology, medical microbiology, neuropathology, and pediatric pathology.

FOR FURTHER INFORMATION. College of American Pathologists, www.cap.org; American Society of Clinical Pathologists, www.ascp.org.

Pediatrics

Status: Major specialty

Projected need: Below average

Securing a residency: Somewhat Competitive

Training programs: Ca. 200

Positions open: Ca. 2,600 (women residents ca. 1,600)

Training period: Three years

Weekly patient contact hours: Average

Attaining patients: Self-referral

Remuneration: Starting below average; median below average

Night and emergency calls: Very frequent

SCOPE. Deals with maintaining the health of infants, children, adolescents, and young adults.

ACTIVITIES. Pediatricians are involved in preventive care as well as diagnosing and treating sick patients. Most pediatricians are employed in group practices. Pediatrics is largely an office-based specialty, but service in a hospital may at times prove necessary.

PROFESSIONAL SATISFACTION. Developing long-lasting trusting relationships with the child and their family is a major consideration. Another factor is being able to contribute to health maintenance rather than only crisis intervention due to acute illnesses.

NEGATIVE ATTRIBUTES. Educating patients' parents in commonsense guidelines of child raising is a challenging task. In addition, the demand by parents to treat patients is excessive.

DESIRABLE PREREQUISITES. Having special ability to relate to children and deal effectively with anxious parents is essential. Awareness of the challenge of treating patients who cannot provide essential medical information is needed. Recognize that there is a very high incidence of night and emergency calls in this specialty. Securing some research experience can prove helpful.

DESIRABLE PERSONAL ATTRIBUTES AND INTERESTS. Check off the desirable attributes and interests of pediatricians you know for certain that you have *in abundance*. Then indicate the total number of checks on the bottom of the list as well as on the summary page the end of this chapter.

_____ Having an easy-going nature
_____ Capable of communicating in a reassuring manner
_____ Highly tolerant of schedule disruptions
_____ Seeks long-term patient and parent relationships
_____ Desires caring for a young patient population
_____ Has good interpersonal skills in dealing with patients
_____ Remains calm when faced with acute illness
_____ Can medically process patients in an efficient manner
_____ Satisfied to have essentially an office-based practice
_____ Can act decisively and confidently when appropriate
_____ Total

RESIDENCY SELECTION FACTORS. In evaluating prospective residents, emphasis is placed on evidence of a willingness to work hard as well as having good interpersonal and communication skills. These should be reflected in letters of recommendation and faculty evaluations and especially in one's personal residency statement.

POSTGRADUATE TRAINING/CERTIFICATION. Residency is three years. About 5% of residency positions are defined as "pediatrics-primary," offering somewhat more outpatient and continuity care experience than the standard program.

Certification can be secured after completing one's residency and passing a written examination.

SUBSPECIALTY OPTIONS. About 40% of residents gain subspecialty fellowship training for two to three years. This takes place in a wide variety of areas including neonatal–prenatal medicine, pediatric cardiology, pediatric medical care, pediatric hematology/oncology, pediatric emergency medicine, pediatric infectious diseases, pediatric nephrology, and pediatric rheumatology. Fellowships are also available in *adolescent medicine, allergy – immunology,* and *pediatric internal medicine.* One of the motivating factors encouraging specialization is that medical care for children is also being provided by family practitioners as well as allied health personnel, such as physician assistants and nurse practitioners.

FOR FURTHER INFORMATION. American Academy of Pediatrics, www.aap.org.

Physical medicine and rehabilitation

Status: Major specialty

Projected need: Significant

Securing a residency: Slightly competitive

Training programs: Ca. 80

Positions open: Ca. 300 (women residents ca. 36)

Training period: Four years

Weekly patient contact hours: Average

Attaining patients: Referral

Remuneration: Starting, below average; median, below average

Night and emergency calls: Rare

SCOPE. Physiatrists serve to evaluate, diagnose, and treat patients suffering from physical disabilities or impairments.

ACTIVITIES. This is to a large extent a hospital-based specialty. These specialists treat patients who have had sports or industrial injuries, suffer from musculorskeletal pain syndromes, are stroke victims, or have other problems which are amenable to rehabilitation. The goal is to elevate pain, improve physical function to an optimal state, and enhance psychosocial adjustment to their condition.

PROFESSIONAL SATISFACTION. Gratification is secured from being able to develop treatment plans for comprehensive rehabilitation for people who need long-term care for chronic problems. For many patients this is the only source for help to improve the quality of their lives.

NEGATIVE ATTRIBUTES. The demand on one's time due to the paperwork requirements and their complexity presents special problems. Limitations in funding to purchase equipment sometimes present frustration.

DESIRABLE PREREQUISITES. Secure a good background in examining and diagnosing musculoskeletal and neurological diseases. This should be in addition to getting a solid base of knowledge in anatomy and physiology. Seek to gain an understanding and appreciation for the nature of chronic illness and its psychosocial impact on patients and their families.

DESIRABLE PERSONAL ATTRIBUTES AND INTERESTS. Check off the desirable attributes and interests for physiatrists you know for certain that you have *in abundance*. Then indicate the total number of checks on the bottom of the list as well as on the summary page at the end of this chapter.

_____ Feels comfortable working primarily with disabled individuals

_____ Tolerates very slow or negligible progress from therapy

_____ Enjoys working with and helping people in great need

_____ Welcomes the challenge of facing complex health problems

_____ Has a realistic approach to solving chronic problems

_____ Capable of coordinating activities to facilitate therapy

_____ Prepared to accept responsibility for people in dire need

_____ Prefers long-term relationships

_____ Likes to be creative and take concrete actions

_____ Can communicate patiently and listen well

_____ Total

RESIDENCY SELECTION FACTORS. Good communication skills and demonstrated ability in the anatomical, physiological, and neurological sciences are important assets in securing a residency appointment.

POSTGRADUATE TRAINING/CERTIFICATION. The four-year residency program includes one year involving an integrated internal medicine program. Many but not all residencies are secured through the NMRP. There are also a small number of double-board combined programs with other specialties, namely, pediatrics or internal medicine and neurology.

Certification can come after completion of a residency and Part I of a written exam. Part II can be taken only after one year of experience as a practitioner in this field.

SUBSPECIALTY OPTIONS. One-year fellowships are available in *spinal cord injury medicine*, leading to a Certificate of Special Qualifications. Certification is also available in *pain management* and *pediatric rehabilitation medicine*.

FOR FURTHER INFORMATION. American Academy of Physical Medicine and Rehabilitation, www.aapmr.org.

Psychiatry

Status: Major specialty

Projected need: Significant

Securing a residency: Strong competitive

Training programs: Ca. 175

Positions open: Ca. 1200 (women residents ca. 600)

Training period: Three years (plus an internship)

Weekly patient contact hours: Below average

Attaining patients: Usually by referral

Remuneration: Starting, below average; median, below average

Night and emergency calls: Moderate

SCOPE. Psychiatrists diagnose and treat patients suffering from mental and emotional disorders and disturbances.

ACTIVITIES. Psychiatrists treat patients whose emotional conditions extend from mildly to very severely disturbed. They practice in a wide variety of settings including private offices and psychiatric hospitals, as well as mental health and substance abuse centers and other sites. A wide variety of approaches and modalities are used in psychiatric treatment, including individual or group therapy and psychoanalytic or behavioral modification approaches, as well as electroshock and psychotropic medications.

PROFESSIONAL SATISFACTION. Generally, psychiatrists find gratification in helping patients with emotional problems by making the appropriate diagnosis and electing the proper treatment approach to remedy the problem. The intellectual challenge of ameliorating the disabling effects of mental illness is very strong among psychiatrists. Restoring people to an acceptable functional state can prove very satisfying.

NEGATIVE ATTRIBUTES. The negative response of some individuals to this profession and the relatively lower reimbursement scale are areas of discontent.

DESIRABLE PREREQUISITES. Gaining a sound background in neurology and pharmacology is essential. Having a potential of learning how to probe deeply into the state of mind of an individual by asking appropriate questions and being able to deal with the responses is important.

DESIRABLE PERSONAL ATTRIBUTES AND INTERESTS. Check off the desirable attributes and interests for psychiatrists you know for certain that you have *in abundance*. Then indicate the total number of checks on the bottom of the list as well as on the summary page at the end of this chapter.

_____ Being a very patient and understanding listener

_____ Having strong oral and written communication skills

_____ Preferring analyzing rather than physically evaluating patients

_____ Enjoying long-term relationships with patients

_____ Tolerating ambiguity and uncertainty

_____ Unperturbed by slow or negligible progress

_____ Objective in attitude when evaluating people

_____ Finding it essential to spend adequate time with individual patients

_____ Not finding technological or procedural approaches appealing

_____ Favoring intellectual challenges as related to behavioral issues

_____ Total

RESIDENCY SELECTION FACTORS. Strong performance in medical school, especially in psychiatry and neurology clerkships, is important.

POSTGRADUATE TRAINING/CERTIFICATION. Programs extend for four years including an internship year. Each program has its own philosophical approach. There also exist a few programs having a combined internal medicine–psychiatry residency.

Certification requires completion of a residency and passing written and oral examinations in psychiatry and neurology.

SUBSPECIALTY OPTIONS. Fellowships and certification of added qualifications are available in *child and adolescent psychiatry* as well as *geriatric psychiatry, clinical neuropsychiatry, addiction psychiatry, forensic psychiatry*, and *pain management*.

FOR FURTHER INFORMATION. American Psychiatric Association, www.psych. org.

Radiology (diagnostic)

Status: Major specialty

Projected need: Positions possibly decreasing

Securing a residency: Strongly competitive

Training programs: Ca. 200

Positions open: Ca. 1000 (women residents ca. 250)

Training period: Four years (after an internship)

Weekly patient contact hours: Above average

Attaining patients: By referral

Remuneration: Starting, well above average; median, well above average

Night and emergency calls: Common

SCOPE. These specialists utilize x-rays and other forms of energy (e.g., ultrasound, magnetic fields) to determine the health status of various body systems.

ACTIVITIES. Work in this field involves interpreting images secured by standard x-ray procedures, ultrasound graphic images, CT scans, MRI images, and information from other instruments. Radiologists are also trained to perform various invasive procedures. This specialty area is distinct from therapeutic radiology, commonly known as radiation oncology (see Chapter 6). Most radiologists are active in hospital-based practices, but increasing numbers are being employed in free-standing clinics.

PROFESSIONAL SATISFACTION. Diagnostic radiologists enjoy the challenges that arise from interpreting x-ray data and working with new technologies. They find interacting with clinicians in diagnostic consultations to be especially intellectually gratifying.

NEGATIVE ATTRIBUTES. Some physicians overuse radiological services, whereas others avoid the consultative services of radiologists, looking upon them as technicians.

DESIRABLE PREREQUISITES. Obtaining a strong foundation in anatomy and anatomical radiology is important. It is also desirable to take electives in radiology and be aware of recent technological advances in this field.

DESIRABLE PERSONAL ATTRIBUTES AND INTERESTS. Check off the desirable attributes and interests for radiologists you know for certain that you have *in abundance*. Then indicate the total number of checks on the bottom of the list as well as on the summary page at the end of this chapter.

_____ Good verbal and written communication skills
_____ Prefers working primarily with peers rather than patients
_____ Enjoys challenges in solving problems
_____ Seeks prompt and definitive diagnostic results
_____ Favors a set schedule of activities
_____ Is a technologically oriented individual
_____ Has a patient and relaxed personality
_____ Prefers the role of being a consultative expert
_____ Favors diagnosis rather than treatment
_____ Likes to work independently
_____ Total

RESIDENCY SELECTION FACTORS. The grades obtained in anatomy and in a radiology elective, as well as USMLE Step 1 scores, are principal considerations in securing an appointment. Membership in AOA and research are very desirable.

POSTGRADUATE TRAINING/CERTIFICATION. Almost all residency programs require completing an initial clinical base or transitional year before beginning radiology training. First- and second-year positions in radiology can be secured through the NRMP. With the number of practice openings decreasing, some of the individuals completing radiology residencies are opting for one-year fellowships.

Certification requires completion of a residency as well as written and oral examinations. One can also secure certification in radiology with special competence in nuclear radiology or radiation oncology, for which six months of additional training is required.

SUBSPECIALTY OPTIONS. Fellowships are available in *nuclear radiology, neuroradiology, pediatric radiology, musculoskeletal radiology*, and *vascular interventional radiology*. They usually extend for one year. Those completing the program will receive a Certificate of Special Competence.

Surgery (general)

Status: Major specialty

Projected need: Average

Securing a residency: Strong competitive

Training programs: Ca. 250

Positions open: Ca. 2000 (women residents ca. 500)

Training period: Five years

Weekly patient contact hours: Above average

Attaining patients: By referral

Remuneration: Starting, above average; median, above average

Night and emergency calls: Common

SCOPE. General surgeons diagnose and treat diseases and injuries of the organs of the abdominal cavity using operative procedures of varying types.

ACTIVITIES. The restriction of general surgery to one body area, primarily the abdominal cavity, has resulted from the spin-off of the various surgical subspecialties. However, general surgeons are also called to treat cases of injury to the trunk, back, and limb musculature. In rural areas they may need to be involved in subspecialty work. Advances in laparoscopic techniques and microsurgery have had a profound impact on this field and improved patient care and outcomes.

PROFESSIONAL SATISFACTION. Gratification is usually attained by directly being able to alter the disease process in a definitive manner that is usually highly favorable to the patient. Facing and overcoming diagnostic and technical challenges also provides for much satisfaction. Patients commonly hold their surgeons in very high regard and express their satisfaction to them, which provides a strong sense of fulfillment.

NEGATIVE ATTRIBUTES. As with other specialties, the paperwork and its detailed need for accuracy are sources of discontent.

DESIRABLE PREREQUISITES. An in-depth educational background in anatomy is essential. This is an especially demanding specialty that requires hard work and long hours. Being aware of this is most important before a commitment is made.

DESIRABLE PERSONAL ATTRIBUTES AND INTERESTS. Check off the desirable attributes and interests for general surgeons you know for certain that you have *in abundance*. Then indicate the total number of checks on the bottom of the list as well as on the summary page at the end of this chapter.

_____ Has team leadership qualities

_____ Capable of thinking quickly and acting decisively

_____ Has superior manual dexterity

_____ Enjoys caring for people from all walks of life

_____ Desires to see treatment results quickly

_____ Prefers action to merely thinking

_____ Has role models to influence career choice

_____ Capable of quick recall of knowledge and information

_____ Has a forceful and optimistic personality

_____ Tends to be a perfectionist

_____ Total

RESIDENCY SELECTION FACTORS. High class rank, as well as impressive recommendations that indicate a willingness to work hard, and having a strong basic science foundation are qualities that are sought in prospective candidates.

POSTGRADUATE TRAINING/CERTIFICATION. This specialty involves a five-year training program. Residency appointments are of two types. One is known as *categorical*, which commits the individual and institution to a full five-year relationship, subject to year-by-year review. These residencies are highly competitive. The other type of residency appointment is called *preliminary*, providing for a one- to two-year mutual commitment. It is designed for those planning a surgical subspecialty appointment after acquiring knowledge in basic surgery. There is less competition for such appointments and no assurance that one can continue in the same program in general surgery if the resident desires to do so beyond the preliminary term.

Certification involves completion of a five-year residency and passing written, oral, and clinical testing examinations.

SPECIALTY OPTIONS. These will be considered separately in Chapter 5, where surgical subspecialties are discussed in detail.

FOR FURTHER INFORMATION. American College of Surgeons, www.acs.org.

Urology

Status: Major medical–surgical specialty

Projected need: About average

Securing a residency: Extremely competitive

Training program: Ca. 125 (women residents ca. 30)

Positions open: Ca. 250

Training period: Five years

Weekly patient contact hours: Above average

Attaining patients: Usually by referral

Remuneration: Starting, above average; median, well above average

Night and emergency calls: Periodic

SCOPE. Urologists diagnose and treat diseases and injuries to the kidneys, ureters, bladder, and urethra. For male patients they are also involved in prostate and genital problems and fertility issues.

ACTIVITIES. Urological surgery has moved largely into ambulatory procedures; consequently inpatient service is usually relatively limited. Urologists have expanded their use of noninvasive procedures by utilizing such techniques as lithotripsy to eliminate kidney stones. Urologists and nephrologists frequently collaborate in treating patients with kidney disease.

PROFESSIONAL SATISFACTION. Working in an area where the disease processes are understood and usually treatable, as well as having opportunities for surgery, is gratifying.

NEGATIVE ATTRIBUTES. Urologists as a group seem generally satisfied with their specialty except for the usual complaints about excessive paperwork.

DESIRABLE PREREQUISITES. Taking a urology elective, securing surgical experience, and being an achiever in medical school are especially helpful.

DESIRABLE PERSONAL ATTRIBUTES AND INTERESTS. Check off the desirable attributes and interests for urologists you know for certain that you have *in abundance*. Then indicate the total number of checks on the bottom of the list as well as on the summary page at the end of this chapter.

_____ Have superior manual dexterity

_____ Desire to see concrete results from their activities

_____ Favor regularly scheduled activities

_____ Prefer action to thinking

_____ Like patient contact and helping patients

_____ Enjoy variety rather than repetition

_____ Have outgoing personality

_____ Can communicate well with people

_____ Capable of being a good listener

_____ Enjoy having expertise in a limited area

_____ Total

Table 3.2 Major specialties and your potential suitability

Specialty	Suitability level
Anesthesiology	
Dermatology	
Family practice	
Internal medicine	
Neurology	
Obstetrics/Gynecology	
Ophthalmology	
Otolaryngology	
Pathology	
Pediatrics	
Physical medicine	
Psychiatry	
Radiology	
Surgery	
Urology	

RESIDENCY SELECTION FACTORS. Having an impressive academic record in medical school, especially in the surgery clerkship, and being able to demonstrate superior manual dexterity are important. Membership in AOA and honors in a urology elective, as well as research, can prove most helpful.

POSTGRADUATE TRAINING/CERTIFICATION. Residency training consists of two years of general surgery followed by three years of urology. The specialty appointment is obtained through the American Urological Association Residency Match, which places most of the residents in the specialty. The preliminary general surgical appointment is then secured by being matched through the NRMP.

Certification requires completing a residency as well as written and oral examinations, plus 18 months of practice.

SUBSPECIALTY OPTIONS. Fellowships are available in *pediatric urology* and special training is also offered in *kidney transplantation, urologic oncology,* and *reproductive surgery.* However, no certification program exists for these subspecialty areas.

FOR FURTHER INFORMATION. American Urological Association; www.AUANET. org

Summary

Having reviewed the major specialties, you are now in a position to assess the extent of your natural potential suitability for any of the 15 major specialties discussed.

The results of your self-evaluation should be indicated in Table 3.2 above. Note the number of your personal attributes and interests you checked off for each of the specialties discussed in this chapter.

Transfer the three highest specialty scores checked off to Form 2.3 of the *Specialty Selection protocol* (see p. 23). If uncertain if the attributes of a major specialty choice are applicable to you, compare them to your own framework profile generated in Forms 2.1 and 2.2 (see pp. 19–20). One or more of these specialties may merit being subjected to a reality check (see Chapter 8).

Should internal medicine or surgery be among the top three choices, evaluate your interest in the subspecialties of these two major areas (see Chapters 4 and 5, respectively). If any of the subspecialties are strong potential career choices, these should also be included among the areas to be listed on Form 2.3.

For completeness, review the other specialty topics described in Chapter 6, Since they offer additional career options.

4 | Medical Subspecialties

Overview

There was a time, more than a century ago, when a senior European professor at a medical school was considered a repository of all the knowledge that existed. Such professors were believed to be qualified to teach a wide gamut of subjects in both the basic sciences and clinical areas of medicine. Initial scientific advances in the early part of the 1900s resulted in the therapeutic option becoming separated into two distinct directions, medicine and surgery. Over time, the volume of knowledge regarding all of the body's principal systems and major illnesses dramatically increased. Consequently subspecialization ultimately became inevitable. This development is an ongoing process, with new areas continually evolving (see Chapter 6). Thus, subspecialists have, by virtue of their advanced training, a high degree of expertise in a specific area. Subspecialty training may be secured in the course of a residency or fellowship. Some subspecialties may be organ-specific (e.g., cardiology or nephrology), whereas others are disease-specific (e.g., oncology or rheumatology). Training in the different subspecialties may vary in length and some may require prior PGY-1 preparation.

Characteristics

Table 4.1 summarizes the characteristics of the medical subspecialties. A detailed discussion of each follows.

Table 4.1 Medical subspecialties

Specialty	Nature of work	Prereq. year(s)	Training area	Training period min.	max.
Allergy and immunology	Treatment of illness due to hypersensitivity to a specific substance or condition	Three	Medicine	Two	Three
Cardiovascular diseases	Diagnosis and treatment of heart and blood vessel diseases	Three	Medicine	Three	Three
Critical care	Treating life-threatening cases	Three	Medicine	One	Two
Emergency medicine	Diagnosis and treatment of acute and life-threatening illnesses	One	Medicine	Two	Three
Endocrinology, diabetes, and metabolism	Treatment of diseases of the glanduler system and many hormonal disorders	Three	Medicine	Two	Two
Gastroenterology	Diagnosis and treatment of diseases of the digestive tract	Three	Medicine	Two	Three
Geriatric medicine	Treating illnesses of the elderly	Three	Medicine	Two	Three
Hematology	Treatment of blood disorders	Three	Medicine	Two	Three
Infectious Diseases	Treating communicable illnesses	Three	Medicine	Two	Three
Nephrology	Diseases of the kidneys	Three	Medicine	Two	Three
Oncology	Treating cancer patients	Three	Medicine	Two	Three
Pulmonary medicine	Disease of the respiratory tract	Three	Medicine	Two	Three
Rheumatology	Diagnosis and treatment of arthritic diseases	Three	Medicine	Two	Three

Note: definitions for capsule and text headings are given on p. 26 of Chapter 3.

The choices

Each of 13 medical subspecialties will be discussed below.

Allergy and immunology

Status: Subspecialty of medicine and pediatrics

Projected need: Somewhat above average

Securing a residency: Not competitive

Training programs: Ca. 70

Positions open: Ca. 224 (women residents ca. 150)

Training period: Two-year fellowship (after a three-year residency)

Weekly patient contact hours: Below average

Attaining patients: Primarily by referral

Remuneration: Starting, below average; median, below average

Night and emergency calls: Infrequent

SCOPE. Allergy and immunology are devoted to the diagnosis and treatment of allergic, asthmatic, and immunological diseases, especially those of a chronic nature.

ACTIVITIES. This largely office-based subspecialty is usually practiced in metropolitan areas. The sources of allergic reactions can be determined by testing the patient with a series of small doses of different stimuli or allergens. Once they are identified, the mode of treatment involves injecting mild doses of allergen to gradually build up the patient's immunity to the causative agent (e.g., dust, specific foods). Because of the number of physicians in other fields who do allergy testing and treatment (e.g., family practice doctors and dermatologists), opportunities have diminished.

PROFESSIONAL SATISFACTION. Satisfaction is derived from being able to assist patients in a meaningful way to overcome their personal allergy problems and improve their lifestyles. Specialists also appreciate the intellectual challenge that exists in this field. The fact that there are long-term relationships established with patients, frequently with several members of the same family, adds to practice satisfaction.

NEGATIVE ATTRIBUTES. Frustration may arise from noncompliant and argumentative patients.

DESIRABLE PREREQUISITES. Securing good, broad-based clinical training in medicine is important.

DESIRABLE PERSONAL ATTRIBUTES AND INTERESTS. Check off the desirable attributes and interests of allergists and immunologists you know for certain that you have *in abundance*. Then indicate the total number of checks on the bottom of the list as well as on the summary page at the end of this chapter.

_____ Enjoys helping people with problems that seriously impact their lives

_____ Likes the challenge of problem solving by applying the scientific method

_____ Is detail-oriented in one's work habits

_____ Has an innate investigative approach to problem solving

_____ Has patience and is compassionate and understanding

_____ Has strong verbal communication skills

_____ Favors long-term patient relationships with individuals and families

_____ Prefers an essentially office-based practice

_____ Favors the basic absence of night and emergency calls

_____ Prefers an organized work schedule

_____ Total

SPECIALTY SELECTION FACTORS. The quality of one's performance during residency training is the principal factor in securing an allergy/immunology fellowship. This will be reflected in faculty evaluations and letters of recommendation.

POSTGRADUATE TRAINING/CERTIFICATION. Specializing in this area requires a two-year fellowship in allergy and immunology, after completion of a three-year residency in internal medicine or pediatrics. The training provided covers both allergy and immunology. Patient care is the primary activity, but there is some emphasis on research.

Certification either in internal medicine or pediatrics and successfully completing a two-year fellowship are prerequisites for certification by the American Board of Allergy and Immunology.

SUBSPECIALTY OPTIONS. Some specialists become involved in teaching, research, and administrative work. Advanced work in clinical and laboratory immunology is possible.

FOR FURTHER INFORMATION. American Academy of Allergy, Asthma and Immunology, www.aaaai.org.

Cardiovascular diseases

Status: Medical subspecialty

Projected need: Limited

Securing a residency: Competitive

Training programs: Ca. 175

Positions open: Ca. 700 (women residents ca. 40)

Training period: Three years plus an internal medicine residency

Weekly patient contact hours: Above average

Attaining patients: Referral

Remuneration: Starting, well above average; median, well above average

Night and emergency calls: Very frequent

SCOPE. This specialty involves the medical treatment of adult patients with heart and vascular diseases.

ACTIVITIES. Responsibilities of these practitioners involve both the diagnosis and treatment of relevant medical problems. The former requires securing an accurate history, performing a thorough physical examination, and, where necessary, ordering or executing specific clinical tests. With advances in technology, cardiologists can be divided into office-based, noninvasive, and invasive practitioners. The latter utilize angiography and angioplasty (balloon procedures), respectively, for the diagnosis and treatment of coronary artery disease. Consequently, invasive cardiologists usually are hospital-based practitioners. Some office-based practitioners also perform angioplasty.

PROFESSIONAL SATISFACTION. Gratification comes from being able to establish a definitive diagnosis and then provide treatment that ameliorates the condition whenever possible. Long-term relationships tend to be established with cardiologists, which usually prove especially satisfying for practitioners in this field.

NEGATIVE ATTRIBUTES. This is a very stressful specialty because of the long hours and need to make critical decisions, as well as having an abundance of paperwork.

DESIRABLE PREREQUISITES. Obtaining a solid grasp of internal medicine will provide a strong base for this specialty.

DESIRABLE PERSONAL ATTRIBUTES AND INTERESTS. Check off the desirable attributes and interests of cardiovascular specialists you know for certain that you have *in abundance*. Then indicate the total number of checks on the bottom of the list as well as on the summary page at the end of this chapter.

_____ Having very sound clinical judgment

_____ Being quick-thinking and an action-oriented person

_____ Prepared to routinely handle emergencies

_____ By nature thorough and detail-oriented

_____ Being patient and a good listener

_____ Appreciating long-term patient relationships

_____ Capable of readily making and accepting critical life decisions

_____ Accepting the burden of a very unpredictable schedule

_____ Possessing strong communication skills and a reassuring personality

_____ Having manual dexterity, especially for invasive techniques

_____ Total

SPECIALTY SELECTION FACTORS. Performance during one's internal medicine residency is a major factor. Recommendations from attendings confirming a willingness to work hard as a team member and having a sound knowledge base are very important.

POSTGRADUATE TRAINING/CERTIFICATION. The three-year cardiology program requires prior completion of an internal medicine residency. The cardiology residency can be scored by means of a NRMP Specialty Match. A substantial number of residency programs contract with prospective candidates on an individual basis.

Certification requires completion of a residency and passing of examinations.

SUBSPECIALTY OPTIONS. These are available in *pediatric cardiology* and *clinical cardiac electrophysiology*. Training is also available in *nuclear cardiology* and *cardiac cauterization*.

FOR FURTHER INFORMATION. American College of Cardiology, www.acc.org

Critical care medicine

Status: Medical subspecialty

Projected need: Significant

Securing a residency: Not competitive

Training programs: Ca. 150

Positions open: Ca. 500 (women residents ca. 125)

Training period: Varies from one to two years after prior training

Weekly patient contact hours: Average

Attaining patients: By assignment

Remuneration: Starting, average; median, average

Night and emergency calls: Significant

SCOPE. Working in this specialty involves management of critically ill medical and surgical patients.

ACTIVITIES. Physicians in this multidisciplinary specialty apply their knowledge of respiratory, cardiovascular, and fluid physiology to establishing and maintaining the stability of critically ill patients. They may also have separate practices in areas of their individual specialties, which may be in internal medicine, pulmonary medicine, or anesthesiology. Critical care is exclusively provided in hospitals, because they have the special facilities used exclusively for patients in a serious medical state.

PROFESSIONAL SATISFACTION. The ability to provide potentially lifesaving medical services that may significantly improve a patient's chances for recovery from acute illness, trauma, or surgery will provide much gratification to practitioners in this field.

NEGATIVE ATTRIBUTES. The substantial stress derived from treating very seriously ill patients and having to make life-altering decisions can prove very challenging.

DESIRABLE PREREQUISITES. A strong base in internal medicine, especially in cardiovascular medicine and respiratory physiology, is very useful.

DESIRABLE PERSONAL ATTRIBUTES AND INTERESTS. Check off the desirable attributes and interests of critical care specialists you know for certain that you have in *abundance*. Then indicate the total number of checks on the bottom of the list as well as on the summary page at the end of this chapter.

_____ Capable of rapidly evaluating serious situations

_____ Quick thinking and decisive and appropriate rapid response to events

_____ Rapid recall of vital information

_____ Able to react effectively even under intense pressure

_____ Team leadership abilities

_____ Prefers hospital-based practice

_____ Capable of integrating information effectively

(continued)

(continued)

_____ Accepts short-term relationships with patients

_____ Capable of dealing compassionately with anxious relatives

_____ Prepared to accept failure in spite of maximal effort on patients' behalf

_____ Total

SPECIALTY SELECTION FACTORS. Performance during one's preliminary residency training is a major factor. This will be reflected in letters of recommendation from attendings regarding the quality of patient management.

POSTGRADUATE TRAINING/CERTIFICATION. Training depends on one's background. Certificates of Special Competency are offered by the American Board of Internal Medicine. Two pathways are availlable: a two-year fellowship following residency or a one-year fellowship after subspecialty training. Anesthesiology and surgery boards also offer certificates. Critical care is also a subspecialty option for those in pediatrics.

SUBSPECIALTY OPTIONS. See above. Critical care is commonly incorporated into a three-year pulmonary diseases fellowship.

FOR FURTHER INFORMATION. Society for Critical Care Medicine, www.sccm.org.

Emergency medicine

Status: Medical subspecialty

Projected need: Above average

Securing a residency: Strongly competitive

Training programs: Ca. 125

Positions open: Ca. 1,200 (women residents ca. 300)

Training period: Three or four years

Weekly patient contact hours: Below average

Attaining patients: Usually self-referral (directly or indirectly)

Remuneration: Starting, above average; median, above average

Night and emergency calls: Significant

SCOPE. This specialty deals with a broad spectrum of injuries and acute illnesses, commonly in a hospital emergency room setting or freestanding clinic.

ACTIVITIES. This specialty involves dealing with people from all age groups. Patients are treated who present a very wide variety of problems. They range from major life-threatening conditions to acute illnesses and complex injuries. It may be necessary to use both medical and surgical modalities to treat patients, many of whom may be in dire need. Physicians must be able to make a quick assessment and tentative diagnosis, usually with limited relevant medical information. If the condition is life-threatening, they need to promptly stabilize the patient. When appropriate, the physician needs to arrange for the patient's admission to the appropriate medical or surgical service at the hospital. Patients with limited financial resources suffering from chronic illnesses may also seek help at an emergency room to ameliorate their condition. A pool of such individuals with nonacute problems can be anticipated.

PROFESSIONAL SATISFACTION. The sense of gratification from work in this specialty lies in the nature of the vital activities associated with it. Also there are the diversity of cases and the fast pace and unpredictability of the type of care that needs to be provided to patients who come or are brought into an emergency room.

NEGATIVE ATTRIBUTES. The high degree of stress due to the nature of the activities as well as the need for both day and night shifts. Lack of continuity of care is another negative feature of this specialty.

DESIRABLE PREREQUISITES. Securing broad experience through a wide variety of medical rotations is strongly advised, as is developing one's manual dexterity. Exposure to E.R. work can be very beneficial in identifying your assets relative to work in this unique area.

DESIRABLE PERSONAL ATTRIBUTES AND INTERESTS. Check off the desirable attributes and interests of emergency medicine specialists you know for certain that you have *in abundance*. Then indicate the total number of checks on the bottom of the list as well as on the summary page at the end of this chapter.

_____ Strong team leadership ability

_____ Capacity for rapid assessment of critical situations

_____ Quick decision-making capacity to respond when necessary

_____ Not easily overwhelmed by demanding circumstances

_____ Can function effectively while tolerating intense stress

_____ Knowledgeable in various relevant disciplines of medicine

_____ Can secure cooperation of others to implement tasks

_____ Accepts awesome responsibilities and outcomes

_____ Capable of making challenging critical life decisions

_____ Favors variable experiences and short-term patient contact

_____ Total

SPECIALTY SELECTION FACTORS. Academic performance and relevant letters of recommendation, especially from attendings in this specialty, can be very meaningful. AOA membership and research experiences can prove valuable in securing a residency appointment in this very competitive specialty.

POSTGRADUATE TRAINING/CERTIFICATION. Most positions are secured at the PGY-1 level through the NRMP, but some can be gained through the PGY-2

Advanced NRMP Match. In the latter case, a year of internship in internal medicine, family practice, or surgery or a transitional year is required.

Certification requires completing a three-year residency and an appropriate examination.

SUBSPECIALTY OPTIONS. The NRMP Specialties Matching Services offers competitive opportunity for fellowships in *pediatric emergency medicine*. Other fellowships are offered in *sports medicine, hyperbaric medicine,* and *medical toxicology*.

FOR FURTHER INFORMATION. American College of Emergency Physicians, www.acap.org.

Endocrinology, diabetes, and metabolism

Status: Medical subspecialty

Projected need: Well below average

Securing a residency: Not competitive

Training programs: Ca. 120

Position open: Ca. 225 (women residents ca. 100)

Training period: Two years after internal medicine residency

Weekly patient contact hours: Average

Attaining patients: Usually by referral

Remuneration: Starting, below average; median, below average

Night and emergency calls: Occasional

SCOPE. Specialists in this area treat patients with illnesses resulting from a variety of dysfunctional hormonal conditions.

ACTIVITIES. These specialists are involved in diagnosing and treating various diseases of a hormonal or nutritional nature. This includes disorders such as diabetes and calcium and lipid imbalances, as well as growth and blood pressure disorders. They also serve as consultants regarding treating postoperative patients and may be involved in research.

PROFESSIONAL SATISFACTION. The fact that relevant patient problems are medically treatable and outcomes are frequently favorable is an attractive aspect of this specialty, as are the wide variety of problems encountered and the intellectual challenge involved in resolving them.

NEGATIVE ATTRIBUTES. Lack of compliance on the part of the patient as regards meetings their responsibilities generates frustration on the physician's part.

DESIRABLE PREREQUISITES. Being highly knowledgeable about the physiology of the body and laboratory test procedures and their validation is essential to developing expertise in this area.

DESIRABLE PERSONAL ATTRIBUTES AND INTERESTS. Check off the desirable attributes and interests of endocrinology, diabetes, and metabolism specialists you know for certain that you have *in abundance*. Then indicate the total number of checks on the bottom of the list as well as on the summary page at the end of this chapter.

_____ Seek a high degree of expertise in an intellectually demanding field

_____ Prefer long-term patient relationships with individuals varying in age

_____ Find complex problem-solving challenging

_____ Have good communication and listening skills

_____ Naturally empathetic to patients with chronic illnesses

_____ Does not expect immediate patient response to treatment

_____ Works with patients in an organized manner

_____ Accepts incremental improvement in health status of patients

_____ By nature intellectually curious as to how things work

_____ Prefers to practice in a large city and not at community hospitals

_____ Total

SPECIALTY SELECTION FACTORS. Impressive achievement during one's internal medicine residency, as reflected by recommendations, is most important. Letters from attendings should reflect a strong knowledge base in medicine and an ability to facilitate resolution of complex problems.

POSTGRADUATE TRAINING/CERTIFICATION. A three-year residency in internal medicine is a prerequisite, followed by two years of subspecialty training in endocrinology, diabetes, and metabolism.

SUBSPECIALTY OPTIONS. Opportunities for basic science or clinical research exist.

FOR FURTHER INFORMATION. Endocrine Society, www.endo-society.org.

Gastroenterology

Status: Medical subspecialty

Projected need: Well below average

Securing a residency: Somewhat competitive

Training programs: Ca. 150

Positions open: Ca. 300 (women residents ca. 50)

Training period: Two years (after completing internal medicine residency)

Weekly patient contact hours: Above average

Attaining patients: By referral

Remuneration: Starting, above average; median, above average

Night and emergency calls: Limited

SCOPE. Practitioners deal with diseases of the digestive tract and its associated organs, namely, liver, pancreas, gall bladder, and its ducts.

ACTIVITIES. The clinical potential of this specialty has significantly increased with the very impressive advances in endoscopy that have taken place. This technique permits direct visualization of the esophagus and stomach, whereas colonoscopy allows visualization of the large intestine. Patient age varies and common illnesses treated are ulcers, colitis, and nutritional disorders.

PROFESSIONAL SATISFACTION. Being able to respond satisfactorily to patient needs is a major source of gratification. This is also derived from the challenges of diagnosis and the appeal of using one's manual dexterity in the use of endoscopic procedures.

NEGATIVE ATTRIBUTES. Particularly frustrating for gastroenterologists are psychophysiological problems, which are hard to manage.

DESIRABLE PREREQUISITES. Getting a sound grounding in internal medicine is essential to success as a gastroenterologist.

DESIRABLE PERSONAL ATTRIBUTES AND INTERESTS. Check off the desirable attributes and interests of gastroenterologists you know for certain that you have *in abundance*. Then indicate the total number of checks on the bottom of the list as well as on the summary page at the end of this chapter.

_____ Is procedure-oriented plus having good manual dexterity
_____ Communicates well and is a patient listener
_____ Action-focused rather than thinking-oriented
_____ Likes to face diagnostic challenges
_____ Communicates well and is a good listener
_____ Enjoys patient contact and assisting them in resolving their problems
_____ Analyzes data and systematically seeks to arrive at a diagnosis
_____ Likes to utilize manual skills in activities
_____ Prefers both office- and hospital-based activities
_____ Seeks a scheduled program of activities
_____ Total

SPECIALTY SELECTION FACTORS. Performance during the internal medical residency, as reflected in letters of recommendation from supervising attendings, is the key factor in securing an appointment.

POSTGRADUATE TRAINING/CERTIFICATION. This subspecialty requires two years of training after completing a residency in internal medicine. One can secure a position through the NRMP Specialty Match one year prior to initiation of subspecialty training.

SUBSPECIALTY OPTIONS. An additional year of fellowship training is available in endoscopic retrograde cholangio-pancreatography (ERCP).

FOR FURTHER INFORMATION. American College of Gastroenterology, www.acg.org.

Geriatric medicine

Status: Primary care medical subspecialty

Projected need: Significant

Securing a residency: Not competitive

Training programs: Ca. 125 (ca. 100 in internal medicine, ca. 25 in family practice)

Positions open: Ca. 500 (women residents ca. 50)

Training period: One year (after completing appropriate residency)

Weekly patient contact hours: Average

Attaining patients: Direct or referral

Remuneration: Starting, below average; median, below average

Night and emergency calls: Occasional

SCOPE. Practitioners are involved with treating both medical and psychosocial problems of senior citizens.

ACTIVITIES. This relatively new subspecialty serves the older segment of the population. These people frequently suffer from multiple chronic problems such as hypertension, diabetes, arthritis, and heart dysfunction. This group needs to be treated especially sympathetically and physicians need a great deal of patience and tolerance when dealing with them.

PROFESSIONAL SATISFACTION. There are two major sources of satisfaction for those working in this specialty. They are being able to treat the whole person and in many cases improving the quality of their lives. Relationships can extend over a long period of time.

NEGATIVE ATTRIBUTES. Reimbursement for services is relatively low and patient care is time-consuming.

DESIRABLE PREREQUISITES. Become well grounded in internal medicine, especially diseases that affect the elderly. Familiarize yourself with the special challenge of taking histories and conducting physical exams of the elderly and with their particular needs.

DESIRABLE PERSONAL ATTRIBUTES AND INTERESTS. Check off the desirable attributes and interests of geriatric medicine specialists you know for certain that you have *in abundance*. Then indicate the total number of checks on the bottom of the list as well as on the summary page at the end of the chapter.

_____ Can relate sympathetically to older individuals

_____ Has patience and is highly tolerant of individual idiosyncrasies

(continued)

(continued)

_____ Willing to treat patients with multiple chronic diseases

_____ Accepts incremental progress in outcomes

_____ Prefers regular schedule of activities

_____ Prepared to graciously accept after-hours calls

_____ Seeks longer-term patient relationships

_____ Willing to handle psychosocial needs of patients

_____ Willing to coordinate activities with other care providers

_____ Quick-acting when necessary to meet acute situations

_____ Total

SPECIALTY SELECTION FACTORS. Performance during clerkship training as manifested by letters of recommendation based on an internal medicine residency is the key factor in securing an appointment.

POSTGRADUATE TRAINING/CERTIFICATION. A basic prerequisite for training in this field is completion of a residency in family practice, internal medicine, or psychiatry. A typical accredited program is two years, but others are of varying lengths.

SUBSPECIALTY OPTIONS. A limited number of programs offer training in *geriatric psychiatry*. Fellowships in this field are listed in the Directory of Psychiatry Residency Training Programs put out by the American Psychiatric Association.

FOR FURTHER INFORMATION. American Geriatric Society, www.american geriatrics.org.

Hematology

Status: Medical subspecialty

Projected need: Average

Securing a residency: Not competitive

Training programs: ca. 135 (ca. 25 in hematology; ca. 115 in hematology–oncology)

Positions open: ca. 200 (ca. 50 in hematology; ca. 350 in hematology-oncology), (Women residents, ca. 80)

Training period: Two-year fellowship (after internal medicine residency)

Weekly patient contact hours: Average

Attaining patients: By referral

Remuneration: Starting, above average; median, average

Night and emergency calls: Occasional

SCOPE. Hematologists diagnose and treat patients with diseases of the blood as well as neoplastic diseases.

ACTIVITIES. This largely office-based specialty deals with a wide variety of blood diseases and treats various body organs associated with these problems. Hematologists treat some of their more seriously ill patients in hospitals. Significant progress has been made in treating patients with these diseases over the past decades.

PROFESSIONAL SATISFACTION. Gratification results from the intellectual challenge of attaining a diagnosis by clinical and laboratory methods and providing appropriate treatment for patients in distress due to their condition.

NEGATIVE ATTRIBUTES. When treatment proves unsuccessful, dealing with the consequences is disheartening.

DESIRABLE PREREQUISITES. Gaining a sound background in cell biology, biochemistry, and laboratory testing, coupled with the development of superior clinical diagnostic skills, is essential.

DESIRABLE PERSONAL ATTRIBUTES AND INTERESTS. Check off the desirable attributes and interests of hematologists you know for certain that you have *in abundance*. Then indicate the total number of checks on the bottom of the list as well as on the summary page at the end of this chapter.

_____ Willing to care primarily for seriously ill patients
_____ Seeks the challenge of difficult diagnoses
_____ Genuinely capable of manifesting compassion to the seriously ill
_____ Concerned with the psychosocial needs of patients and their families
_____ Willing to accept schedule disruptions graciously
_____ Action-oriented and quick-acting as circumstances warrant
_____ Comfortable with only incremental progress from therapeutic measures
_____ Being a good listener and communicating well
_____ Detail-oriented and lab testing-focused in formulating diagnoses
_____ Prepared to accept negative outcomes in spite of intense efforts
_____ Total

SPECIALTY SELECTION CRITERIA. An impressive performance during a preliminary internal medicine or pediatric residency will strongly influence attaining a desired subspecialty residency. This should be reflected in evaluations and recommendations by supervising attending physicians.

POSTGRADUATE TRAINING/CERTIFICATION. There are two pathways available to those selecting specialty training in this field. Both require completion of a three-year residency in internal medicine or pediatrics. One path involves two years of subspecialty training in hematology, while the other consists of three years of training in combined hematology–oncology programs. Note that there are some programs exclusively devoted to oncology (see p. 72).

SUBSPECIALTY OPTIONS. See two options noted above.

FOR FURTHER INFORMATION. American Society of Hematology, www. hematology.org.

Infectious diseases

Status: Medical subspecialty

Projected need: Below average

Securing a residency: Somewhat competitive

Training programs: Ca. 140

Positions open: Ca. 300 (women residents ca. 120)

Training period: Two years (after internal medicine residency)

Weekly patient contact hours: Average

Attaining patients: By referral

Remuneration: Starting, below average, median, below average

Night and emergency calls: Limited

SCOPE. Practitioners are involved in the diagnosis and treatment of contagious diseases.

ACTIVITIES. In spite of the advances in vaccination against bacterial infections and immunization, as well as the development of antibiotics, infectious diseases are still rampant. This is especially true for HIV/AIDS and drug-resistant strains of tuberculosis. Work in this field is both office and hospital-based, and frequently involves consultations. Many specialists are engaged in research.

PROFESSIONAL SATISFACTION. The intellectual challenge of arriving at a diagnosis and the ability to assist and even cure people are particularly gratifying. Consulting work is also very appealing.

NEGATIVE ATTRIBUTES. Establishing diagnoses in this specialty is very time-demanding and generates pressure and stress, as do the unforeseen calls for consultations.

DESIRABLE PREREQUISITES. Securing a strong foundation of basic medical knowledge is essential for this specialty. One needs to be alert to details and be conscientious about keeping up with current literature.

DESIRABLE PERSONAL ATTRIBUTES AND INTERESTS. Check off the desirable attributes and interests of infectious diseases specialists you know for certain that you have *in abundance*. Then indicate the total number of checks on the bottom of the list as well as on the summary page at the end of the chapter.

_____ Enjoys the challenge of complex problems

_____ Willing to expend long hours at work

_____ Can relate well to referring physicians, patients, and their families

_____ Highly observant and very detail-oriented personality

_____ Willing to accept schedule disruptions

(continued)

(continued)

_____ Highly patient and logical regarding problem-solving

_____ Enjoys caring for patients, even if progress is slow or negligible

_____ Careful to protect one's own well-being when practicing

_____ Has a positive outlook on life and its problems

_____ Recognizes the strong possibility of negative outcomes

_____ Total

SPECIALTY SELECTION FACTORS. Performance during an internal medicine residency as reflected in recommendations by supervising attendings is critical in determining your potential for an appointment.

POSTGRADUATE TRAINING/CERTIFICATION. Two-year fellowship appointments can be secured after completing an internal medicine residency. Fellowships can be secured via the NRMP Specialties Matching Services.

SUBSPECIALTY OPTIONS. Opportunities for work in HIV/AIDS research are available in many locations.

FOR MORE INFORMATION. Infectious Disease Society of America, www.infsociety.org.

Nephrology

Status: Medical subspecialty

Projected need: Below average

Securing a residency: Not competitive

Training programs: Ca. 125

Positions open: Ca. 350 (women residents ca. 100)

Training period: Two years (after internal medicine residency)

Weekly patient contact hours: Above average

Attaining patients: By referral

Remuneration: Starting, above average; median, average

Night and emergency calls: Frequent

SCOPE. Nephrologists deal with patients having kidney diseases and disorders of the urinary tract.

ACTIVITIES. Most patients seeking the services of nephrologists suffer from chronic diseases. The major activities in this specialty are managing dialysis and treating transplant patients. This largely office-based practice also involves considerable consultative work.

PROFESSIONAL SATISFACTION. There are two major features that provide for gratification for work in this field. One involves the challenge of the diagnostic and treatment aspects; the other is that successful treatment can, in many cases, be lifesaving.

NEGATIVE ATTRIBUTES. Caring for chronically ill patients can produce considerable stress. In addition, excessive regulations add to the burden of work in this specialty.

DESIRABLE PREREQUISITES. It is very desirable to obtain some experience working with a practicing nephrologist. This exposure can be very informative as to what one anticipates in this field.

DESIRABLE PERSONAL ATTRIBUTES AND INTERESTS. Check off the desirable attributes and interests of nephrologists you know for certain that you have *in abundance*. Then indicate the total number of checks on the bottom of the list as well as on the summary page at the end of the chapter.

_____ Enjoys the challenge of problem-solving

_____ Has a detailed and precision-oriented nature

_____ Favors long-term patient contact

_____ Enjoys helping patients with serious medical problems

_____ Able to treat chronically ill patients in a sympathetic manner

_____ Favors long term patient relationships

_____ Capable of facing physical and emotional challenges

_____ Has good communication and listening skills

_____ Has a strong logical approach to complex problems

_____ Willing to persevere even in the face of severe obstacles

_____ Total

SPECIALTY SELECTION FACTORS. Letters of recommendation from supervising attendings during one's internal medicine residency have a decisive impact on being selected for an appointment in nephrology.

POSTGRADUATE TRAINING/CERTIFICATION. Initially one must satisfactorily complete a three-year internal medicine residency. This is then followed by a two-year fellowship in nephrology. To secure a fellowship the programs need to be contacted directly.

SUBSPECIALTY OPTIONS. Not relevant.

FOR FURTHER INFORMATION. American Society of Nephrology, www.asn-online.org.

Oncology

Status: Medical subspecialty

Projected need: Somewhat low

Securing a residency: Somewhat competitive

Training programs: Ca. 30

Positions open: Ca. 100

Training period: Two years (after an internal medicine residency)

Weekly patient contact hours: Average

Attaining options: By referral

Remuneration: Starting, average; median, average

Night and emergency calls: Occasional

SCOPE. This specialty deals with the diagnosis and treatment of neoplastic diseases.

ACTIVITIES. Oncology is only partially an office-based specialty, because it has considerable hospital responsibilities. Specialists may be affiliated with large medical centers as well as community hospitals. The negative impact of this disease on the various body organs has called for varying approaches to treatment. Consequently, oncologists have developed areas of special expertise. Many hematologists are also involved in oncology.

PROFESSIONAL SATISFACTION. Significant strides have been made in oncology. Consequently, when possible, extending life and ameliorating pain of the chronically ill can prove gratifying, even in the face of frequent terminal outcomes.

NEGATIVE ATTRIBUTES. The principal frustration stems from the result of failure when one has made a maximal effort to succeed.

DESIRABLE PREREQUISITES. Serious self-evaluation to determine your ability to work in this very stressful specialty is critical. So is the willingness to frequently make life-and-death decisions. One needs to have the ability to assist both patients and their families in chronic, critical situations that may extend for a long period of time.

DESIRABLE PERSONAL ATTRIBUTES AND INTERESTS. Check off the desirable attributes and interests of oncologists you know for certain that you have *in abundance*. Then indicate the total number of checks on the bottom of the list as well as on the summary page at the end of this chapter.

_____ Having an optimistic nature is most imperative

_____ Anxious to help patients in dire need and provide support to their families

_____ Prepared to face very emotionally challenging problems with most patients

_____ Possess the psychosocial skills needed to communicate with cancer patients

_____ Prepared to be flexible in the face of changing circumstances

_____ Strongly favors continuous education to stay up to date

_____ Recognizes the strong inherent possibilities of failure and frustration

_____ Potentially capable of being very patient and intensely compassionate

_____ Capable of decision-making with limited information

_____ Able to act objectively under the stress of treating the critically ill

_____ Total

SPECIALTY SELECTION FACTORS. As with other subspecialties, appointments are greatly influenced by input from internal medicine residency supervisors such as the chairperson and department head and attendings, as reflected in their letters of recommendation.

POSTGRADUATE TRAINING/CERTIFICATION. Completing an internal medicine or pediatric residency is a prerequisite for undertaking a one-year oncology program. Many programs offer combined three-year hematology–oncology training fellowships.

SUBSPECIALTY OPTION. Combined hematology–oncology program noted above, (see also p. 68).

FOR MORE INFORMATION. American Society of Clinical Oncology, www.asco.org.

Pulmonary medicine

Status: Medical subspecialty

Projected need: Below average

Securing a residency: Somewhat competitive

Training programs: Ca. 35

Positions open: Ca. 75 (women residents ca. 30)

Training period: Two years (after an internal medicine residency)

Weekly patient contact hours: Average

Attaining patients: By referral

Remuneration: Starting, below average; median, average

Night and emergency calls: Occasional

SCOPE. Pulmonologists diagnose and treat diseases of the respiratory system.

ACTIVITIES. This is both an office- and hospital-based specialty. It deals mostly with patients having chronic lung diseases including cancer, asthma, emphysema, and a variety of occupational illnesses. There are a number of standard procedures associated with pulmonary medicine, including bronchoscopy, mechanical ventilation management, and endotracheal intubation.

PROFESSIONAL SATISFACTION. The intellectual challenge of a specialty and a willingness to remain active in internal medicine can contribute to professional satisfaction. Gratification also comes about by virtue of the variety of patients seen for diagnosis and treatment.

NEGATIVE ATTRIBUTES. The stressful nature of dealing with critical care situations and incidents of negative outcomes is troublesome.

DESIRABLE PREREQUISITES. Securing a strong foundation as a medical student in physiology, microbiology, and radiology is strongly advised.

DESIRABLE PERSONAL ATTRIBUTES AND INTERESTS. Check off the desirable attributes and interests of pulmonary medicine specialists, you know for certain that you have *in abundance*. Then indicate the total number of checks on the bottom of the list as well as on the summary page at the end of this chapter.

_____ Desires to face challenging problems

_____ Likes patient contact and assisting them

_____ Is mechanically inclined

_____ Has a detailed and precision-oriented personality

_____ Favors decision-making rather than merely thinking

_____ Has good communication skills and patience to listen

_____ Prepared to work patiently with chronically ill individuals

_____ Has manual dexterity to meet the specialty's needs

_____ Has intellectual curiosity to address problems

_____ Favors an organized work schedule

_____ Total

SPECIALTY SELECTION FACTORS. Performance during internal residency training as judged by attendings during your internal medical residency will be decisive in being selected for a fellowship.

POSTGRADUATE TRAINING/CERTIFICATION. Following satisfactory completion of a three-year internal medicine residency, upon acceptance, one undertakes a pulmonary medicine fellowship. These can be secured through the NRMP Specialty Match.

Certification can be acquired upon satisfactory completion of a fellowship and passing appropriate exams.

SUBSPECIALTY OPTIONS. Additional training can be taken to secure expertise in _critical care medicine_ or _pediatric pulmonology._

FOR FURTHER INFORMATION. American College of Pulmonary Physicians, www.chestnet.org.

Rheumatology

Status: Medical subspecialty

Projected need: Below average

Securing a residency: Not competitive

Training programs: Ca. 100

Positions open: Ca. 175 (women residents ca. 90)

Training period: Three-year fellowship (after an internal medicine residency)

Weekly patient contact hours: Below average

Attaining patients: By referral

Remuneration: Starting, below average; median, below average

Night and emergency calls: Occasional

SCOPE. Rheumatologists are involved in the diagnosis and treatment of diseases of the joints and soft tissues.

ACTIVITIES. Physicians practicing in this essentially office-based specialty, for the most part, treat patients suffering from arthritis. Other patients may have a variety of musculoskeletal or autoimmune diseases. Their medical problems may be acute or chronic. Considerable advances have been made in this field in recent years. Specialists may be called in for consultative work and their practice may also involve internal medicine along with rheumatology, rather than being engaged full time in the latter.

PROFESSIONAL SATISFACTION. Gratification commonly stems from diagnostic challenges. Arthritic problems frequently respond to medical treatment. Rhumatologists provide amelioration of pain and hence an improvement in the quality of patients' life. This is obviously satisfying for practitioners in this field.

NEGATIVE ATTRIBUTES. None are specific to this field. Those existing are communication problems with patients and administrative tasks typical of many other specialized areas.

DESIRABLE PREREQUISITES. Securing a strong base in biochemistry, immunology, and radiology is very desirable. Some other relevant areas in which to secure experience are orthopedics and rehabilitation.

DESIRABLE PERSONAL ATTRIBUTES AND INTERESTS. Check off the desirable attributes and interests of rheumatologists you know for certain that you have *in abundance*. Then indicate the total number of checks on the bottom of the list as well as on the summary page at the end of this chapter.

_____ Prepared to work primarily with geriatric patients

_____ Willing to provide long-term care

_____ Satisfied with incremental progress to therapeutic measures

_____ Favors an organized work schedule

_____ Has considerable patience and good communication skills

_____ Has a detail- and precision-oriented personality

_____ Enjoys patient contact in an office setting

_____ Willing to handle complex problems

_____ Exacting and detail-oriented individual

_____ Not especially attracted to procedural approaches in medical care

_____ Total

SPECIALTY SELECTION FACTOR. The impact of recommendations from the internal medicine residency will significantly influence your potential for gaining a fellowship.

POSTGRADUATE TRAINING/CERTIFICATION. A three-year residency in internal medicine must be completed satisfactorily prior to initiating a fellowship in rheumatology. One needs to contact the program directly to apply for a position.

Table 4.2 Medical subspecialties and your potential suitability	
Subspecialty	**Suitability level**
Allergy and immunology	
Cardiovascular diseases	
Critical care medicine	
Emergency medicine	
Endocrinology, diabetes, and metabolism	
Gastroenterology	
Geriatric medicine	
Hematology	
Infectious diseases	
Nephrology	
Oncology	
Pulmonary medicine	
Rheumatology	

SUBSPECIALTY OPTIONS. There are opportunities for specialized training in *pediatric rheumatology.*

FOR FURTHER INFORMATION. American College of Rheumatology, www.rheumatology.org.

Summary

Having reviewed the medical subspecialties, you are now in a position to assess the extent of your natural potential and suitability for any of the thirteen that have been discussed. The results of your self-evaluation should be indicated on Table 4.2. Note the number of your personal attributes and interests you checked off for each of the medical subspecialties discussed in this chapter.

Transfer the three highest-ranked subspecialties to the appropriate column of Form 2.3 of the *Specialty Selection Protocol.* (see p. 23). If uncertain if the attributes of a prospective subspecialty choice are applicable to you, compare them with your own framework profile generated in Forms 2.1 and 2.2. (see pp. 19 and 20). One or more of your choices may later merit being subjected to a reality check (see Chapter 8).

5 | Surgical Subspecialties

Overview

Surgery has been the major alternative treatment modality to medicine since the profession was placed on a sound scientific footing. The introduction of anesthesia and the multitude of advances made in this field have dramatically enhanced the opportunities for the performance of surgery. Recognition of the critical importance of antisepsis, combined with the introduction of antibiotics, has allowed highly successful outcomes of surgical intervention. Consequently, advances in surgery have had a profound impact on the quality of health and have contributed significantly to the extension of life.

As a result of fundamental advances in patient care, as well as major technological breakthroughs, it became possible to apply therapeutic surgical approaches in all body areas. Consequently, a significant number of surgical subspecialties have evolved. Surgery is also a component of several major specialties, such as ophthalmology, otolaryngology, obstetrics/gynecology, and urology. The introduction of microsurgical, laparoscopic, and laser techniques has further expanded the potential of the field significantly and diminished the inherent risk of surgery for most patients.

Characteristics

Table 5.1 summarizes the characteristics of the surgical subspecialties. A detailed discussion of each of them follows.

Table 5.1 Surgical subspecialties

Specialty	Nature of work	Prereq. year(s)	Training area	Training period min.	max.
Colon and rectal surgery	Treatment of diseases of the lower bowel	Three	General surgery	Two	Two
Hand surgery	Treatment of injuries to the hand and forearm	Five	General surgery	One	One
Neurological surgery	Surgery of the brain, spinal cord, and peripheral nerves	One	General surgery	Five	Six
Orthopedic surgery	Treatment of skeletal deformities and injuries to bones and joints	One	General surgery	Three	Four
Plastic surgery	Surgery to repair or restore injured, deformed, or destroyed parts of the body.	Four	General surgery	Two	Three
Thoracic surgery	Surgical treatment of chest diseases	Four	General surgery	Two	Two
Vascular surgery	Surgery of blood vessels	Five	General surgery	Two	Two

Note: See definitions for capsule summaries described on pg. 26.

The choices

Seven surgical subspecialties will be discussed below.

Colon and rectal surgery

Status: Surgical subspecialty

Projected need: Above average

Securing a residency: Competitive

Training programs: Ca. 50

Positions open: Ca. 60 (women residents ca. 10)

Training.: One year (after a five-year general surgery residency)

Weekly patient contact hours: Above average

Attaining patients: By referral

Remuneration: Starting, above average; median, well above average

Night and emergency calls: Occasional

SCOPE. Colon and rectal surgeons apply their skills in the diagnosis and treatment of problems associated with the large intestine, rectum, and anal canal, as well as the perineal region.

ACTIVITIES. The major diagnostic technique used by these specialists in performing their activities is endoscopy. When appropriate, they apply their surgical skills to resolving problems amenable to such treatment. Work in this field is divided between office- and hospital-based settings.

PROFESSIONAL SATISFACTION. Gratification is afforded from being able to perform surgery that results in enhancing patients' well-being and frequently being able to resolve serious problems.

NEGATIVE ATTRIBUTES. These include long hours, paperwork, and dealing with negative outcomes. These dislikes are also common for other surgical natures.

DESIRABLE PREREQUISITES. Determine your liking for surgery and seek to gain exposure to colon and rectal surgery. Strong manual dexterity skills in general surgery are especially needed in this field. Being decisive and having an even temperament are valuable assets for a successful practice in general and this subspecialty in particular.

DESIRABLE PERSONAL ATTRIBUTES AND INTERESTS. Check off the desirable attributes and interests of colon and rectal surgeons you know for certain that you have *in abundance*. Then indicate the total number of checks on the bottom of the list as well as on the summary page at the end of this chapter.

_____ Has superior manual dexterity

_____ Desires a high degree of professional medical expertise

_____ Strongly prefers prompt concrete results from one's efforts

_____ Enjoys patient contact even if it is short-term

_____ Meticulous and thorough work habits are standard

_____ Favors a structured professional work schedule

_____ Can act decisively and quickly when necessary

_____ Anxious to use manipulative skills regularly

_____ Comfortable with working in a limited area

_____ Likes challenging medical situations

_____ Total

SPECIALTY SELECTION FACTORS. Evaluation of your residency performance by means of letters from supervising attendings during general surgery training will strongly influence securing a fellowship in this field.

POSTGRADUATE TRAINING/CERTIFICATION. The postgraduate training period is among the longest, involving a five-year general surgery residency plus a one-year colon and rectal surgery fellowship.

Certification in this subspecialty requires prior certification in general surgery and satisfactory completion of fellowship training in the specialty.

SUBSPECIALTY OPTIONS. Not relevant.

FOR FURTHER INFORMATION. American Society of Colon & Rectal Surgeons, www.fascrs.org.

Hand surgery

Status: Surgical subspecialty

Projected need: Average

Securing a residency: Competitive

Training programs: Ca. 50

Positions open: Ca. 100 (women residents ca. 28)

Training.: One-year fellowship (after a five-year general surgery residency)

Weekly patient contact hours: Average

Attaining patients: By referral

Remuneration: Starting, average, median, average

Night and emergency calls: Occasional

SCOPE. Hand surgeons are concerned with the diagnosis and treatment of disorders of and injuries to the hand and forearm.

ACTIVITIES. Advances in microsurgical techniques have had a profound impact on the potential of the subspecialty of hand surgery. This mostly outpatient surgical practice area has become very important, especially in light of the high incidence of sports injuries. Some practitioners have such a high degree of expertise that they can undertake surgical reimplantation of limbs after major accidents.

PROFESSIONAL SATISFACTION. This stems primarily from the highly valuable service surgeons provide individuals by means of their surgical skills in restoring functional use of hands and arms.

NEGATIVE ATTRIBUTES. This subspecialty has drawbacks similar to those of others in surgery, but due to its limited scope it is difficult to establish oneself at the offset.

DESIRABLE PREREQUISITES. A good background in muscloskeletal anotomy and neuroanatomy as well as neurology is a strong asset. Superior manual dexterity talents and being able to make quick judgments are very desirable. Being calm under pressure and having good communication skills will prove very useful.

DESIRABLE PERSONAL ATTRIBUTES AND INTERESTS. Check off the desirable attributes and interests of hand surgeons you know for certain that you have *in abundance*. Then indicate the total number of checks on the bottom of the list as well as on the summary page at the end of this chapter.

_____ Gains satisfaction from working with one's hands

_____ Acts decisively and quickly when necessary

_____ Prefers professional medical expertise in a limited area

_____ Prefers an organized professional schedule

(continued)

(continued)

_____ Seeks readily apparent results from treatment

_____ Desires challenging opportunities

_____ Is very patient by nature

_____ Has meticulous work habits

_____ Total

SPECIALTY SELECTION FACTORS. Performance during surgical residency as reflected in letters of recommendation from supervising attendings will provide a major basis for fellowship selection in hand surgery.

POSTGRADUATE TRAINING/CERTIFICATION. Completion of a residency in general surgery, orthopedic surgery, or plastic surgery is a prerequisite for securing a fellowship in hand surgery. These can be obtained through the NRMP Specialty Match.

SUBSPECIALTY OPTIONS. Not applicable.

FOR FURTHER INFORMATION. American Association of Hand Surgery, www. handsurgery.org.

Neurological surgery

Status: Surgical subspecialty

Projected need: Average

Securing a residency: Strongly competitive

Training programs: Ca. 100

Positions open: Ca. 150 (women residents ca. 15)

Training.: Six to seven years (after first postgraduate year)

Weekly patient contact hours: Above average

Attaining patients: By referral

Remuneration: Starting, well above average; median, well above average

Night and emergency calls: Common

SCOPE. Covers the diagnosis and surgical treatment of diseases of and injuries to the brain, spinal and peripheral nerve injuries and abnormalities, and injuries to associated structures.

ACTIVITIES. Neurosurgeons utilize both operative and nonoperative approaches in their treatment protocols. Like anesthesiologists, they are involved in pain management cases. Newer innovative approaches such as stereotactic surgery and fetal tissue transplantation are opening new vistas for the treatment of a variety of neurological diseases.

PROFESSIONAL SATISFACTION. This frequently comes from dramatic postoperative patient outcomes. The challenge of resolving complex technical issues surgically, especially in a highly confined area is, particularly appealing to neurosurgeons.

NEGATIVE ATTRIBUTES. As in other surgical subspecialties, paperwork is frowned upon. The consequences of negative outcomes having a very profound effect on lowering the quality of life is troublesome.

DESIRABLE PREREQUISITES. A strong foundation in neuroanatomy and neurology is an essential basis for this specialty. A high degree of manual dexterity is very important.

DESIRABLE PERSONAL ATTRIBUTES AND INTERESTS. Check off the desirable attributes and interests of neurological surgeons you know for certain that you have *in abundance.* Then indicate the total number of checks on the bottom of the list as well as on the summary page at the end of this chapter.

_____ Manual dexterity is very well developed

_____ Extremely patient personality, especially when under stress

_____ Capable of devoting meticulous attention to detail

_____ Has a high degree of self-confidence

_____ Can work well under intense pressure

_____ Seeks perfection in work being done

_____ Enjoys working with one's hands

_____ Desires to observe significant results from one's efforts

_____ Likes working with and caring for seriously ill patients

_____ Prepared to patiently solve complicated and challenging problems

_____ Total

SPECIALTY SELECTION FACTORS. Evidence of superior ability in neuroanatomy, neurology, and neurophysiology is very valuable. Also, it is helpful to gain experimental experience in animal work in this field, in addition to clinical exposure. Having a strong interest in neuroscience, surgery, and research is a major asset in securing a residency appointment.

POSTGRADUATE TRAINING/CERTIFICATION. Residency positions can be secured through the Neurological Surgery Matching Program, which is sponsored by the Society of Neurological Surgeons. Rank Order Lists are submitted in mid-January with the results announced around the end of the month. Students need initially to sign up for the NRMP PGY-1 Match for an internship position.

Certification involves completing a residency, passing a written exam, and after two years of practice an oral exam.

SUBSPECIALTY OPTIONS. Not relevant.

FOR FURTHER INFORMATION. American Association of Neurological Surgeons, www.aans.org.

Orthopedic surgery

Status: Surgical subspecialty

Projected need: Below average

Securing a residency: Extremely competitive

Training programs: Ca. 150

Positions open: Ca. 600 (women residents ca. 55)

Training.: Five years

Weekly patient contact hours: Average

Attaining patients: By referral

Remuneration: Starting, above average; median, well above average

Night and emergency calls: Moderate

SCOPE. Orthopedic surgeons seek to restore maximal function to diseased, deformed, or injured segments of the musculoskeletal system.

ACTIVITIES. Practitioners utilize, in addition to surgery, medications and physical and occupational therapy in their work. Ambulatory surgery has increased significantly in this specialty. In addition to treating fractures and other injuries, major technological advances allow treatment for joint degeneration and congenital skeletal deformities.

PROFESSIONAL SATISFACTION. Using clinical judgment and skill to solve a wide variety of interesting and challenging orthopedic problems is most gratifying. Being in a field that is actively making significant advances is especially appealing.

NEGATIVE ATTRIBUTES. Paperwork associated with compensation and disability cases and a variety of liability claims is time-consuming.

DESIRABLE PREREQUISITES. Completing an orthopedic surgery clerkship, if possible at a site of a potential residency, is strongly advised, because it provides a reliable source for evaluating your potential.

DESIRABLE PERSONAL ATTRIBUTES AND INTERESTS. Check off the desirable attributes and interests of orthopedic surgeons you know for certain that you have *in abundance*. Then indicate the total number of checks on the bottom of the list as well as on the summary page at the end of this chapter.

_____ Being an action-oriented individual

_____ Capable of acting decisively when necessary

_____ Has good hand–eye coordination for meticulous work

_____ Capable of applying a biomechanical approach to problems

_____ Possessing good oral and written communication skills

_____ Enjoys caring for people and improving their health status

(continued)

(continued)

_____ Accepts disruption in one's daily schedule

_____ Favors challenging situations that unexpectedly arise

_____ Responds decisively to situations that need prompt attention

_____ Enjoys obtaining prompt response to one's efforts

_____ Total

SPECIALTY SELECTION FACTORS. Because of its very highly competitive nature, high USMLE scores, research experience, AOA membership, and an impressive clerkship evaluation in this field will facilitate securing a residency.

POSTGRADUATE TRAINING/CERTIFICATION. Most residency appointments at the PGY-1 level are filled through the NRMP. Training usually involves a one-year transitional internship and four years of orthopedics. The initial year can be in general surgery or another approved medical/surgical specialty.

Certification requires completion of a residency, 22 months of experience, and passing a written examination.

SUBSPECIALTY OPTIONS. One-year fellowships are available in a wide variety of areas, including *hand surgery, reconstructive orthopedics, musculoskeletal oncology, pediatric, orthopedic surgery, sports medicine, surgery of the spine,* and *joint replacement surgery.*

FOR FURTHER INFORMATION. American Academy of Orthopedic Surgeons, www.aaos.org.

Plastic surgery

Status: Surgical subspecialty

Projected need: Below average

Securing a residency: Extremely competitive

Training programs: Ca. 90

Positions open: Ca. 180 (women residents ca. 40)

Training.: Two or three years fellowship (following a surgery residency)

Weekly patient contact hours: Average

Attaining patients: By referral

Remuneration: Starting, above average; median, well above average

Night and emergency calls: Significant

SCOPE. Plastic surgery involves treating patients using operative methods for both reconstructive and cosmetic purposes.

ACTIVITIES. These practitioners utilize their skills to correct body disfigurations arising from trauma or congenital sources. The potential of this field has expanded with the development of microsurgical and liposuction techniques. A very substantial amount of plastic surgery is carried out on an outpatient basis.

PROFESSIONAL SATISFACTION. This is derived from meeting a challenge and using one's aesthetic and surgical skills to achieve visible results that provide patients with a high degree of personal satisfaction.

NEGATIVE ATTRIBUTES. Some patients are not satisfied because of unrealistic expectations. Some problems are unsolvable and thus one cannot always respond to patient needs.

DESIRABLE PREREQUISITES. A high level of achievement in one's surgical clerkship and a good anatomical base are necessary.

DESIRABLE PERSONAL ATTRIBUTES AND INTERESTS. Check off the desirable attributes and interests of plastic surgeons you know for certain that you have *in abundance*. Then indicate the total number of checks on the bottom of the list as well as on the summary page at the end of this chapter.

_____ Has good judgment as to what is defined as being attractive
_____ Naturally gifted with a keen sense of proportion
_____ Having superior hand–eye coordination
_____ Skilled in oral communication with patients
_____ Possessing patient and meticulous work habits
_____ Being sensitive to psychosocial issues of appearance
_____ Favoring challenging situations involving clinical judgment
_____ Prepared to act after only giving careful forethought to the situation
_____ Prepared to wait to see tangible results of one's efforts
_____ Seeks to provide patient satisfaction with one's efforts on their behalf
_____ Total

SPECIALTY SELECTION FACTORS. Achievement during prior surgical residency training and one's academic accomplishments in medical school are key factors in fellowship attainment. The more surgical experience one has, the more favorable are chances to secure an appointment.

POSTGRADUATE TRAINING/CERTIFICATION. Traditionally residents complete a three-year general surgery residency, followed by a two-year plastic surgery fellowship. Some plastic surgery programs are three years in length and others accept those who have completed otolaryngology or orthopedic surgery residencies. Because programs vary, it is essential to submit an "Evaluation of Training" form (obtained from the Specialty Board).

Certification requires passing the Surgery Boards, completing a fellowship and then a written exam, and having two years of experience plus an oral exam.

SUBSPECIALTY OPTIONS. After completing a plastic surgery residency, additional training can be obtained in *hand surgery, craniofacial surgery, microsurgery,* or *burn surgery*.

FOR FURTHER INFORMATION. American Academy of Facial & Reconstructive Surgery, www.aafprs.org.

THORACIC SURGERY

Status: Surgical subspecialty

Projected need: Average

Securing a residency: Somewhat competitive

Training programs: Ca. 90

Positions open: Ca. 150 (women residents ca. 10)

Training.: Two-year fellowship (after general surgery residency)

Weekly patient contact hours: Below average

Attaining patients: By referral

Remuneration: Starting, well above average; median well above average

Night and emergency calls: Modest

SCOPE. Practitioners employ surgery to treat diseases or injury to the chest wall and the contents of the chest cavity, namely the heart, the lungs, and their associated vessels.

ACTIVITIES. One of the common operations that cardiothoracic surgeons perform is coronary artery bypass procedures. Those procedures are less complex than heart valve replacement surgery. Work in this area is very stressful and time-consuming. Transplant surgery is practiced by specially trained thoracic surgeons. If the use of artificial hearts proceeds at some future date beyond its current experimental stages, this dynamic field will have a potential need for many more residents.

PROFESSIONAL SATISFACTION. Specialists in the field gain much gratitude and recognition from their patients. This is because patients usually experience dramatic improvement in their condition as a direct consequence of the surgery.

NEGATIVE ATTRIBUTES. The complications that lead to unfortunate outcomes and the need to communicate this to families are stressful.

DESIRABLE PREREQUISITES. A solid anatomy background and surgical clerkship training are essential. Also, gaining experience in this specialty is quite valuable.

DESIRABLE PERSONAL ATTRIBUTES AND INTERESTS. Check off the desirable attributes and interests of thoracic surgeons you know for certain that you have *in abundance*. Then indicate the total number of checks on the bottom of the list as well as on the summary page at the end of this chapter.

_____ Utilizes a logical stepwise approach to resolving problems

_____ Enjoys working with one's hands professionally

_____ Possess superior manual dexterity

_____ Maintains a calm demeanor even under intense stress

(continued)

(continued)

_____ Exhibits patience, determination, and stamina

_____ Quick-thinking and acting in the face of unexpected difficulties

_____ Demonstrates leadership qualities when performing services

_____ Enjoys solving complex medical problems

_____ Seeks a visible response to one's intense surgical efforts

_____ Prepared to make major decisions regarding a person's longevity

_____ Total

SPECIALTY SELECTION FACTORS. The evaluation of performance during one's general surgery residency will significantly influence securing a fellowship in thoracic surgery.

POSTGRADUATE TRAINING/CERTIFICATION. There is a need to complete a three-year general surgery residency prior to undertaking a fellowship in thoracic surgery. This is obtainable through the NRMP Specialties Matching Service.

Certification requires initial board certification in general surgery. Completion of the subspecialty fellowship, plus passing written and oral examinations, is also necessary.

SUBSPECIALTY OPTIONS. Some further training options are available in *transplant surgery.*

FOR FURTHER INFORMATION. Society of Thoracic Surgeons, www.sts.org.

Vascular surgery

Status: General surgery subspecialty

Projected need: Below average

Securing a residency: Extremely competitive

Training programs: Ca. 90

Positions open: Ca. 100 (women residents ca.10)

Training.: One-year fellowship (following a four-year surgical residency)

Weekly patient contact hours: Average

Attaining patients: By referral

Remuneration: Starting, above average; median, above average

Night and emergency calls: Occasional

SCOPE. These practitioners diagnose and treat diseases of the arterial, venous, and lymphatic systems by surgical approaches.

ACTIVITIES. Vascular surgeons are engaged in treating patients whose arteries may be injured or are clogged and thus are generating circulatory problems. Newer methods of microsurgery permit repair of torn, damaged, or bulging blood vessels (aneurysms). Surgeons affiliated with large medical centers are usually involved full-time with work in this specialty. Other specialists who are affiliated with smaller institutions may be engaged in both vascular and general surgery to maintain a fully active practice.

PROFESSIONAL SATISFACTION. Gratification is received in seeing a prompt response, which is often dramatic, to surgical intervention with the restoration of proper blood circulation.

NEGATIVE ATTRIBUTES. As with other surgical fields, administrative work is unpopular and the demand for very careful surgical technique can prove stressful.

DESIRABLE PREREQUISITES. Attaining a solid grounding in anatomy and surgery is essential. Also, if possible, completing an elective in the field is quite valuable.

DESIRABLE PERSONAL ATTRIBUTES AND INTERESTS. Check off the desirable attributes and interests of vascular surgeons you know for certain that you have *in abundance*. Then indicate the total number of checks on the bottom of the list as well as on the summary page at the end of the chapter.

_____ Being detail-oriented and patient by nature
_____ Having meticulous work habits even when working under stress
_____ Possessing superb manual dexterity
_____ Having a compassionate and optimistic personality
_____ Utilizing a logical and precise approach in problem solving
_____ Quick thinking and responding promptly to unforeseen challenges
_____ Preferring an organized professional work schedule
_____ Favoring having expertise in a limited area
_____ Enjoying working with one's hands professionally
_____ Total

SPECIALTY SELECTION FACTORS. As with other surgical subspecialties, performance during one's general surgery residency, as reflected in letters of recommendation, will significantly impact one's chances of securing a vascular surgery fellowship.

POSTGRADUATE TRAINING/CERTIFICATION. Successfully completing a four-year general surgery residency and then a one-year fellowship in vascular surgery is the norm. One can apply for a fellowship through the NRMP General Vascular Match.

Certification requires passing the General Surgery Boards and then exams in vascular surgery.

SUBSPECIALTY OPTIONS. Not relevant.

FOR FURTHER INFORMATION. American Association of Vascular Surgeons, www.vascsurg.org.

Table 5.2 Surgical subspecialties and your potential suitability

Subspecialty	Suitability level
Colon and rectal surgery	
Hand surgery	
Neurological surgery	
Orthopedic surgery	
Plastic surgery	
Thoracic surgery	
Vascular surgery	

Summary

Having reviewed the surgical subspecialties, you are now in a position to assess the extent of your natural potential suitability for any of the surgical subspecialties discussed. The results of your self-evaluation should be indicated in Table 5.2. Note the number of your personal attributes and interests you checked off for each of the surgical subspecialties discussed in this chapter.

Transfer the two highest-ranked specialties checked off to Form 2.3 of the *Specialty selection protocol.* (see p. 23). When uncertain if the attributes of a prospective subspecialty choice are applicable to you, compare them with your own framework profile generated in Forms 2.1 and 2.2. (see pp. 19 and 20). One or more of your choices may merit later being subjected to a reality check (see Chapter 8).

6 | Other Subspecialties

Overview

The previous two chapters discussed the medical and surgical subspecialties. There are, however, a number of subspecialties that do not fit into either of these categories. Nevertheless, these are areas that merit serious consideration by medical students planning their future careers.

It should be noted that two specialty areas, Pathology and Pediatrics, have a large number of subspecialties. Six of each of these will be identified and are shown in Table 6.1 (see also Table 2.1).

Characteristics

Table 6.2 summarizes the characteristics of the other subspecialties. A detailed discussion of each of them follows.

The choices

Each of the following six other subspecialties will be discussed below.

Aerospace medicine

Status: Preventive medicine subspecialty

Projected need: Above average

Table 6.1 Some subspecialty areas associated with pathology and pediatrics

Pathology subspecialties	Pediatric subspecialties
Blood banking	Pediatric endocronology
Chemical pathology	Pediatric cardiology
Dermopathology	Pediatric hematology
Immunopathology	Pediatric orthopedics
Medical microbiology	Pediatric nephrology
Neuropathology	Pediatric Pathology

Securing a residency: Extremely competitive

Training programs: Four years (half being military)

Positions open: Ca. 40

Training.: Three years (after internship)

Weekly patient contact hours: Average

Attaining patients: Self and by referral

Remuneration: Starting, above average; median, above average

Night and emergency calls: Infrequent

SCOPE. Aerospace physicians provide relevant medical guidelines and care for individuals involved in aviation and space travel.

Table 6.2 Other subspecialties

Specialty	Nature of work	Prereq. Year(s)	Training area	Training period min.	max.
Aerospace medicine	Care for individuals involved in space travel	One	Preventive medicine	Two	Two
Nuclear medicine	Use of radioactive substances in diagnosis and treatment	Three	Medicine or radiology	Two	Three
Occupational medicine	Seeks to care for and eliminate occupational hazards	One	Clinical base	Two	Three
Public health and general preventive medicine	Prevention of disease by the promotion of health	One	Clinical base	Two	Two
Radiation oncology	Treating malignant disease by radiation therapy	One	Clinical base	Three	Three

Note: definitions for capsule and text headings are given on p. 26 of Chapter 3.

ACTIVITIES. Personel serviced by these physicians are both flight and ground crews. Employers are NASA, the FAA, the aerospace industry, and the military. Areas of service in this specialty include clinical medicine, research and development, and administration. Certification of pilots as to their eligibility for flight duty is a large part of their activity.

PROFESSIONAL SATISFACTION. The challenge of devising solutions to complex biomedical and technological problems arising from space travel provides gratification to those engaged in work in this field.

DESIRABLE PREREQUISITES. Being a pilot is very helpful for members of this specialty, in order to appreciate the stress of flight. Having a grounding in medicine, statistics, and epidemiology is a valuable asset.

DESIRABLE PERSONAL ATTRIBUTES AND INTERESTS. Check off the desirable attributes and interests of aerospace specialists you know for certain that you have *in abundance*. Then indicate the total number of checks on the bottom of the list as well as on the summary page at the end of this chapter.

_____ Enjoys working with people

_____ Has a strong special interest in aviation

_____ Can work at length on a single challenging problem to seek its resolution

_____ Has a liking and aptitude for physics, physiology, and psychology

_____ Prepared to think problems through to obtain a solution

_____ Enjoys the challenge of solving complex problems

_____ Approaches problems in a consistent methodical manner

_____ Has both patience and determination over the long haul

_____ Is prepared to face unforeseen challenges as a routine occurrence

_____ Maintains an unbiased approach to problem solving

_____ Total

SPECIALTY SELECTION FACTORS. One's overall performance in medical school as well as achievements in physiology and relevant electives carries significant weight. Having a pilot's license is a distinct asset.

POSTGRADUATE TRAINING/CERTIFICATION. The residency program extends for one to three years after completing an internship. Certification requires a fourth year of training, practice, or research.

SUBSPECIALTY OPTIONS. None.

FOR FURTHER INFORMATION. Aerospace Medical Association, www.asma.org

Nuclear medicine

Status: Subspecialty of radiology

Projected need: Average

Securing a residency: Slightly competitive

Training programs: Ca. 100

Positions open: Ca. 65

Training.: Two years (after two-year residency)

Weekly patient care contact: Average

Attaining patients: By referral

Remuneration: Starting, above average; median, above average

Night and emergency calls: Rare

SCOPE. This specialty involves using radioactive materials for diagnostic and therapeutic purposes.

ACTIVITIES. Work in this field involves arranging for insertion of the appropriate amount of radioactive material into the patient's bloodstream and studying its interaction with specific organs. This approach serves to access information relative to organ function in addition to structure. Aside from such *in vivo* studies, specialists perform radioimmuno assay tests on blood and urine samples.

PROFESSIONAL SATISFACTION. Much gratification is provided by being able to assist clinicians in definitive manner in formulating diagnoses. Another element is the varying nature of the cases and the challenges they each present.

DESIRABLE PREREQUISITES. Having a strong interest and good foundation in mathematics, physics, statistics, computer science, and radiation biology is very desirable. Important is a strong interest in instrumentation. Being innovative, curious, and adaptive are character treats that favor working in this field.

DESIRABLE PERSONAL ATTRIBUTES AND INTERESTS. Check off the desirable attributes and interests of nuclear specialists you know for certain that you have *in abundance*. Then indicate the total number of checks on the bottom of the list as well as on the summary page at the end of this chapter.

_____ Interested in instrumentation

_____ Has a strong interest and background in the physical sciences

_____ Naturally anxious to learn new things

_____ Being detail-oriented

_____ Adapts well to change

_____ Enjoys working independently

_____ Oriented toward visual data observation

_____ Has an energetic personality

(continued)

(continued)

_____ Enjoys being on the cutting edge of technology

_____ Seeks definitive answers to significant medical problems

_____ Total

POSTGRADUATE TRAINING/CERTIFICATION. Residency involves two years of training after completion of two years of training in internal medicine, radiology, pathology, or some other acceptable specialty.

Certification involves completion of a two-year residency and passing a written examination.

SUBSPECIALTY OPTIONS. None.

FOR FURTHER INFORMATION. Society for Nuclear Medicine, www.snm.org.

Occupational medicine

Status: Preventive medicine subspecialty

Projected need: Above average

Securing a residency: Slightly competitive

Training programs: Ca. 40

Positions open: Ca. 75

Training.: Two to three years after internship

Weekly patient contact hours: Average

Attaining patients: By referral

Remuneration: Starting, below average; median, below average

Night and emergency calls: Rare

SCOPE. This specialty focuses on the health aspects of specific occupations affected by hazard sources.

ACTIVITIES. Specialists are employed by industry, government, hospitals, teaching institutions, and occupational health clinics. Their service as protectors of the health of the employed is why they are linked to the field of preventive medicine. They succeed by utilizing their knowledge of the impact of both mechanical and psychological stress on employees.

PROFESSIONAL SATISFACTION. This comes about by being able to help a group of people collectively, by designing solutions to challenges, by serving in a management capacity, and also from having a fixed schedule.

DESIRABLE PREREQUISITES. Have a well-rounded medical background with special knowledge of orthopedics and psychiatry.

DESIRABLE PERSONAL ATTRIBUTES AND INTERESTS. Check off the desirable attributes and interests of occupational specialists you know for certain that you have *in abundance.* Then indicate the total number of checks on the bottom of the list as well as on the summary page at the end of this chapter.

_____ Has acute observational talent
_____ Strong oral and written communication skills
_____ Able to work well as part of an organizational team
_____ Skilled in coordinating activities
_____ Finds problem-solving to be a challenging activity
_____ Doesn't seek direct patient medical care
_____ Prefers working on a fixed schedule
_____ Desires solving group problems
_____ Patiently awaits long-term outcomes
_____ Favors creative opportunities to improve health care
_____ Total

SPECIALTY SELECTION FACTORS. Performance in medical school and during one's internship will be the determining factors.

POSTGRADUATE TRAINING/CERTIFICATION. Specialization requires three years of training after an internship. Programs vary, with the recommended Three-year program consists of a clinical year followed by an academic year leading usually to a master's in public health, and by then a year of supervised practical training and field work. The two-year program involves combining the academic and practical aspects into a one-year unit.

Certification involves completing a three-year residency to be followed by one year of practice, teaching, research, or special training.

SUBSPECIALTY OPTIONS. None.

FOR FURTHER INFORMATION. American College of Occupational and Environmental Medicine, www.acoem.org.

Public health and general preventive medicine

Status: Preventive medicine subspecialty

Projected need: Significant

Securing a residency: Slightly competitive

Training programs: Ca. 85

Positions open: Ca. 10

Length of training: Three years (after internship)

Weekly patient care contact hours: Average

Attaining patients: By referral

Remuneration: Starting well below average; median, below average

Night and emergency calls: Rare

SCOPE. Specialists deal with general health promotion and disease prevention.

ACTIVITIES. To accomplish their goals specialists work with individuals, communities, and even the population of the entire country when dealing with various health problems. Their work consists of securing health status information, formulating public health policies, and facilitating implementation of these policies. Public health physicians are employed by all levels of government, private health agencies, and academic institutions. Preventive medicine physicians primarily hold administrative, health care research, and teaching positions.

PROFESSIONAL SATISFACTION. Gratification is obtained from the widely divergent nature of the challenges that arise and need to be met in the course of work in these fields.

DESIRABLE PREREQUISITES. Securing a sound foundation in medicine is very important. Having an interest in politics and economics is helpful. Courses in epidomology, statistics, and health policy are especially beneficial. Practitioners tend to be of an optimistic nature.

DESIRABLE PERSONAL ATTRIBUTES AND INTERESTS. Check off the desirable attributes and interests of public health and general preventive specialists you know for certain that you have *in abundance*. Then indicate the total number of checks on the bottom of the list as well as on the summary page at the end of this chapter.

_____ Idealistically inclined with a sense of mission to improve health

_____ Finds solving complex problems especially appealing

_____ Works well as part of a team of professionals

_____ Capable of coordinating projects

_____ Can be creative in problem resolution

_____ Patient in regard to long-term issues

_____ Has good writing skills

_____ Does not prefer patient care contact

_____ Prepared to make major decisions affecting many people

_____ Works in an objective, systematic manner to achieve goals

_____ Total

SPECIALTY SELECTION FACTOR. Performance in medical school, the nature of social activities, and career goals are the key considerations in selection.

POSTGRADUATE TRAINING/CERTIFICATION. Residency consists of a three-year program following an internship (usually in internal medicine). The first year involves clinical training; the second is devoted to obtaining a master's degree, usually in public health, and the third to proctor-supervised experience. It should be noted that there is no matching program in preventive medicine, so one needs to apply directly to individual programs.

Certification requires completion of a fourth year of practice, teaching, or research and passing a written examination.

SUBSPECIALTY OPTIONS. None.

FOR FURTHER INFORMATION. American Association of Public Health Physicians, www.aaphp.org.

Radiation oncology

Status: Subspecialty of radiology

Projected need: Average

Securing a residency: Highly competitive

Training programs: Ca. 77

Positions open: Ca. 100 (ca. 15 first-year; ca. 85 second-year)

Length of training: Three years (after internship)

Weekly patient contact hours: Above average

Attaining patients: By referral

Remuneration: Starting, above average; median, well above average

Night and emergency calls: Little

SCOPE. These specialists utilize radiation therapy to treat malignant and other diseases.

ACTIVITIES. This field emerged as a distinct discipline from prior association with diagnostic radiology. This was the result of the generation of an enormous amount of valuable new information relative to the application of radiation therapy to the treatment of cancer.

PROFESSIONAL SATISFACTION. Those strongly interested in radiology but wanting substantial patient contact can find it in this field. The challenge of determining a treatment protocol for the patient's specific needs and requirements and then monitoring their progress enhances the satisfaction of working in this field. Being involved as a clinical consultant in a field that is rapidly advancing technologically is especially challenging.

DESIRABLE PREREQUISITES. Taking a radiology elective and having an interest in mathematics and physics are important.

DESIRABLE PERSONAL ATTRIBUTES AND INTERESTS. Check off the desirable attributes and interests of radiation oncology specialists you know for certain that you have *in abundance*. Then indicate the total number of checks on the bottom of the list as well as on the summary page at the end of this chapter.

_____ Prefers an organized professional work schedule

_____ Has empathy for the seriously ill

_____ Favors longer-term patient relationships

_____ Has a patient and relaxed personality

_____ Is detail-oriented and precise

_____ Enjoys having expertise in a limited area

_____ Communicates well with others

_____ Has a pleasant and optimistic personality

_____ Prefers an organized activity schedule

_____ Desires to think problems through before acting

_____ Total

POSTGRADUATE TRAINING/CERTIFICATION. Residency is a three-year program after completion of an internship. The internship and PGY-2 appointments need to be obtained separately.

Certification requires completion of an accredited residency and passing a qualifying examination.

SUBSPECIALTY OPTIONS. None.

FOR FURTHER INFORMATION. Society of Nuclear Medicine, www.snm.org.

Summary

Having reviewed the group of nonmedical and nonsurgical subspecialties discussed, you are now in a position to assess the extent of your potential suitability for any of them. The results of your self-evaluation should be indicated in Table 6.3. Note the number of your personal attributes and interests you checked off for each of the subspecialties discussed in this chapter. Transfer the highest ranked specialty checked off to Form 2.3 of the *Specialty selection protocol*. (see p. 23). The prospective specialty choices you have made warrant more detailed evaluation (see Chapter 2) and may merit being later subjected to a reality check (see Chapter 8).

Table 6.3 Other subspecialties and your potential suitability

Subspecialty	Suitability level
Aerospace medicine	
Nuclear medicine	
Occupational medicine	
Public health and general preventive medicine	
Radiation oncology	

Emerging subspecialties

The established specialties discussed in this and the three preceding chapters are almost all recognized by the American Board of Medical Specialties. However, medicine, being a dynamic science, always has new vistas that are being explored. This results in the slow emergence of new specialty areas that can prove to be of particular interest to medical students and residents, particularly those who are not fully committed to a specialty. Physicians interested in these areas will enroll usually in postresidency fellowship programs to secure specialty training. Two of the emerging areas, namely, critical care and geriatric medicine, have advanced to the point that they deserved consideration in Chapter 4, along with other medical subspecialties. There are seven other areas, however, that show enough promise so that they are early-stage emergent subspecialties and merit being briefly discussed. Three other areas, namely, adolescent medicine, corrective medicine, and palliative medicine/hospice care, are just beginning to develop and these are therefore merely mentioned at this point.

Addiction medicine. Physicians associated with this specialty devote themselves part- or full-time to treating individuals with alcohol or drug dependency problems. Those involved in this work have a background in family medicine, internal medicine, psychiatry, or other primary care areas. Physicians interested in addiction medicine can take postresidency fellowship courses in addiction psychiatry and can secure a Certificate of Added Qualifications in this field. For further information contact the American Society of Addiction Medicine, www.asam.org.

Hospitalists. Physicians in this specialty are involved exclusively with inpatients who are admitted or transferred to a hospital/medical center by their primary doctor for treatment. Upon discharge their office-based physicians will again assume full responsibility for these patients. This emerging subspecialty is favored by the managed care industry as a means of securing greater cost savings in medical services. Hospitalists are especially useful at institutions where a shortage of house staff exists. Most hospitalists are internists, although a small number are family practice physicians and pediatricians. Training usually involves completing an internal medicine or family practice residency. There are a number of programs that have special hospitalist tracks. There are also a few fellowships available in this area. For further information, contact the National Association of Inpatient Physicians, www.naiponline.org.

Medical management. Although medical managers have existed for a long time, it is only recently that medical management is emerging as a distinct subspecialty, with the encouragement of managed care organizations. These specialists help meet the need of medical institutions to comply with a host of governmental regulations and changing health care plans. It is common for some physicians to assume administrative positions in the latter part of their professional careers, although others do so at various stages of their professional lives. Courses in medical management are available through the American College of Physician Executives, the American College of Managed Care Medicine, and various MPH and MBA programs. For additional information, contact the American Medical Directors Association, www.amda.org

Pain medicine. Pain management specialists are active in efforts to prevent pain and are involved to treating persons in pain. They can have important consultative function at various stages of patient care. This field can be considered a subspecialty of anesthesiology, neurology, psychiatry, and physical medicine and rehabilitation. These physicians work at hospitals and pain management clinics. They are receiving greater recognition because other doctors are coming to realize that these physicians are especially qualified to help patients with various pain problems. Training involves a one-year fellowship offered by anesthesiology departments. For additional information, contact the American Academy of Pain Medicine, www.pain.med.org.

Sports medicine. Specialists in this field diagnose and treat nonoperative sports injuries. Thus these physicians are distinct from subspecialists in orthopedic sports medicine. Sports medicine specialists, in addition to providing acute treatment, focus on prevention and rehabilitation. Many of these physicians serve as team medical directors, offer physical fitness evaluations, and work directly with professional athletes. This field is considered a subspecialty of orthopedic surgery, and training involves completion of an orthopedic surgery residency, followed by exposure to primary care medicine (family practice) and a one-year fellowship in sports medicine. For further information, contact the American Orthopedic Society for Sports Medicine, www.sportsmed.org.

Trauma surgery. This is one of the fastest-growing areas of surgery. The rapid spread nationwide of trauma centers has heightened the demand for surgeons who are especially qualified to respond to patients with multiple injuries. Trauma surgeons also serve to manage both the initial and postoperative care of injured patients. Training involves a one- or two-year fellowship after a general surgery residency. For further information, contact the American Association for the Surgery of Trauma, www.aast.org.

Women's health. Different programs have set varying goals for this emerging subspecialty. Many focus on training physicians to provide the special care needed by women, in the belief that heretofore this area was deficient. Others are concerned with developing active proponents, teachers, and researchers for this relatively new field. There is also a goal of making primary care physicians cognizant of women's health issues that lie outside of obstetrics/gynecology. Training involves two possible pathways. One option is completing a special two-year fellowship after completing a residency in family practice, internal medicine, obstetrics/gynecology, or psychiatry. The other is a three-year combined women's health–family practice or internal medicine program. For further information, contact the American Medical Women's Association, www.emwa-doc.org.

The popularity of these emerging specialties should increase over time. They offer new outlets for physicians-in-training to consider when planning their professional careers.

PART TWO

SECURING A RESIDENCY

U PON COMPLETION OF THE SPECIALTY SELECTION PROCESS, YOU CAN MOVE on to the next phase, namely, securing a residency. At the outset, you should recognize that you need to make choices as to which residency programs to apply to among those available in your specific field. However, there may be a major obstacle to being accepted in the field you prefer. Competition among applicants, although varying among different specialties, frequently is very intense. Moreover, competition for placement has also increased because the number of residency openings in some areas has been gradually diminishing due to fiscal pressures.

The challenging situation regarding securing a residency appointment raises the question, what can you do to significantly improve your chances? The answer is that it is essential to learn how best to market yourself and thus enhance your potential in the eyes of prospective program directors. How to achieve this vital goal is the subject of Part Two of the book. It covers in detail the various components associated with enhancing your chances of securing a residency.

It is true that competition makes obtaining a residency a challenge. This obstacle, however, can be successfully overcome, as proven by the fact that generally over 90% of NRMP candidates do secure residency positions. During your lengthy residency selection process you should bear in mind that you were faced with a comparable competitive situation when you applied to both college and medical school, and you obviously were successful. This should serve as a source of encouragement while you are awaiting Match Day.

The following four strategies should facilitate your securing a suitable residency.

1. Sell yourself. This means that as a medical student you should seek to secure as many assets as possible that will make obtaining a suitable residency easier. This should involve seeking the assistance of a suitable mentor/advisor, aiming to obtain honors in a clerkship and/or elective relevant to the specialty area of your interest, and completing a special rotation or externship in this field. Attaining such goals will enable you to submit a resume of attractive credentials that will start things off in the right direction.

2. Start early. Attaining your goal requires having a plan and putting it into effect in an orderly, systematic, and consistent manner. Thus, starting to think about your future residency plans even while in your freshman year in medical school is not premature. More serious consideration by the sophomore year is essential.

3. Be realistic. It is essential to be as objective as you can and also take your advisor/mentor's advice into consideration. If he/she thinks your credentials are especially attractive, then you should consider trying to gain a residency even in a highly competitive program. In other words, don't undersell yourself, but if justified "go for the gold."

4. Act conscientiously. Recognize that the specialty you select and the program where you train will strongly impact your professional career for the duration of your practice. Thus you should make time to give the attainment of an appropriate appointment thoughtful consideration and follow through in a consistent and timely manner on all aspects of the lengthy process.

7 | Laying the Groundwork

Overview

The stability of an edifice in large part depends upon the foundation that it rests on. This is equally true for attaining a suitable residency. This will depend on quite a number of factors, and several of those are under your control. Two of these factors are (1) whether the decisions you make regarding securing a residency are determined by sound advice and (2) if your record is good enough to warrant an invitation for an interview in a specific specialty. These two issues, namely, securing an appropriate advisor/mentor and generating a credible academic record, will be the focus of the discussion in this chapter.

Selecting an advisor/mentor

Making the appropriate choice of a person to turn to for guidance as a medical student is critical for your future success. This individual may turn out to be more than a counselor: he/she can serve in multiple roles as taskmaster, cheerleader, critic, and confessor. This person may be able to help you in a host of ways:

■ Serve as an outlet to discuss your concerns, both short- and long-term.

■ Steer you in a suitable direction when you are uncertain or faced with a choice.

■ Keep you focused on the tasks ahead so that you don't deviate unproductively.

■ Provide valuable and current information based on their knowledge and experience.

■ Provide encouragement along the long and challenging road to attaining a residency.

■ Guide you through personal difficulties that may arise during medical school.

■ Help you obtain early clinical experience, which will facilitate gaining exposure to the world of medicine.

■ Call your attention to valuable research opportunities.

■ Indicate how you can gain the most from clinical opportunities that come your way.

■ Guide you through the complexities involved in selecting a specialty.

■ Lead you through the residency Match process.

■ Help secure you interviews for possible residency positions.

■ Try to protect you from becoming overwhelmed by your obligations.

■ Help protect your mental and/or physical health from impairment due to a poor lifestyle.

The following criteria can be used for selecting an advisor/mentor. Try to secure the services of an individual who has *many* of the following attributes:

■ Has a personality that is compatible with yours, so that you hit it off and feel comfortable in their presence.

■ Can serve as a role model, both personally and professionally.

■ Is known to be patient and open-minded.

■ Is someone you can confide in, because you can trust that your revelations will go no further.

■ Offers a reasonable degree of accessibility when counseling is necessary.

■ Will not pressure you to accept the advice given either directly or subtly.

■ Has broad connections due to involvement in regional and national affairs.

■ Will help you achieve your goal, irrespective of which specialty you ultimately choose.

■ Has a successful track record of counseling individuals seeking residencies.

Securing an advisor/mentor

Being aware of what type of person to look for is one issue. The next challenge is finding one and securing their willingness to serve as your advisor/mentor. This person should preferably be a member of the school's clinical teaching faculty and be highly competent both professionally and as a guidance counselor. Such individuals are likely to be dedicated to student welfare and willing to provide assistance, assuming that they are not overly committed to their other responsibilities.

At a medical school, the individuals who best know which faculty have an established reputation for clinical teaching are the third- and fourth-year students. You can try to meet such students in the school library or hospital cafeteria. Indicate your status and problem and invite their input. Parenthetically, you can ask if any of the especially prominent faculty members are also known as helpful advisor/mentors. Try to obtain a reasonable sampling of opinions, so that you can come up with a useful short list of prospects. Attempt to obtain this information early on in your medical school career. You can even make an effort to do so as a senior premed, after you have been admitted and have committed yourself to attend by sending in a deposit. In other words, the earlier this issue is settled the better. Having an advisor/mentor will make it less likely you will stumble because of being uninformed or misinformed.

Some institutions have a formal advisory system and each department can provide you with a list of prospective advisors. The dean's office, which is responsible for sending out supporting material for residency appointments, may prove helpful. It may assist your efforts toward securing a suitable advisor/mentor if you make yourself known to relevant faculty. This can be done by participating, if you have free time, in ward rounds or clinic sessions, or observing surgical procedures. Naturally, you should dress appropriately for the occasion. It is remotely possible that you may even end up becoming an unofficial member of a treatment team. Seek to generate a favorable impression by reflecting the characteristics of a thoughtful, compassionate person. Be sure to always act in an appropriate manner, but not by being excessively complimentary to a potential advisor/mentor. Participation in such activities should provide an opportunity to allow you to judge your possible personal compatibility with a prospective counselor.

Once you have formulated and prioritized a short list of suitable advisor/mentors, make an appointment to speak with one or more of them. If good rapport is established, determine the individual's willingness to guide you through medical school and toward a suitable residency appointment. If the person is not available, ask for an alternative suggestion. If the person suggested is on your short list, seek them out or hold the name in reserve if you prefer to try someone else.

Before you suggest that an individual serve as your advisor, seek to ascertain if the prospective candidate is broad-minded and flexible about the choice of a specialty. If they express a narrow view, by emphasizing their own specialty as being far superior to all others, gracefully withdraw with a remark, such as that you will pursue the selection of an advisor after you have gotten further into the educational process. To be committed to a pathway prematurely can prove disastrous and may create a difficult relationship later on. However, if you have a serious idea as to your future plans, it is obviously beneficial to have an advisor/mentor who has some relationship to the potential field you are considering, since they should be up to date about the current state of affairs regarding competition for securing an appointment in the field.

It is important, after selecting your advisor/mentor, to maximize the benefit you can obtain from such an individual. To do so, bear in mind the following:

■ *Establish a relationship*. It is absolutely essential that your advisor/mentor get to know you well and that you become well acquainted with him or her. Developing a positive relationship will enable you to speak your mind freely and express your emotions during every trying phase of your medical education. Moreover, your advisor/mentor will undoubtedly write about you at great length to the dean's office, where a composite letter of recommendation will be formulated. Much of the content of that letter may come from the evaluation that the advisor/mentor submits, because such individuals are especially knowledgeable about a prospective specialty applicant.

■ *Arrange meetings*. To achieve your goal of establishing a relationship, arrange for your initial meeting early and subsequent ones as frequently as is mutually desirable. Obviously you should demonstrate the courtesy of scheduling an initial appointment for a meeting in advance. At that time, ascertain your advisor/mentor's schedule of availability and discuss a time table for periodic visits and how to handle emergency situations.

■ *Prepare the groundwork*. It is vital that you maximize the benefits of your contacts with your advisor/mentor. This can best be done by preparing, in advance, a list of issues and questions you may wish to discuss or seek advice about. If you wish to obtain input regarding to some material you prepared, such as a personal statement or resume, submit your draft in advance and then you will more likely obtain thoughtful criticism.

■ *Maintain contact*. It is your responsibility to keep your advisor/mentor up- to-date on all relevant activities and future plans. Discuss your criteria for selecting residency programs to apply to. Inform him of any pending interviews. If he has a contact there, perhaps he can place a phone call that may prove to your advantage. Upon your return, provide your advisor/mentor with feedback that can prove useful to other applicants.

■ *Maximize your advisor/mentor assistance*. It is up to you to take advantage of the expertise that can be provided at appropriate interludes in the residency application process. Feel free to ask for specific suggestions as to which programs you should apply to rather than simply reviewing your list. Ask if you can obtain a thorough evaluation of your personal statement, rather than just general comments. Request a mock interview, rather than merely general advice on the subject.

Ascertain your advisor's advice on a time frame for your planned program toward securing a residency. When you reach the point where you have made a tentative or definitive choice of your specialty, arrange a meeting with your advisor to inform them of what it is. If it is in your advisor's field, they will then undoubtedly proceed to give you the sound advice that you need on how to proceed. If the advisor is not in your selected field, obtain a suggestion as to which faculty member in that specialty can be of special assistance to you. Inquire if your advisor can place an introductory call to that person on your behalf. Above all else, make sure your advisor's status relative to your activities remains intact. This should be the case even if you will be obtaining guidance from someone else devoted exclusively to your potential future residency plans.

Grades to strive for

Medical school is a very demanding experience that requires absorbing a large amount of complex material over a short period of time. Given the hectic pace of most educational programs, it is essential that you optimize the attainable results from your academic efforts.

Residency programs have their own criteria for evaluating candidates for residency appointments. The goal of a residency director is to gain an in-depth assessment of a candidate's potential. *Prior* to extending an interview invitation. For this purpose, what is utilized as a frame of reference is medical school grades, Board scores, faculty recommendations, and performance assessments of clerkships and electives taken in the specialty you are applying for.

Grades reflect your ability to memorize facts, retain information, and, where necessary, apply data to solve problems and make decisions. When a school uses a pass/fail grading system, in part or exclusively, you can only compensate by focusing particularly on areas where your strengths lie, by securing strong written evaluations from faculty. Most schools, however, use letter grades to evaluate their students. Under such circumstances, securing recognition by being awarded an A (or its equivalent of High Honors or Outstanding) in a specific subject will clearly attract attention. It distinguishes you from others regarding your potential in this specialty. Thus, although few are capable of getting honors in several subjects during a specific year, a special effort should be directed to maximize your achievement in the subjects most beneficial to you. Therefore, when seeking to specifically achieve high honors in your medical school studies, your priorities should be in the following order:

Third-year required clerkships

Subspecialty clerkships

Basic science courses

Senior elective courses

Each of these categories will be discussed individually:

Third-year required clerkships. Grades (and evaluations) in these areas are key factors used to compare prospective residents. They will be available to residency program directors by the time they are making decisions regarding granting interviews. Therefore, if you are considering specializing in one of the third-year core subjects, a special effort should be made to be a high achiever in the selected area. If your interests are uncertain, as they may well be, then you should focus on performing impressively on your internal medicine and surgery clerkships, because they are the basis for many subspecialty areas of training.

The timing as to when an internal medicine or surgery clerkship should be taken, assuming the choice is yours, depends on the extent of your prior clinical exposure during your basic science years. If this is very limited, then choose from the other clerkship areas in order to become clinically acclimated, before undertaking such demanding and critical rotations. However, if you have had adequate exposure to feel comfortable with patient care responsibilities, then time these two clerkships early on, when most convenient. If one of the other third-year rotations (e.g., pediatrics or psychiatry) is a reasonable possibility for subsequent postgraduate training, take it at the time when you feel you will have the most success. This may be just following a rotation of lesser interest, which you think you will do well in, and thus it can serve as a suitable warm-up clerkship prior to a key one, the premise being that nothing breeds success like success!

Subspecialty clerkships. These are usually taken during your senior year. Depending on your ultimate career choice, the importance of completing a subspecialty rotation should not be underestimated. You should take such an elective early on in your senior year, if you seriously think that the field presents a realistic residency possibility for you. Of greater importance is where the clerkship is taken. If you wish to maximize the effect on your residency selection potential, a subspecialty clerkship should be completed at a major teaching hospital. It is also preferable if you are working under an attending physician or department chairperson who has name recognition among residency program directors. Your advisor/mentor may be able to facilitate getting such a clerkship for you. Securing honors in a subspecialty clerkship may open up potential doors to an especially attractive residency appointment.

Basic science courses. If your career goal is or might be an academic one, where research plays a pivotal role, or if it is geared toward pathology, then honors in a basic science area can be decisive. Even for the vast majority of medical students, who wish to have a clinical career, such an honors grade can also have a special positive impact if it is in a course that has relevance to a prospective specialty. Thus, honors in neuroscience will benefit those with thoughts of specialization in neurology, neurosurgery, or psychiatry. The same is true for achieving striking success in anatomy for those possibly interested in general surgery, a surgical subspecialty, or surgical pathology.

If, on the other hand, you have not set your sights on any specific field, which is understandable at an early stage in your studies, you may nevertheless devote extra time and effort to one subject per year (or even each semester, if possible) to see if you can achieve an honors grade in it. For those with strong chemistry backgrounds this may be in courses such as biochemistry and pharmacology. Securing some honors grades even in peripheral courses may prove to be a potential asset, because it adds distinction to your academic record. Caution needs to be taken to avoid overextending yourself in a quest for honors, and then having to make up for it, jeopardizing your overall performance.

Senior elective courses. These grades, in areas outside of your specialty, carry the least weight. This is because there appears to be a problem of grade inflation associated with senior electives. As a consequence, there is a tendency to discount them. However, you should recognize that even a senior elective will nevertheless contribute to your knowledge base.

If you have taken a senior elective in your prospective specialty and have done well, you should take advantage of this fact by having an updated transcript sent out to residency programs to which you applied.

Aside from taking an elective to gain an honors grade in the area of your specialization and thus enhance your residency potential, there are a number of other considerations relative to completing electives:

■ A major incidental benefit of taking an elective in your field of interest is that it can serve to reaffirm your decision or give you reason to reconsider your conclusions and review your options. Similarly, if uncertain of your choice in general or between two specialty options, taking an elective can help clarify the situation. It can open your mind to entirely new possibilities. Clarify the situation and maintain an open mind to new possibilities.

■ Although securing additional elective experience in your prospective specialty is useful, it should be balanced by other electives to round out your background. This may prove to be an appealing quality in the record of a prospective candidate for a postgraduate appointment.

■ You take a senior elective in the first semester of your last year. This will allow time for evaluations and letters of recommendation sent in your behalf for this rotation to have an impact on your residency appointment.

■ To view an elective as a vehicle to secure an honors grade in order to compensate for mediocre or poor performance in a clerkship is probably excessively optimistic. Consult your advisor/mentor as to how best to respond to such a situation.

■ Because your specialty training should provide you with adequate expertise in your field of choice, it is advisable when selecting electives to pick those that will augment your background. Thus, if you are considering a surgical specialty (or subspecialty), you may wish to supplement it with electives in critical care, emergency medicine, or radiology, which can in time prove helpful. Similarly, if you are planning a career in primary care, then additional courses in emergency medicine, pediatrics, and dermatology would be appropriate. If your interests are narrowly focused then some exposure to family medicine can be an asset at some future date.

■ Some seniors may choose to take electives on subjects that have stimulated their academic curiosity. This results from the realization that they will not have another opportunity to explore areas of special interest at a later date.

■ Where some especially prominent individual is offering an elective, one may wish to grasp this unique opportunity to obtain in-depth and up-to-date information from an authority.

■ Some consideration should be given to taking a nonscience elective, such as business management or medical ethics, which may prove useful in the future.

■ You may wish to consider taking an elective in a subject that is of special interest to you, such as research, a legislative internship, on working with the medically disadvantaged at home or abroad. Permission from the school administration needs to be given for all such activities. If you can justify your proposal, it may be approved and can prove to be meaningful both personally and professionally.

■ Although some seniors seek to take an elective at an institution they may be anxious to join as residents, this may not be the wisest course. Although such a decision can serve as an "extended interview," its negative aspects (e.g., need to relocate, being in competition with institutional students, mandating the need for an impressive performance) are contraindications to undertaking such a course of action.

■ An out-of-town elective, if chosen, should preferably not be scheduled during November or December. Your chances to obtain optimal clinical exposure during this time would be reduced. Also, during any such elective opportunity, make the most of it by taking the initiative and attending departmental grand rounds and conferences. It will serve to enhance your status with the program supervisor and may earn you an especially favorable recommendation that can be of future benefit.

■ You should schedule your residency interviews so that they are appropriately distributed among the electives you take so that you do not have an excessive number during any one elective, which can create difficulty for you to meet your responsibilities.

Attaining honors

Several key elements are associated with attaining honors. As noted, it is a valuable asset to secure honors in at least one clinical rotation. To do so requires an effort to make yourself knowledgeable in a manner that will impress both your attendings and the house staff. This involves becoming familiar with the cases of patients covered by your treatment team in an in-depth manner. You should acquire an understanding of the details of any procedures specific to the rotation that you are scheduled to observe or carry out. During rounds you may wish to relate some esoteric information that will indicate that you have done homework on the subject. Four other desirable steps that you should take to enhance your performance are as follows:

Be prepared. Every clerkship rotation is an experience in itself. Not only is the subject matter significantly different, but so usually are the entire clinical ambience, working style, and required knowledge base. To readily integrate yourself into a program, you should try to become familiar with the operation of each rotation in advance. Departmental offices frequently have guidance directives that will inform you of the range of your responsibilities you may face as a medical student during the clerkship. The office secretary should be able to provide you with information on the makeup of your treatment team, the time and place of the initial meeting, the conference and lecture schedule, a list of readings (both required and recommended), the nature of the on-call schedule, the exam protocol (written, oral, and their number), and if there will be any obligations to give presentations, as well as other vital information.

You may find it worthwhile to discuss in advance the nature of the rotation and characteristics of the treatment team members with fellow classmates who have already completed a rotation in this specialty. But you should realize that their responses are subjective opinions, based on individual personal experiences, and thus may well be biased.

Make yourself available. There are always routine tasks ("scut work") that need to be done and that interns or residents may prefer not to do. If your schedule allows, offer to do some scut work in a graceful manner. The positive impression you leave on your superiors will likely pay off when the time comes for a written evaluation in your behalf.

Be upbeat. Your colleagues and coworkers prefer a congenial atmosphere as the site of their employment. You can make your contribution by acting courteously and thoughtfully, even under the trying circumstances of an extended night call. Being a pleasant person to have around is something people take note of, since they feel better sharing the burden of patient care under such circumstances.

Do well on the final. Most rotations have a written or oral final exam. Determine, if possible, its general contents from those students who have already completed the rotation. Use all available free time to prepare for it. Reading assignments or suggestions given at the outset of the rotation should prove valuable in preparing for these tests, as will appropriate supplementary readings relative to patient care.

Board scores and your residency

As far as the Boards are concerned, medical schools have varying requirements for promotion to the third year and for graduation. Many schools require passing only the USMLE Step 1, whereas others require passing both Steps 1 and 2 in order to graduate. Residency directors are urging applicants to meet their school requirements early so they are not caught in a bind if a matched resident fails to graduate because of poor Board scores.

As to the value of Board scores, it is a widespread practice to use them, especially Step 1, as a critical assessment tool. There are three reasons for doing so (even though the exam was obviously not designed for this purpose).

1. The USMLE, by its nationwide use, allows objective comparison of applicants from different schools, each having its own curriculum, grading scheme, and standards.

2. The utilization of pass/fail grading systems and frequently bland dean's letters sent out in behalf of applicants provides a limited means of properly evaluating candidates based on the supporting data available. Hence the greater importance of USMLE scores in assessing a candidate's potential.

3. The caliber of a residency program is reflected by the success of its residents on specialty board exams. These results are published and thus are available to all interested parties. The fact that there is a correlation between doing well on the USMLE and on the specialty board exams is a further inducement for using the Step 1 scores as a means of defining future potential.

In light of this situation, it is this clear that Step 1 of the USMLE, although oriented essentially to the basic sciences, is a *critical* element in securing a residency. This is because most seniors do not take Step 2 until after the residency selection process has been completed.

The obvious corollary to this situation is that you should invest the time and effort to maximize your performance on the USMLE, especially Step 1. It is needed for graduation, for obtaining a residency (including its type and quality), and for securing a license. Finally, it should be noted that the minimum scores that need to be obtained to be in contention for a residency appointment depend on how competitive a program is.

Evaluations and their role

Your grades and USMLE Step 1 scores are the two quantitative components that influence residency selection outcomes. They define your performance in a quantitative manner. However, by themselves these two parameters cannot provide the entire picture of a candidate's ability and potential. Your image as a prospective physician-in-training is fleshed out by the tone and contents of the dean's letter, which in turn is strongly influenced by the evaluations submitted from faculty members. These can serve to define the character, skills, personality, and potential of each individual applicant. They may add the element of depth to a bland image, thereby intimating what the person would be like as a resident. Evaluation comments can provide the color that can enhance or weaken the impression provided by grades. They can be reflected in and will usually be consistent with the summary statement at the end of a dean's letter. This, in turn, will influence the decision as to granting an interview.

In light of the importance of evaluations, it is obvious that for a medical student, a special effort must be made to leave a favorable impression on supervisors and colleagues. It should be noted that these comments regarding securing honor grades are applicable to the issue of securing favorable evaluations as well.

8 | Getting Started

Overview

The next step after making appropriate prospective choices of a specialty, and then prioritizing your options, is planning for securing a residency appointment. This process requires careful thought and strategic planning. At this point, it will be necessary to secure information about programs offering training in your selected field of interest. This should be carried out in an organized manner, so that your efforts can prove maximally effective. If possible, set aside some fixed time segments that can be devoted exclusively to securing a residency. This will (a) enable you to remain up-to-date with the status of your activities in this area, (b) facilitate meeting deadlines, and (c) allow you to respond in a timely fashion to any issues that may arise. By staying on top of things, you will maximize your chances of achieving success in this vital endeavor.

Specialty reality check

Applying the *Specialty selection protocol* as outlined in Chapter 2, you should have narrowed down your prospective specialties or to a prioritized list of the most suitable ones (see Form 2.4), (see p. 22). It is vital, however, to determine if these choices are realistic before you proceed to act further.

There are both subjective and objective aspects of carrying out a specialty reality check. These will be briefly outlined.

Subjective approach. You need to judge the validity of the factors that have influenced your choice of prospective specialties. This requires asking and answering the following questions:

- Are any of the role models who may have influenced you significantly represented among the specialties you have chosen?
- Are the relevant professional activities you may have observed during the course of your clinical rotations representative of typical experiences of practice in the specialties?
- How do you feel about the professional and emotional rewards and frustrations inherent in your prospective specialty options?
- Do your colleagues who know you well feel that your specialty choices are an appropriate one for you?

The answers to these questions should be sought from attendings and colleagues and be coordinated with the results of the following objective approach.

Objective approach. From this prospective, there are two issues to be focused on when carrying out your reality check, namely, (a) how competitive is the prospective specialty and (b) how competitive a candidate are you? As to the former question, the intensity varies somewhat from year to year. Nevertheless, many specialties have lengthy track records for consistently attracting numerous candidates and thus are known as being highly competitive. Under these circumstances, one should obviously seek to obtain the most recent data on this issue to be aware of the likely prospects. Obviously, in general terms competitiveness is influenced by the number of openings there are for a specialty, as compared with applicants, for each year. A perspective on this issue can be secured by reviewing the three groupings in Table 8.1. This table classifies specialties and subspecialties into groups based on competition to secure a residency appointment.

An insight as to the second issue, namely, how competitive you are, can be obtained by completing Form 8.1. As objectively as possible, you should estimate your level of academic performance in comparison to that of your classmates. Do the same regarding your USMLE Step 1 scores. When determining your medical school and USMLE performance, bear in mind the caliber of the student population at your school. This is because the competition for residency positions is both regional and nationwide.

Finally, candidly estimate how *faculty* evaluate your personal abilities as related to those the specialty calls for. In other words, honestly judge how your traits will be reflected in the dean's letter and recommendations sent in your behalf to residency programs. These attributes are enumerated in item 5 for each of the specialty descriptions found in Chapters 3, 4, and 5. Apply his evaluation in each area on your prioritized list of specialty choices (see p. 22). It would be desirable for you to check the objectivity of your assessment with your mentor. You should realize that few if any of the candidates for residency positions have high ratings in all categories. Rather, it is the overall appeal of your strengths relative to what the program seeks that will make the difference.

Form 8.1 Your competitive status assessment

Specialty _____

Your level (check one)

Performance	High	Average	Low
Academic	_____	_____	_____
USMLE Step 1	_____	_____	_____

Specialty attributes (list)	Faculty designated attributes (check)
1. _____	1. _____
2. _____	2. _____
3. _____	3. _____
4. _____	4. _____
5. _____	5. _____
6. _____	6. _____
7. _____	7. _____
8. _____	8. _____
9. _____	9. _____
10. _____	10. _____

Total matching attributes. After completing Form 8.1, you can judge the merit of your choice of a specialty by seeing into which of three groups your assessment fits best, using the criteria outlined in Table 8.2.

Correlating the information now available to you will facilitate your validation of your choice of a specialty. This can be done using Form 8.2.

Form 8.2 Specialty validation

Prospective specialty (Form 2.4)	Competitiveness of specialty (Table 8.1)	Your competitiveness (Table 8.2)
1. _____	_____	_____
2. _____	_____	_____
3. _____	_____	_____

Obviously, if your competitive ranking is high, then your potential in competing for an appointment is quite favorable. If the ranking is only average or modest, then correlation with a less competitive specialty of interest may be desirable and may enhance your chances of success. Those in the latter two categories should carefully

Table 8.1 Competition for specialty positions

Group 1 Intense	Group 2 Above average	Group 3 Moderate
Colon & rectal surgery	Aerospace medicine	Allergy & immunology
Dermatology	Family practice	Anesthesiology
Emergency medicine	Internal medicine	Cardiology
Neurological surgery	Internal medicine – pediatrics	Child and adolescent psychiatry
Obstetrics & gynecology	Ophthalmology	Child neurology
Orthopedic surgery	Pediatrics	Critical care medicine
Otolaryngology	Plastic surgery	Endocrinology, diabetes, and metabolism
	psychiatry (adult)	
Pediatric surgery	Radiation oncology	Gastroenterology
Surgery (general)	Thoracic surgery	Geriatric medicine
Urology	Trauma surgery	Hand surgery
	Vascular surgery	Hematology
		Infectious diseases
		Medical genetics
		Nephrology
		Neurology
		Nuclear medicine
		Occupational medicine
		Pathology
		Physical medicine and rehabilitation
		Preventive medicine
		Public health & general preventive medicine
		Pulmonary diseases
		Radiology (Diagnostic)
		Rheumatology
		Sports medicine

review their options with their advisor/mentors before deciding on the best course of action.

Securing information

A variety of important issues associated with securing information relative to residency programs will be discussed in this section.

Organizing data. Most medical students apply to a relatively substantial number of residency programs. This requires obtaining and properly storing a considerable amount of paperwork. Organizing material is best done by designating a labeled

Table 8.2 Ranking classification of competitiveness

Group 1: High	Group 2: Average	Group 3: Low
High grades	Average grades	Modest grades
High scores	Average scores	Modest scores
7–10 attributes	5 or 6 attributes	1–4 attributes

folder for each program and keeping all pertinent information about each program in it. This should include a residency program assessment form (Form 9.1, p. 126). All these folders can most conveniently be stored in an organized manner in a large file box. If you regularly file all information received where it belongs, it will be there for you when you need it. This will certainly be valuable at the time when you are applying for admission to a program and prior to interviews.

What you want to know. Having chosen the specialty you seek training in, you need to find out which programs best meet your specific needs. It is thus essential that you obtain information that will allow you to familiarize yourself with the nature of each program. Such literature should provide details about the physical and clinical aspects of each program and afford some basis for making comparisons between programs.

Where to get information. As far as specialty program information is concerned, information sources will be described in terms of primary, secondary, and other sources.

Primary sources

AMA-FREIDA (AMA FELLOWSHIP AND RESIDENCY ELECTRONIC INTERACTIVE DATABASE ACCESS). This computerized directory is sold to medical school libraries and enrolled students are granted free access to utilize it. FREIDA is a Windows-based program and thus it is user-friendly. Each program listed in this database has about 90 items grouped into 10 categories. Because of the overwhelming amount of information available, you should first determine what specific information you are looking for, prior to initiating your search. Since the data in this electronic directory are more than half a year old, you may wish to confirm any critical or questionable information at the time of your interview to determine if it is currently accurate.

NRMP DIRECTORY (NATIONAL RESIDENCY MATCHING PROGRAM DIRECTORY). This program directory is an essential source of information about NRMP PGY-1 programs as well as specialty matches. It contains program numbers needed to prepare a Match Rank Order List as well as the Match schedule of activities. This directory is published annually by the NRMP. The address of this organization is listed in Appendix (see p. 348).

Secondary sources

"GREENBOOK" (GRADUATE MEDICAL EDUCATION DIRECTORY). This book is issued annually by the AMA. It lists all ACGME-approved residency training programs. This directory has largely been supplanted by the FREIDA database (see above). Of special value, however, is Section 11. Under the heading "Program Requirements," one can find useful information on a program's philosophy, scope, training prerequisites, expected training content, composition of teaching staff, and facilities. Of interest in this directory is an appendix that delineates the requirements for certification by the appropriate specialty boards.

COUNCIL ON TEACHING HOSPITALS DIRECTORY. This book is published by the AAMC. It contains information on more than 400 hospitals that are members of the Council of Teaching Hospitals (a section of the AAMC). This source can provide information on the workings of the hospital and thereby on the type and quality of residency training being offered.

AMERICAN HOSPITAL ASSOCIATION GUIDE TO HEALTH CARE. An annual publication of the American Hospital Association, it describes over 7000 of its member hospitals. This book can provide information about hospitals that you can conceivably be assigned to during the course of your training, because of their affiliation with the residency program that you may become associated with.

COUNCIL OF TEACHING HOSPITALS SURVEY OF HOUSE STAFF STIPENDS, BENEFITS, AND FUNDING. This annual publication will provide a guide to salaries and benefits in different geographic regions by type of hospital and training year. Since it is not tactful to request this information at the time of your interview, you can secure an approximate idea as to remuneration from this source.

THE TRANSITIONAL YEAR PROGRAM DIRECTORY. This annual publication of the Association for Hospital Medical Education describes the characteristics of *transitional* PGY-1 year programs. It serves as a supplement to the FREIDA database. This source book is of special interest to those seeking information about this type of residency program (see Chapter 1).

PHYSICIAN DISTRIBUTION AND MEDICAL LICENSURE IN THE UNITED STATES. An AMA publication based on physician surveys that provides detailed statistics on many practical aspects of each specialty.

ANNUAL REPORT ON GRADUATE MEDICAL EDUCATION. This appears annually in a December issue of *JAMA* and contains useful information about house staff position supply and demand.

Other sources

PROGRAM OFFICES. Having acquired information on potential suitable programs, you can send off a fax, e-mail, or postcard to individual residency programs that you are interested in, requesting literature about the programs. Some dean's offices have preprinted cards specifically designed for this purpose. Any responses should be kept in the file you set up for each of the programs. Be sure that the information you receive relates to the year you wish to initiate your residency. The

information obtained will vary widely in both appearance and detail and will probably not be suitable for making comparisons between programs. It may supplement
the information you gain from the FREIDA database because it is more recent.
Thus can help you narrow down your choices of programs to apply to and thereby
make the program selection process easier.

PROFESSIONAL SOCIETIES. These can provide general information about their
specialties. Some of their published directories of residency programs in individual
specialties can be quite useful. Specialties providing such resources include family
practice, internal medicine, psychiatry, preventive medicine, physical medicine and
rehabilitation, and urology.

JOURNALS. Some journals contain advertisements listing residency openings.
These are commonly found in *The New Physician* but may also appear in the *New
England Journal of Medicine* and *JAMA*. Advertising for residents may suggest that
a program is having difficulty filling its slots, and such openings should therefore
be very carefully screened.

RESIDENCY FAIRS. Medical schools and even hospitals may schedule fairs in
which residency directors very frequently participate. Personal interchange and
acquisition of literature can provide you with useful information about possible
suitable openings and offer an opportunity to get direct responses to any questions
you may have.

INDIVIDUAL CONTACTS. A variety of individuals can provide information that may
prove helpful in your search for information. This includes your medical school's
dean of students, who, based on prior years of experience, is usually knowledgeable
as to the current difficulty in securing residencies in different fields. This possibly
includes having familiarity with potential residency slots that are or will become
available. Your specialty advisor may be aware of the situation with programs in
relevant geographic areas. Similarly, your mentor may be in a position to be of
direct benefit to you in your search because of personal contacts at his/her dis-
posal. Finally, your school library should have valuable resources that may be worth
tapping and thus consulting with a reference librarian can prove beneficial.

THE INTERNET. The Internet has become a readily accessible and quite valuable
up-to-date source of information about residency programs. Thus information may
be posted on Web sites of both specialty societies and individual residency programs. The AMA Web site is a good place to initiate your search, as are the Web
sites for the AAMC and *The New Physician*. Web sites for individual specialties are
provided at the end of each areas description (see Chapters 3, 4 and 5).

9 | Residency Program Selection

Overview

Based on the sources of information regarding residencies provided in Chapter 8, a significant number of programs in your specialty should come to your attention. Their number needs adjustment relative to your own competitiveness, how difficult it is to secure a position in the specialty you have chosen, and personal considerations. This entire issue will be discussed in the first section of this chapter. Next will come a section entitled *Strategy for applying*, to facilitate obtaining interviews. This subject will be followed by considering how you evaluate a program at an interview, so that you can properly prepare a Rank Order List for the Match, after all your interviews have been completed.

Selecting prospective programs

In this section, a procedure is presented on how to carry out a *preliminary* screening of residency programs to see if they meet your basic needs. This is done by determining if the training institution is suitably located and if it is the type of appointment that you seek. Other significant personal issues should also be checked at this point. By this means you should formulate a group of prospective residency programs, which then can be reduced to a reasonable level, as is discussed of p. 125.

Once you have reduced the prospective residency program number to a reasonable number, the interview invitations you receive will allow you to proceed further and formulate a Rank Order List for the Match. The process of actually preparing a Rank Order List will be discussed in Chapter 12.

Strategy for applying

Previously, emphasis was placed on the components needed to enhance your chances to secure an interview. You now need to proceed beyond the procedural requirements. What is necessary at this point is an action plan that will facilitate achieving your goal.

The basic strategy being recommended is very straightforward and simple: *submit your application early*. This advice is based on the fact that the value judgments made by program directors regarding granting interviews generally tend to become increasingly tough as time goes on. This change is generated by the growing number of applications that are submitted for evaluation during the course of the selection processes. To further achieve your aim of securing an early review of your credentials, you should (a) expedite preparation of all the materials that you must generate yourself and (b) arrange for material from other sources (e.g., a transcript from the Registrar's Office and recommendations sent from the Office of the Dean of Students and by faculty) to be forwarded in a timely fashion.

Because most programs have deadlines for receipt of supporting material, it is best not to assume that your file is complete. Rather, check and see if this really is the case by calling the residency program office periodically. If something is missing, identify what it is. Where possible, promptly have a duplicate sent off and where comparable documents were sent to other programs, see if they were received. In any case, bear in mind that Dean's letters customarily are not sent out until November 1, so expect them to be there only after that date.

A well-known technique used by students to get final exam grades as early as possible after a test, without having an agonizing wait for a Registrar's report, can also be applied to determine the completeness of your residency application file. This involves sending a semicomplete, self-addressed postcard along with application material being submitted to the residency program. You can thereby request that they return it to you after placing a confirmation mark in front of a statement that your file is now complete. You should attach a brief note with the card, requesting and thanking them for their cooperation regarding this matter. The receipt of such a card can be a clear signal to follow up with a call to the department office inquiring if you should schedule an interview. If necessary, feel free to call subsequently and politely to inquire about the status of your application, without

Table 9.1 Residency application management

Competitive ranking	No. of program inquires	No. of residency applications	No. of interviews desirable
high	20–30	6–14	5–10
average	25–35	10–20	7–12
low	30–40	15–25	10–15

embarrassment or feeling that you are being too pushy. Your obvious interest in the program may pay off unexpectedly with an invitation to present yourself for an interview. The motto for attaining a residency should be: prepare promptly, submit early, and follow up regularly!

An important part of the strategy of applying is to determine how many programs you should apply to. By now you most probably have identified to your satisfaction the specialty you seek to enter. Securing a place in a suitable postgraduate training program has two aspects. It involves determining (1) the number of programs to apply to and (2) the number of programs that it is desirable to be interviewed at. The decision as to these two questions hinges on three factors. These are (a) the extent of competitiveness in the specialty you seek a residency in (see Table 8.1), (b) the school you are coming from, and (c) your strength as a candidate. You should bear these three elements in mind when formulating your application strategy, using the suggested guidelines shown in Table 9.1. (Note: Your competitive ranking should be determined from Table 8.2.)

The process of peeling down programs to a desirable number should be done most thoughtfully. You should not reject a program

■ Until you adequately review available information to determine that for some valid reason it is not suitable for your needs.

■ Because you feel that you will be unable to get appointed, since you feel that you are not a strong enough candidate for that program.

■ Due to unfavorable comments made about a program by a fellow student, whose validity you have not corroborated.

To achieve your goal of selecting suitable programs, it is necessary to determine what are your most basic priorities for use when evaluating specialty program's merit. The criteria will obviously vary for each individual and are a very subjective issue. Thus considerable thought needs to be given as to what your own priorities are. These should be identified on Form 9.1. Respond by noting E–essential or A–acceptable for each of the criteria listed below.

Form 9.1 Basic criteria for program acceptability

1. Location   Rating

    Region: Identify _____

    Cities: Identify _____

2. Clinical training: Institution: Identify type

   _____ University medical center

   _____ Middle level hospital

   _____ Community hospital

3. Other features

   _____ Availability of suitable housing for yourself and family

   _____ Availability of educational facilities for children

   _____ Availability of job opportunities for spouse

   _____ Cost of living in the area

   _____ Transportation ease to the training site

   _____ Social and entertainment opportunities available

   _____ Additional features:

   _____ _____

   _____ _____

   _____ _____

Once you are ready to complete this form, do so using a pencil. This is because after completing it, you should view the result as a first draft. It should then be reconsidered with your spouse (and perhaps your family), your advisor/mentor, and maybe close friends at your medical school. Be prepared to modify your responses as circumstances necessitate.

Bear in mind that you can personalize Form 9.1 by either adding criteria of importance to you or deleting those that are insignificant. Assign a rating of *E* or *A* to any new criteria added.

Note: A detailed evaluation of the individual program criteria is presented in the first section of this chapter.

Evaluating a residency program

The majority of PGY-1 residents are selected by means of the *Match*. This term denotes that an agreement has been arrived at between the residency program and the applicant, relative to offering and accepting a residency appointment, respectively. It was activated because both parties found it mutually beneficial to do so. The residency program believes it will obtain the services of the type of resident that it seeks to employ. The prospective residents, on the other hand, feels that the designated program will provide the training that will ensure their competency as a future practitioner in the specialty chosen and will ultimately make them eligible for Board certification upon meeting designated requirements.

The need to prepare for the Match makes it necessary that residency applicants determine what qualities they prefer in a program. Consequently, you must carefully evaluate prospective programs, in order to be able to formulate a suitable list of programs to apply to in light of your personal interests.

A wide range of factors are important in evaluating a residency program. These will be summarized in Form 9.2, and should be applied to individual programs. Each prospective resident (in consultation with family, as appropriate) can determine if a criterion is absolutely essential or merely desirable.

Location. This factor plays a critical role in the choice of every individual's residency plans. One can get some general idea of the nature of medicine in a geographic area from conversations with attendings from various locations. One of the general reasons people choose a specific location is that the likelihood of ultimately ending up practicing there is higher. In addition, different regions of the country have various concentrations of residency opportunities. The five areas having a high concentration of training programs are:

(a) Atlantic states: New York, New Jersey, and Pennsylvania

(b) Central states: Illinois, Ohio, Indiana, Michigan, Minnesota, and Wisconsin

(c) South Atlantic Coast states: Florida, North Carolina, Tennessee

(d) Pacific Coast state: California

(e) Southwestern state: Texas

Other factors restricting the choice of a specific location are considerations relative to the needs of a spouse, children, or parents. Some medical students are influenced by the physical characteristics of a region. Given the limited free time usually available to a resident for nonprofessional activities, it probably is not desirable to place too much weight on this issue. There is a natural inclination to seek a residency at the institution where one is a medical student. This is because one's familiarity with the facilities is a strong reassuring element. Nevertheless, this is not advisable because psychologically the faculty will tend to view you as a medical student rather than as a resident. This can make performance more challenging because a subjective opinion of you may have been established. Going to a different institution and demonstrating your abilities starting with a clean slate may prove to be beneficial.

Clinical training. This is the key feature that helps determine if you will have a successful residency experience. This factor is composed of a number of elements that in sum will determine how well prepared you emerge to practice your specialty.

These elements include (a) the nature of the institution, (b) the number of patients treated, and (c) the number of procedures carried out in the specialty. Although patient volume is important, what is really meaningful is the ratio of patients to residents. A proper balance between them is critical to avoid getting too little experience in an overstaffed situation or, on the other hand, being exposed to inadequate supervised experience in an understaffed institution.

Clinical exposure. It is very valuable to find out about the diversity of patients and diseases that you will see at the training facility. A wide range of typical cases for your specialty is what best prepares you as a resident for professional life. The type of institution the residency program is affiliated with can provide information on this important issue.

Setting. The issues of patient volume and level of responsibility are basically determined by the type of institution that sponsors the program. Ideally the goal should be to secure a position at a midlevel institution, namely, somewhere between a large urban medical center and a small community hospital. This should provide you with both the experience and supervised training to meet your future needs. Any gap in training at such an institution can conceivably be filled by short residency stints away from the home base.

Securing information on the extent of professional exposure to and activity in ambulatory care sites is also essential, because considerable medical services are currently being provided in such settings. Inquire as to the rate of hospital admissions at the institution's emergency services facilities. It should be about 15% or more to reflect adequate patient volume.

Responsibility. It is important to ascertain the extent of responsibility as a resident that will be delegated to you in managing patient care. This means determining which of the medical orders you can write and which need prior approval by a superior before they can be executed. Your educational and training goals should be to obtain graduated increased responsibility for patient care. To be excessively engaged in scut work for your supervisors, will not enhance your career goal. On the other hand, to be prematurely placed in a position of responsibility for patient care without adequate training and experience is equally undesirable.

Many specialties have standard diagnostic or therapeutic procedures associated with them. Specialty societies usually can provide information as to what these are (see Appendix 1). It is important to learn if you will obtain adequate exposure to and training in such procedures in the course of your residency. Securing information on the extent of training opportunities in a specific program, be they diagnostic (e.g., colonoscopy) or therapeutic (e.g., surgery), is best obtained from residents at the time of your interviews. Seek also to determine if ancillary personnel are available to handle routine tasks such as drawing blood. It is important to establish that your exposure will adequately prepare you to enter practice with a sense of confidence that you are able to accept the responsibilities that lie ahead.

On-call and work schedule. There is wide variability in this overtime activity among residency programs. It depends on the specialty, institution, service, and postgraduate year. Being on-call every third night is common, but in some programs it may be more often than others. Thus, seek to obtain a clear picture of the on-call schedule from residents in the programs you are considering. This is essential to protect your long-term interests. Once you have this information, evaluate if you can anticipate the demands such overtime service will make on your lifestyle and if they are acceptable. This is especially true for surgical residencies. Working an excessive number of hours is not unusual in some specialties. As to a resident's work schedule, the standard recommended target goal of 80 hours per week maximum (averaged over four weeks) is not always met.

Reputation. Prior to considering the possibility of postgraduate training at *any* program, you should determine if it is certified. This means that the residency program has met the standards established by the certifying board of the specialty. A Residency Review Committee established by the specialty board conducts, on a regular basis, on-site inspections and evaluations to see if a program meets the mandated training requirements. This ensures that, at the very least, the minimum acceptable conditions for the specialty are being met.

For those planning a career in academic medicine or anticipating the need for fellowship training in a subspecialty, an appointment at a prestigious institution is certainly beneficial. The majority of residents who enter a general or specialty practice can feel reassured that conscientiously completing a certified program will provide them with the essential training necessary for their future professional work. Thus a program's reputation need always not be at the top of the list of factors to consider when making a Rank Order List.

An institution's standing is usually the result of the quality of its faculty and its research. While a high reputation is an appealing feature, it should not be considered more important than what the program personally has to offer you. Some programs have name recognition due to the high standing they have been accorded by physicians over the years. This status should not be taken at face value. Their current reputation should be investigated in depth, rather than relying upon hearsay. Up-to-date information on a program's quality can best be secured by securing interviews at various institutions. This also allows comparisons to be made between what programs offer.

To really judge a program you should focus on the faculty and how they can be of benefit to you. This means ascertaining the faculty commitment to patient service as clinical educators, beyond merely making appearances at rounds. In other words, determine if attendings are available for guidance when you need them. This will clue you in as to the support you can count on in terms of personal assistance and/or advice, which may help you overcome unanticipated challenges during your residency. The extent of formal teaching by attendings, in whatever format (e.g., formal lectures, group conferences, and bedside teaching), should also be ascertained. The bottom line is to investigate the degree of involvement of faculty in the professional well-being and growth of residents. If it is inadequate, then naturally your training may suffer. Finally, determine if there is stability in the faculty or if there is a high turnover rate and consequently mostly youthful members make up the service. Their teaching experience under these conditions is inevitably limited when compared to well seasoned attendings.

Curriculum. In evaluating programs, their curricula can be one good source for comparison. This is especially relevant when you need to find out (a) what are the services you will be assigned to, (b) in what order this will take place, (c) and for how long, each will take place. In addition, most current information regarding possible intraspecialty rotations can be ascertained during your interview. It is also useful to inquire about the extent of interaction of residents with other specialties.

From both the program literature and your interview, you should seek to ascertain the breadth of training the program offers in your field of interest. You may also wish to become, when relevant, aware of extent of exposure to subspecialty fields provided as part of the training. This will allow you to determine the extent of your interest in the possibility of a fellowship following completion of your residency.

Education as a resident is also secured by means of conferences. Their numbers may vary widely from almost daily to once or twice a month. This is another means of making comparisons between programs. It is important to learn how much time will be available to you to attend professional conferences. Discussions with residents should enable you to elucidate the policy of the program regarding this issue. It is useful to try to find out how effective such conferences are in reality in enhancing your fund of specialty knowledge.

Work atmosphere. The curriculum is but one aspect of a residency program, albeit a vital one. It partially contributes to the nature of the working atmosphere. It is, however, important to try to gain a sense of the interrelationship and camaraderie among the staff, both professional and ancillary. Again, this can best be uncovered during the course of an interview with both residents and support personal. It will indicate to you how pleasant a place it is to secure your training. A stressful atmosphere can significantly impede your training and patient care. The reverse is certainly true for a congenial situation and this is the type of situation you obviously seek.

Research. Participation in research as part of a residency program is becoming increasingly popular. It offers a variety of advantages and can open up new intellectual horizons for many. To benefit the most in this area, it is important to secure the support of an experienced researcher/mentor who is willing to guide you in what for most is a new and uncharted pursuit of knowledge. If you have research interests, you should inquire about the availability of space, funding potential, and especially subjects of current interest among faculty. In addition to the aforementioned needs, it is obviously essential to ascertain how much time can potentially be made available to residents for research. Programs use different schedule mechanisms to make research opportunities available. Thus this issue should be looked into.

Facilities. The nature and modernity of the facilities of the institution where you would serve as a resident can have a marked impact on your performance. You should inquire from residents if they feel that their facilities are adequate, superior, or substandard. Determine how well maintained the institution is and how convenient essential services are. An aged structure with a shabby interior will certainly not enhance the working environment. The quality and efficiency of patient care can be influenced by the quality of the surroundings.

Clinical laboratory services. These include getting necessary lab reports in a timely fashion. Having such support certainly is essential to facilitating a prompt and effective response by house staff and attendings to the urgent medical needs of patients. It is therefore, very desirable to learn about the availability, efficiency, and reliability of the hospital's labs. A resident is expected to provide lab data to the treatment team in a timely fashion and is held accountable for doing so.

Computerization. Because time is of the essence in a resident's daily activities, being able to obtain computerized records of lab results and patient backgrounds is a significant asset. Although this is most likely the case, you should nevertheless make appropriate inquiries to be certain that such an arrangement exists.

Library. This is an important support source for your medical education. It should offer up-to-date reference texts, access to prominent current journals in your field, appropriate online reference sources, and photocopying equipment. You should evaluate this resource site during the course of your visit to the institution for an interview.

On-call sites. Although these facilities are used only for limited periods of time, they should provide a suitable place to get a well-deserved rest break at night, when time permits. It should have the minimum amenities to meet your personal needs. The nature of these facilities merits your attention during the course of your site visit. They may reflect the degree of consideration an institution is prepared to extend for the well-being of its residents.

Security. The safety of one's working environment is something that should not be taken for granted. This is true even for hospitals, where unfortunately physicians have not been immune to being physically attacked. This is especially valid in emergency treatment facilities. You should become aware of the seriousness with which personal safety is viewed at the institution. This can best be done by making *discrete* inquires from residents as to the facility's safety record. Inquiries as to the nature and effectiveness of the security provided at the institution are also in order.

Parking. This essential feature is available to a varied extent at most institutions. Its accessibility and cost (which frequently is subsidized) obviously merit looking into. Also, find out if parking poses a possible hazard to personal safety when leaving the institution at night. Prospective female residents should determine if there is a need for an escort when leaving the institution at night and the opportunity to secure such assistance.

Compensation. This important issue will be considered in terms of salary and benefits. These items vary among institutions and in different sections of the country. Church-affiliated institutions pay somewhat more than state-supported ones. There are also variations in salary level, depending on the type of hospital. When progressing through the varied levels of a residency program, one can expect on average a 10% increase in relation to the cost of living. The offer of especially high salaries by a program should raise concern as to whether this may be due to their being unable to attract personnel, and thus such a situation merits thorough evaluation before making a commitment.

Benefits. This nonsalaried component of compensation, is a significant element in your remuneration package. You need to determine precisely what these benefits are and how much residents must contribute to the various items making up the package. Health insurance companies offer group health programs for residents, sponsored by their institutions. You should inquire whether your spouse and children are covered (or could be added); what benefits your coverage provides; and your direct contribution (as a payroll deduction) and co-payments for various medical services. The extent of coverage varies by regional location of the institution. Prescription drug benefits are provided by most programs and many also provide dental benefits.

Other health benefits that are offered to a variable extent are psychiatric services, a potentially valuable asset for residents working under stress, and vision care (glasses, contact lenses). Sick leave coverage is another benefit that you should inquire about during the course of your interview at residency sites.

Nonhealth benefits are also offered to residents to a variable extent. These may include life insurance, disability insurance (important in light of the HIV/AIDS issue), parking and housing subsidies, and meals when on-call and when working, as well as child care. One benefit that is standard and fully paid for by the institution is liability (malpractice) insurance. It is wise, however, to inquire as to how much coverage is provided and the kind of policy offered (limited coverage, or a more comprehensive occurrence policy). Other important factors to be taken note of are vacation time and, for women, maternity leave after pregnancy.

Moonlighting. Residents are generally paid relatively modest salaries and often have large debts, stamming from medical school. If you contemplate moonlighting to supplement your income, you should inquire as to what is the institution policy regarding this. Careful thought needs to be given before undertaking such after-hours work, because of the extra demands that it places on individuals. (See also Chapter 13.)

Summary

It is critical to evaluate all programs that you visit thoroughly. Form 9.2 is designed to help you achieve this goal.

Form 9.2 Residency interview assessment form

Program Director _____   **Phone #** _____

Name of Institution _____

Address _____   **Fax #** _____

_____   **E-mail** _____

1. Location
   Region of country   _____
   City size   _____
   Rural, urban, inner city   _____

2. Clinical training
   Patient volume   _____
   Staffing level   _____
   Patient/staff ratio   _____

3. Clinical exposure
   Patient types   _____
      Typical   _____
      Atypical   _____
   Disease types   _____
      Typical   _____
      Atypical   _____

4. Setting: Hospital type
   Large urban   _____
   Ambulatory care   _____
   Emergency admissions   _____

5. Responsibilities
   Diagnostic procedures   _____
   Therapeutic procedures   _____
   Scut work   _____
   Private patients treatment _____

(continued)

Form 9.2 *(continued)*

6. On-call schedule
   Average _____
   Excessive but tolerable _____
   Very excessive _____

7. Reputation and faculty
   Institutional status _____
   Program quality _____
   Stability of faculty _____
   Commitment of faculty _____
   Quality of faculty _____
   Faculty-resident relationships _____

8. Curriculum
   Organization _____
   Conferences (number and caliber) _____
   Interspecialty interaction _____

9. Work atmosphere
   Congenial _____
   Stressful _____

10. Research
    Ongoing level _____
    Opportunities _____

11. Support services availability
    Adequate _____
    Superior _____
    Substandard _____

12. Facilities
    Adequate _____
    Superior _____
    Substandard _____

13. Clinical laboratory services
    Availability _____
    Efficiency _____
    Reliability _____

14. Computerization
    Laboratory results _____
    Patient records _____

15. Library
    Reference texts _____
    Current journals _____
    On-line services _____
    Photocopy equipment _____

16. On-call sites
    Adequate _____
    Superior _____
    Inferior _____

17. Security
    Adequate _____
    Superior _____
    Inferior _____

18. Parking
    Availability _____
    Cost _____
    Security _____

19. Compensation
    Salary _____
    Salary scale _____

20. Benefits
    Personal medical insurance _____
    Family medical insurance _____
    Prescription drug insurance _____
    Dental insurance _____
    Resident contribution _____
    Liability insurance _____
    Vacation allowance _____
    Maternity leave _____

10 | Applying for a Residency

Overview

Having selected your future specialty, and chosen prospective programs of genuine interest, you are now at the next key juncture, namely, submitting your applications to secure a residency appointment. Thus, at this point, preparation of all the material to be submitted in support of an application for a PGY-1 position is essential. To attain your goal, it is important to be a salesperson, with the aim of presenting yourself in the most favorable light possible. This means providing appropriate accurate and complete responses to all questions and issues raised during the application process. To do so, you need to carefully read each application, preferably more than once. Be certain that your responses to all questions are clear and up-to-date.

In the individual residency program files that you create for yourself, note all (a) deadlines that need to be met and (b) material that the program specifically requests. By this means you help ensure that the processing of your application will not be delayed because needed information or material is unavailable to the program director. Do not assume that you will be notified by a residency program that some document is missing or that your application is incomplete. They may well *not* do so and consequently you can lose out in the application process by default. Copies of all communications and logs of all phone calls should be kept in the relevant program file. A meticulous approach to record-keeping is essential to stay on top of things. This is important, because you will certainly be applying to multiple institutions, whereas at the same time you are fully preoccupied with your clerkship and elective responsibilities as a third- and fourth-year medical student.

Four important factors are associated with applying for a residency. Crucial to attaining success are being (a) organized, (b) neat and pleasant, (c) thorough, and (d) timely. Each of these elements will now be considered.

Being organized. Whether by downloading from Web sites, or from responses to requests from residency programs for descriptive literature, you can anticipate accumulating a torrent of information. Consequently, setting up a file system is a key element in efficient and productive handling of the paper flow. By placing incoming material in the appropriate file as soon as possible after receipt, you will be assured that it will not be misplaced and that it will be available promptly when needed at a later date. Associated with this issue is good record-keeping so that you know what has transpired and when with regard to each residency program. You will thus not be dependent solely on your memory for details of past activities and you will be able to respond promptly to any situation that may develop. Consequently, you will thus be able to focus more fully on your clerkship responsibilities and not overburden your memory with details that are readily available.

Being neat and pleasant. Your contact with the residency program will initially be by mail, e-mail, fax, and phone. You should realize that the first impressions you will be making therefore come about indirectly by these communications. Thus, in all written communications, you should employ, whenever possible, a computer and laser printer because of the positive impact the attractive appearance of your messages will have. If circumstances require you to use longhand, you should make a special effort to print neatly so that what you write is readily legible. Residency directors have reported on the potential strong negative impact of lack of neatness has on a candidate's chances because of the possible implications that can be drawn. It has been reported that this deficiency may in some cases contribute to failure to secure a residency.

You need to be equally careful and tactful with all your verbal communications not only with the director, but also with residency office personnel. Thus, when speaking with a program secretary on the phone, make sure that you are polite and coherent. Know exactly what you wish to say or ask. Obviously this is even more valid for any occasion in which you speak to the program director. The bottom line is that when you write or speak, make sure to leave a positive impression, because you will never know its potential impact on the image you are generating.

Being thorough. When completing ERAS or responding to an inquiry, carefully ascertain what information is being sought. Check to see if your response is the proper one. If a lengthy reply is called for, prepare and proofread your draft before sending in your final copy. You need to avoid any embarrassment resulting from the submission of incomplete or inappropriate information.

Being timely. Residency programs need to process a multitude of applicants. They thus usually adhere strictly to their established schedules, to be sure that (a) applications can be responded to efficiently, (b) interviews can be properly scheduled, and (c) responses can be sent out in an orderly manner. To facilitate these activities it is essential for applicants to respond to all requests from programs promptly and meet all deadlines set. Making sure that this is accomplished is *your* responsibility.

In summary, you should not merely look upon a residency appointment as a significant educational and training opportunity, but act as if you are applying for an important professional position. This means that you need to put your best foot forward to achieve your goal, especially in the face of the competition.

Your application

When you applied to medical school, you undoubtedly utilized AMCAS for the bulk of your applications. This service is sponsored by the Association of American Medical Colleges. The procedure involved completing only one application, which was then sent to multiple institutions where you wished to be considered for admission. The same organization also sponsors the Electronic Residency Application Service (ERAS). It utilizes an identical approach and it has been phased in gradually for most specialties. ERAS is appealing to applicants because it provides an efficient and time-saving means of applying for a residency. ERAS transmits residency application materials and supporting credentials from applicants and medical schools to residency program offices over the Internet. This service thereby also facilitates the placement activities of both medical schools and residency programs, in addition to helping medical students secure postgraduate appointments. Institutions participating in ERAS are all U.S. medical schools, the NBME, and the ECFMG.

The ERAS program began in 1995 and currently it has the following participating specialties:

Anesthesiology

Dermatology

Diagnostic Radiology

Emergency Medicine

Family Practice

General Surgery

Internal Medicine – Emergency Medicine

Internal Medicine – Pediatrics

Internal Medicine – Psychiatry

Nuclear Medicine

Obstetrics and Gynecology

Orthopedic Surgery

Pathology

Pediatrics

Pediatrics – Emergency Medicine

Pediatrics – Physical Medicine and Rehabilitation

Pediatrics – Psychiatry

Physical Medicine and Rehabilitation

Psychiatry – Family Practice

Radiation Oncology

Transitional Year

Urology

Almost all the programs in these specialties select their residents through ERAS. In addition, all Army and Navy PGY-1 residencies also do so.

Application Supplies. To facilitate preparation of the online ERAS application, an ERAS student workstation kit is provided. This includes (a) a student data diskette, (b) a special instruction manual, and (c) a worksheet.

Securing Assistance. To facilitate use of the ERAS program, a button is provided to get to a help screen. This will provide you with guidance to a path for seeking answers to any questions that may arise. It also provides access to the glossary of terms utilized in the program.

The ERAS process has 12 steps that must be carefully followed. These steps are briefly summarized under three headings.

1. *Secure Information.* Determine the programs that may be of interest to you by contacting them by mail or visiting their Web sites. Ascertain for certain that they participate in ERAS.

2. *Secure Material.* Obtain your ERAS student workstation kit (see above). To do this, you need to contact your school's dean's office.

3. *Secure a Deadline.* It is imperative to check the processing schedule at your school to ensure that you do not miss their deadlines. Your medical school is responsible for getting the supporting material sent off in a timely fashion.

Your personal statement

This important component of the application presents a significant challenge. Many students tend to put off drafting their statements and consequently their applications may be delayed. The goal of writing a personal statement is not to have the program judge your literary skills, but rather to see if you can provide valuable information about yourself in a concise and coherent manner. What is sought is insight into your level of personal and professional growth at this stage in your career.

The importance of the personal statement seems to depend upon the specific program that you are applying to. There is evidence to suggest that it has a greater impact, for example, on ob/gyn program directors than on family practice ones. Generally, its importance apparently ranks below that of other parameters such as USMLE scores, grades, and recommendations, both for selecting interviewees and for ranking candidates. However, the impact of the personal statement should not be underestimated and its preparation deserves your careful attention, because it may be just the element that tilts the decision on acceptance into a program in your favor.

Bear in mind, when writing your statement, that your readers may well be physicians, who generally are conservative by nature. Thus the tone and word choices should be appropriate to such an audience. The addition of any non-ERAS application statement should be enhanced by using good quality paper and a laser printer. In either case the grammar and spelling of your statement need to be carefully checked. The maximum length should be a single full page.

Your statement allows you to get your personal message *directly* to the program's director. You should use it as a vehicle to seek to convince the reader that you are an attractive candidate and that, at the very least, you merit an interview so that you can be judged at first hand. It is helpful to make an inventory of your assets prior to undertaking preparation of your personal statement. In doing so emphasis should be on (a) your abilities and character, (b) your academic and career accomplishments, (c) the reasons for selecting the specialty, (d) the motive for choosing the specific program that you are applying to, (e) your tentative future plans, and (f) an impressive summary. These issues will now be elaborated on.

Personal Attributes. These should be presented in the form of accomplishments, such as your overall college and medical school record, especially if you can demonstrate a strong level of consistency in your performance. Additionally, relate any special achievements in clerkships and electives, as well as any research or other evidence that demonstrates your intellectual potential, especially that is relevant to the residency position you seek. Because the application will have a place to list your specific achievements, you need not repeat them on the personal statement.

Motivation. As to your reasons for choosing the specialty, carefully consider all relevant factors. These may include some very positive personal experiences, such as having skills or talents that are particularly suited for the specialty. Other factors may be the special gratification provided by practicing in this field or being influenced by a role model. Note that to indicate in your statement that you are attracted by the appealing lifestyles of specific practitioners in the specialty or that their level of income are attractive factors, obviously is inappropriate and is potentially self-defeating.

It is appropriate to identify the characteristics of the specialty that you find appealing. These should be correlated with personal attributes that you have. Where possible, support the relationship between the specialty references and your own abilities by past educational and training experiences.

Program Selection. Regarding your rationale in the selection of a residency program, it is best to respond in general terms. You may wish to indicate the highly favorable comments you heard about their program (e.g., from your advisor/mentor or former residents): its desirable location, its dedicated faculty, and the superior training opportunities and facilities it offers. In responding to this question, avoid customizing the essay, which would make it unsuitable for use with all programs.

Career Goals. Your future plans should be described only in general terms. But you need to bear in mind the nature of the institution where the program is located. If, for example, research is a major feature, this aspect should be a possible significant consideration when describing your future career plans. If your tentative goals are focused on clinical or academic medicine or working in an underserved area, this should be indicated in an appropriate manner and be supported by providing convincing evidence.

Concluding Remarks. You may wish to use your personal statements, if space permits, to discuss briefly such matters as your family, your hobbies, and any of your community service activities. Should there be any relevant issues regarding yourself or your background (e.g., a close member of your family being a physician) that merit being mentioned, this is the appropriate place to do so. Avoid raising any controversial subjects.

Your AMCAS essay may provide you with a source for color, to give your essay a personalized touch and thus an especially appealing quality. However, make sure to avoid any suggestions that you are an odd or atypical individual, because they usually are looking for candidates who will fit into the group. Finally, you may wish to end your statement with a concluding paragraph in which you summarize your potential as a resident in terms of your willingness to work hard and be a team player and your desire to apply your ample talents and skills to the best of your ability. Aim to establish that you will be a solid asset to the department and thus worthy of being sought after. The end product should reflect the considerable effort that you put into preparing your statement. (See sample statements in Appendix 3).

Your recommendations

Residency programs require several letters of recommendation in support of your application. These include a letter from your medical school administration, known as the dean's letter. Other letters should come from the faculty and attendings, who get to know you from your course work and clerkships. These important communications reflect how people view you both professionally and personally.

Dean's Letter. This is not, strictly speaking, a recommendation, but rather an academic evaluation that is sent out for all fourth-year medical students applying for residencies. These detailed letters include your educational history, a description of your academic performance, and usually direct quotations from written evaluations submitted by attendings who have served as supervisors of your clinical rotations.

Be aware that you may be able to influence the quality of your dean's letter in your favor. Thus, you should inquire as to exactly who is the person writing dean's letters at your school. Most probably it is the dean of students, but it need not necessarily be so. It is common practice to be invited to meet with whomever is the letter writer. If and when this takes place, you should obviously make a strong effort to leave a favorable impression. You can also inquire if you can see the letter after it is drafted. You may then try, if essential, to have changes made, but only if factual errors are present. If you are sure that an attending physician who supervised you holds you in exceptionally high regard, consider suggesting that this person, in addition to writing in your behalf, personally speak with the dean of students about you. It is also important to submit all required information to the dean's office in a timely fashion. To expedite matters you may even provide the dean's office with preaddressed labels to be used to send the letters to residency program offices that you are applying to.

Other recommendations. Usually three letters are requested, with one frequently expected to come from the medical school's department chairperson of the relevant specialty. Even where it is not required, it can prove very valuable to secure such a letter. You can do this best by arranging an appointment with the chairperson. Seek his/her advice as to which programs to apply to. Inquire if the chairperson would be willing to write a recommendation on your behalf; if so, leave a copy of your resume and express your gratitude for their forthcoming assistance. The chairperson has ready sources in the department from whom to obtain information relative to your abilities and past performance. Thus the letter can prove to be especially helpful because of the status of the writer.

Other letters should come from clinical faculty members with whom you have had close professional contact, especially in your field of interest or one related to it. A letter from a faculty member under whom you worked directly on a project can prove especially beneficial. You may also wish to choose as a reference source a rotation supervisor for whom your clinical work was outstanding. Letters from mentors or advisors can prove equally valuable. Having indicated what are desirable sources for recommendations, it is also worthwhile noting that there are inappropriate ones as well. These include house staff, relatives, and clergy; it will not serve your best interests to seek assistance from them.

Your resume

This is an important document that should provide a synopsis of your educational background and life experiences. It should be sent to all of the programs you will be applying to. You may attach it to the end of your personal statement, when filing an ERAS application, unless specifically advised otherwise. You should include it with all non-ERAS applications whether requested or not. Careful attention should be focused on both the resume's contents and appearance, because impressions do count. The makeup of a suitable resume will now be discussed.

Contents. Personal information should include

1. Your name, full address, phone number, e-mail address, and fax number.

2. Your objective. Briefly state the rationale for submitting your resume.

3. Your education. Start with medical school and include enrollment and anticipated graduation date. Next, list all graduate and undergraduate schools attended, with degrees, dates of attendance, and majors. Providing GPAs and class rankings at these institutions is optional, but if exceptionally high, it should be noted.

4. Honors/awards received. Describe these separately for medical and other schools. Include scholarships, memberships in honor societies, and election to organizational offices.

5. Research publications. List in reverse chronological order (i.e., most recent first) any articles or abstracts in which your name appears. Note the full title of the journal, the volume, including the inclusive page numbers, and the year of publication. In this segment briefly describe any as yet unpublished research projects being worked on. Identify the location of the laboratory and the name of your supervisor.

6. Professional organizations. Identify any national organizations you belong to, even if you are only a student member, (e.g. American Medical Association, American Medical Students Association).

7. Extracurricular activities. Indicate any relevant activities you have been active in, such as a volunteer ambulance service.

8. Supplementary personal information. Indicate if you are married, and if so, if you have children. If you are a citizen (native-born or naturalized), this should also be noted.

9. References. Indicate that you will provide suitable references, upon request.

Finally, note that:

■ Your resume should be designed to be easily readable. For the reader to spend excessive time to decipher a poorly designed resume can prove frustrating and diminish one's chances for gaining an interview.

■ Be sure that there are no gaps in the chronological order of your educational advancement. If interruptions exist, explain the circumstances involved clearly (e.g., a sabbatical after a college).

■ Make sure that your resume provides a full and clear picture of your accomplishments and potential.

■ Bear in mind that your resume should be able to serve as a ready reference source for you and an interviewer, to bring forth vital information in response to questions that may arise.

Appearance. The two formats that are usually utilized are as follows:

10. One involves identifying varying typestyles for different headings and noting the facts beneath them.

11. Another consists of having the heading placed on the far left, in column-like format, and the responses on the right.

Whatever your choice of resume format, it should be aesthetically appealing and concise. The appearance will give the reader an initial impression and you wish to make it as favorable as possible.

Guidelines for preparing your resume. Guidelines can be summarized as follows:

12. Your resume should be one page in length (or at most two).

13. Make sure all information is accurate, concise, and clear.

14. Place your name, address, and phone number on top (not the word *Resume or Curriculum Vita*).

15. Make sure your resume is neat in appearance and attractive in design.

16. Use an inkjet or laser printer for the final copy to maximize a favorable impression that you wish to make.

17. Use action words in any descriptive sections (e.g., under *Objective*, indicate that you are "seeking superior postgraduate training in the field of _____").

18. Use 20- or 24-point bond paper. Most applicants select white, but some, to make their resumes stand out, use ivory or gray. Others using white will select a textured finish to give the paper a special feel.

19. The overwhelming majority of applicants use $8\frac{1}{2} \times 11''$ paper. However, some use $7\frac{1}{4} \times 10\frac{1}{2}''$ or $11 \times 17''$ folded in half to draw attention to their resumes. In the falter case the text would be on the inside and the name and address on the outside.

20. Select computer graphics that will make your resume look distinctive and eye-catching. Use 10 or 12 point for your font size. You may use type of differing heights to create emphasis. Similarly, type styles can be varied if you prefer, especially in the choice of headings. The varying style should be an appropriate match for the font chosen for the body of the text. To call attention to vital information you may use italics, bullets, or other symbols.

21. If appropriate, you may wish to make reference to knowledge of foreign languages that you may have and any military service.

22. Show a draft of your resume to your advisor/mentor, note the reaction, and then respond appropriately.

Your transcript

Residency programs expect to receive transcripts of your medical school record. They will use this document to judge the direction and level of your performance and, by inference, your intellectual potential. Your achievements are largely recorded in some coded format. There is no standard mode for doing so and, consequently, interpreting the data can generate confusion and misunderstanding. This is because identification of levels of student performance varies widely due to the use of different terms and symbols.

If you have an impressive record, it is in your best interest to ensure that the true nature of your achievements is brought to the attention of the residency program. This certainly can enhance your chances to secure an appointment. To maximize a favorable impression, it can be in your interest to prepare a transcript fact sheet that will serve to supplement your resume. Such a sheet should

a. Clearly identify the courses in which you have received honors or top grades and note how they are identified on your transcript.

b. Identify courses in which you received good or B grades. Identify the comparable grades on your transcript.

c. Explain any unusual markings that appear on your transcript. Thus a course with a letter P should be clarified as being a passing grade or a course in progress.

d. Explain any *incomplete* on your record fully, clearly, and carefully.

e. Where recognition for achievement was granted to you by noting an award on the transcript, you should briefly discuss its nature.

f. Regarding your class rank, if you are in the upper 50%, this should be noted on the fact sheet (even if not recorded on your transcript).

Finally, it is important to note that, if your record has improved significantly during your lower senior year you should have an updated supplementary transcript sent out to the program office (preferably with a note indicating that it is an updated version).

You can arrange to send your transcript to the program office even before they receive your application. So do not hesitate to get transcripts out early.

Note. See appendices 2 and 3 for sample resumes and personal statements respectively.

11 | The Residency Interview

Overview

The interview is usually the most decisive component of the residency selection process. The personal exchange that takes place at the hospital or medical center will be critical in determining how you are ranked by the program you are applying for. Thus, a maximal effort should be expended to achieve a successful outcome.

Having possibly been exposed to interviews when trying to get into college and most certainly when seeking admission into medical school, you are obviously not a novice as regards this trying experience. With your successful background in gaining acceptance into college and medical school, you should be more self-confident and at ease about the outcome of upcoming interviews. However, adequate preparation is, nevertheless, essential to help ensure similar success at this stage in your career.

You should realize that it is quite natural for your anxiety to increase as you approach the interview phase of the residency application process. This is understandable, because you find yourself in a highly competitive situation. It is important to recognize at this point that there are no ideal candidates for residency appointments. Rather, the chances for securing an appointment are dependent on the extent of the competition, the specialty in question, and the specific program within that specialty.

A wide variety of criteria are used in evaluating candidates (e.g., grades, class rank, evaluations). It should be recognized at the outset that the process is not a fully objective one. The interview provides a valuable vehicle to judge if the applicant fits into the program. This needs to be determined by both the program director and the applicant, so that a mutually beneficial match results.

The definition of "fit" refers to being able to perform effectively as a member of a house staff treatment team. Recommendations reflecting performance in specialty clerkships and electives, clerkship grades, and class rank are among the important rating criteria. They can unlock the door to securing an interview, but your performance at this event can make all the difference in determining if and where you will receive an appointment.

Scheduling interviews

A key element facilitating your success is *strategic timing* of your interviews. Rationally one would think it might be worthwhile to secure practice interview experience early on at a residency site of little interest. Such a preparatory effort can be obviated by the mock interview approach discussed below. You will thereby achieve a comparable result of obtaining interview experience, with less effort and expense.

A strong case can be made for scheduling your interviews *as late as possible*. This is because, at that particular point in the selection process, (a) interviewers have a more realistic view of the applicant pool, (b) ratings based on evaluation of interviewers tend to be higher, and (c) you are likely to be remembered better by interviewers the later you have contact with them. This approach to the timing of your interviews should be given thoughtful consideration, in view of its potential positive effect on your efforts to secure a residency appointment.

Preliminary preparation

Being successful at an interview can be greatly facilitated (a) if your thoughts are well organized in advance, (b) if you are adequately prepared to express your views, and (c) if you remain calm and relaxed during the entire interview process. The best way to achieve these three goals is by preparing yourself by means of a mock interview. This approach, along with practical preparations for the interview process, is discussed in this section. In addition, the interview-enhancing suggestions to be offered will help provide you with a greater potential for a positive outcome.

The four areas to be considered in terms of preliminary preparation are (1) a mock interview, (2) practical preparations, (3) interview enhancement steps, (4) and generating a positive image.

(1) Mock interview. This is a close imitation of the real thing, and can serve as a dress rehearsal for it. You should prepare for a mock interview just as you would for a real site visit. This means you should dress up, carry your essential documents, and review answers to typical questions beforehand. To maximize the realistic quality of your mock interview experience, your specialty advisor and/or mentor should, if possible, serve as interviewer. Alternatively, experienced faculty interviewers who are specialists in your prospective field of specialization, or even the school's dean of students, can do so. If necessary, enlist the assistance of some of your colleagues who have already gone through the interview process. Tell any interviewer that you anticipate challenging questions and expect a candid evaluation of your performance, to maximize the benefit you get from the experience.

A mock interview should be arranged only after you feel adequately prepared for it. Develop a list of possible questions that might be asked (see last section). You can also draft an outline of appropriate written responses to these questions. Then practice your verbal responses and have others evaluate your comments. Some schools may have career counseling services that can provide assistance in this area. You should recognize that a serious approach to the mock interview scenario is essential, so that it serves as a vital part of your preparation for the actual interview experiences you anticipate facing.

In summary:

■ A mock interview should give you more confidence, help keep you more relaxed, facilitate being better organized, and consequently enable you to leave a more favorable impression.

■ You should undertake a mock interview only after you have appropriately and adequately prepared for this experience.

■ The mock interview should be carried out in a manner that imitates the actual interview as closely as possible.

■ Seek knowledgeable interviewers, who will help provide a realistic environment.

■ Request that you be challenged at the mock interview with reasonably difficult questions and that you be treated like an actual interviewee.

■ Secure candid feedback on all aspects of the interview process. This includes your dress, your responses to questions, how effectively you impressed your interviewers, and especially how you can improve the impression you give.

■ If possible, audiotape or, better yet, videotape the mock interview. You can thus pinpoint areas that need improvement or even radical change.

■ Practice responses to questions using a tape recorder during any free time, or even only in your mind, when a suitable opportunity arises.

(2) Practical preparations. A variety of practical considerations are associated with the interview process. These are related to travel arrangements, travel tips, housing, appropriate dress, and interview enhancement steps. Each of these issues will be considered separately.

TRAVEL ARRANGEMENTS. It is reasonable to anticipate receiving multiple interview invitations in response to a batch of applications for a residency position that you sent out. It is in your best interest, in terms of saving time, effort, and money, to see if, when scheduling, you can cluster some of these interviews. This may be carried out either geographically or timewise. One of the benefits of early submission of residency applications is that prospective programs will have more interview dates to offer you to choose from. When fortunate enough to receive several interview offers that possibly can be clustered, it behooves you to seek the cooperation of program secretaries to facilitate your arranging doing so in this manner. This can frequently be arranged, so don't hesitate to politely ask to set up interviews at appropriately convenient dates.

In formulating clustered travel plans, care needs to be taken to avoid scheduling an excessive number of interviews over a very short time span. This can be counterproductive, because it will not allow adequate time to fully evaluate the events that transpired at each individual site. You may also need some postinterview time at the site to see more of the facilities, or activities, and/or to obtain informal input from residents in the evening. If necessary, time may be needed to check out the community in which the hospital is located as to its suitability for you and your family.

Seek to find out if it is possible to secure special fares for the sites you wish to visit. The Internet can facilitate securing airline tickets at reduced rates. It is worthwhile using this resource as a potential cost-saving mechanism. You may also wish to investigate the value of joining an airline frequent flier club and using its affiliated hotels and car rental outlets. This arrangement may also prove to be monetarily profitable and time-saving.

TRAVEL TIPS. The following suggestions can make flying more efficient and possibly more fiscally advantageous.

■ Schedule your flight, if you can, for the early morning or late night to enhance your chances of on-time departure and arrival.

■ Seek to get an aisle seat as close to the front exit as possible. This will facilitate your departing the plane as early as possible and getting to your destination on time. This will lower your anxiety about arriving on time.

■ Try to restrict your luggage to a single carry-on plus a garment bag, if necessary. This will also save time waiting to collect checked-in luggage. To facilitate storing your luggage in the cabin, seek to board the plane early, ensuring access to the maximum overhead storage space.

■ Unless you need to go directly from the plane to your interview site, be dressed casually and comfortably during the plane flight. This will allow you to nap or sleep, without worrying about creasing your clothes. Resting can be facilitated by a set of foam earplugs and an eyeshade. Securing on-flight rest can be beneficial to your interview performance.

■ If a meal will not be served on the flight, make sure to take a snack and drink along. If food will be served and you require a special meal, order it when booking your trip.

■ If your flight is canceled, it is best to promptly call your travel agent, rather than competing with others at the ticket counter seeking to reschedule. Keep the agent's and other vital phone numbers (e.g., program office, housing location) readily available.

HOUSING. This potentially can be a major expense, since it may prove necessary to stay overnight at the interview site. Possible sources for low-cost housing include the following:

■ Local hotels. Rates in these facilities very widely. Making inquires at various appropriate facilities can be helpful. Program secretaries may be able to provide you with sources of relatively inexpensive housing in the vicinity of the interview site. They usually have lists of such places, as well as names of residents who are willing to accommodate guests in their homes (particularly students from their former medical school.)

■ AMSA operates a housing program for its members. Its Membership Services Department can provide detailed information as to what may be available in specific cities.

■ The National Organization of Student Representatives may have provided your school's student affairs office with a booklet listing medical students who have volunteered guest housing at their schools for perspective residents.

■ The AMWA office has a list of bed and breakfast sources that can provide accommodations at modest expense.

APPROPRIATE DRESS. Your lifestyle is your own personal affair; nevertheless, your attire sends a message of who you are. The basic rule regarding appearance at residency interviews is to dress up and do so conservatively, to accommodate the attitudes of many prospective interviewers. When your initial appearance makes a favorable impression, it facilitates setting a positive tone for the balance of the interview. Your attire should not make you stand out and detract from the essential goal of the interview, namely, finding out your personal compatibility with the program. So dress appropriately and enhance your chances for successful interviews.

For *men* a solid or pinstripe navy or gray suit is most desirable. The suit should be well pressed and have a good fit. It need not be excessively expensive or the latest style. The shirt should be long-sleeved and white or pale blue and the collar should fit appropriately. A solid color tie with a simple repeating design goes well with the recommended suit and shirt. The bottom line is to dress conservatively by avoiding bright colors and weird designs. With this outfit, wear comfortable, shined black or brown shoes. For adequate comfort, these should not be new. They should be worn with a pair of appropriate solid-colored socks.

Careful personal grooming is most essential. This means having trimmed nails, and having your hair cut to an appropriate length, which adds to giving you a professional look. The impression you should aim for is that the interviewer should feel, "This is what I would like a physician to look like."

Being conservatively dressed also applies to *women*. This involves wearing a skirted suit when you go for your interview. The style should be that worn by a professional businesswoman. Don't be concerned with what is chic; rather make sure the outfit consists of a skirt that extends below the knee and has a long-sleeved blazer jacket. The preferable color choices for an outfit are light gray, medium blue, and dark maroon. The outfit should fit well, be free of creases, and preferably not be made from silk. Your shoes should be very comfortable, and closed in front and in back. The color should appropriately match your suit. The shoes should not have excessively high heels. Keep your jewelry simple, restricting it to a plain watch, ring, necklace, or brooch. A purse is unnecessary; utilize a carrying case of some sort. This can be used to carry your personal necessities, including your resume, personal statement, and makeup kit. Although you naturally wish to enhance your appearance, don't do so by putting on *excessive* makeup. Avoid elegance in clothes and in your hairstyle. What you seek is to convey is an image of a mature professional, which is what most interviewers seek in a future colleague.

(3) Interview enhancement steps. The following suggestions refer to ways to help achieve successful interview outcomes:

■ *Overcome weaknesses.* You should at the outset realize that no applicant for a residency is the perfect candidate. Thus it is advisable that you review letters of recommendation or evaluations that may be available to you from your pre-medical school days or from medical school faculty who supervised your rotations or electives. These may provide clues as to any of your inherent deficiencies that leave a negative impression on people. Seek to find out what they are and if they are currently valid and can be overcome or at least be masked, so that they are not evident during your interviews. If a problem is identified, don't be reluctant to ask your advisor/mentor for candid advice on this subject, so that you can learn how best to handle it.

■ *Arrive rested.* Arrange to get a good night's sleep before your interview session. This can be achieved by departing on the preceding day and securing overnight housing near the interview site. As a consequence, you will tend to be more relaxed, calm, and self-assured.

■ *Appear neat.* Protect the condition of your dress clothes by carefully packing your travel bag in an organized manner. This means folding clothes along their natural crease lines. Smaller items should be rolled up and placed on the sides to minimize mobility of the central contents. Shoes also should be put on the side, in plastic bags, and placed in your travel luggage.

■ *Obtain a schedule.* If you weren't sent a schedule of your interview site activities, obtain one by fax from the residency program office. This will help you anticipate what to expect and facilitate the proceedings going more smoothly. You can request a schedule a day or two before your interview, at the same time confirming your appointment. By this means you will ensure that there have been no last-minute changes that might upset your interview activities and plans.

■ *Arrive early.* The faculty members assigned to interview you are busy people. Thus if you foresee coming late, minimize the negative impression your lateness will make by calling ahead to the program office. Obviously you should make every effort to be on time. If a schedule is not obtainable, at least confirm the time when your interview should begin, to make sure that you will not be late. It is also in your best interest to arrive early, so that you become somewhat acclimated to your surroundings at the very outset. This should make you feel more comfortable by the time the interview begins.

■ *Check appearance.* When dressed and ready to be interviewed, visit a rest room at the institution that is nearest to the program office to give yourself a last-minute look-over. Make any adjustments necessary to enhance your appearance.

■ *Utilize free time.* Your schedule may allow some free-time slots during your varied activities. Maximize the potential benefit of such opportunities by visiting the institution's library, wards, and adjacent clinical facilities, to the extent that time permits.

(4) Generating a positive image. You need to recognize that the impression you leave will not be determined *solely* at formal interview sessions. Rather, you will be observed from the time you walk into the program office until you depart from the hospital. Thus, during all your interactions with staff, residents, and any other applicants, be outgoing and friendly. You are being evaluated as to how it would be to have you present full-time as a resident at the institution. You should thus leave all those who you meet, with a firm impression that it would be nice if this were the case. Special attention should be taken at the lunch that you will participate in. Do not overeat and be sure to use good table manners.

The importance of selling yourself stems from the well-known aphorism "If you don't toot your own horn, nobody will toot it for you." This also applies to securing a residency appointment. You need an appropriate time to *diplomatically* call attention to a number of your personal attributes that you feel may be significant in the interviewer's eyes. Thus, a major effort should be placed on demonstrating that you have, among others, the following five attributes:

- *Enthusiasm.* Demonstrating a genuine and strong interest both in the specialty and in the program you are interviewing at is an obvious means for enhancing your chances.

- *Self-confidence.* Coming across as having inner strength (but not arrogance) is a sought-after quality in applicants.

- *Dedication.* A clear impression of a firm commitment to achieving professional excellence as a team member is an important message to convey.

- *Communication skills.* Speaking in an analytical manner so that your thoughts come across logically and effectively will also have a positive impact.

- *Integrity.* The interviewers should gain a perception that your ethical standards are high and you can be relied on as a person with a sense of discretion, good judgment, and reliability.

Seek to relate an experience from your background that demonstrates *some* of these attributes. This will provide convincing support for your effort to sell yourself as a person who will be an asset to their program.

Finally, you should not rush departure from the interview site. Plan your return flight so that there is adequate free time available after your scheduled activities have concluded. This will enable you to adjust your schedule in the event that your interviews run late. In addition, you might want to use any extra available time to observe facilities you could not see before, or meet informally with residents. They can provide you with vital information about the program and/or the community you may wish to live in.

Preinterview essentials

The night before your interview, it would be wise to review the following topics, on the basis of material that you prepare in advance.

Know your specialty. Your interviewers are aware that you seek to become clinically knowledgeable in a specialty. While recognizing your lack of technical expertise, they nevertheless do expect you to be well aware of the general nature of the specialty. This means information about the levels of remuneration for practitioners, standard procedures used, subspecialty options, relationships with other specialists, specialty board requirements, major new advances, the name of the prominent specialty journals in the field, and prospects for the future.

Most of these issues are discussed in Chapters 3, 4, 5, and 6, where the individual specialties are described in detail. The goal you face is to be able to demonstrate that you have a strong commitment to the specialty based on your innate potential, past exposure, and basic academic and personal knowledge of it.

Review your background information concerning the following issues.

Know your program. Prepare a summary of information about the program in advance of your trip from the literature that was sent to you, as well as any updates that you may have gotten from a Web site, your advisor, or fellow students. Chapter 8 provides a section dealing with securing information. It can be helpful to secure background on the program director and department faculty. This can be obtained by carrying out a search as to their interests as reflected in their publications. Notes that you may have gathered from speaking with other interviewees should be reviewed to pick up any useful tips. In responding to questions about the program, obviously you should demonstrate a strong interest in it, but support your reasons with facts. Such an approach should certainly resonate well with interviewers.

Interview protocol. From the moment of entering the interview site, be cognizant of the following critical elements:

■ *Know your interviewer.* The program secretary should be asked to provide you with the names of prospective interviewers. If a name is difficult to pronounce, check it with the secretary so that you can do so properly.

■ *Bring essential material.* The evening before your interview, make sure you have available (a) a brief summary of information about the program, along with the name and phone number of the program secretary and the names of prospective interviewers; (b) your residency interview assessment form (Form 9.2); and (c) some lightweight reading material of importance that you can use during any waiting interludes that may take place the course of your site visit. This should include information about the program and its faculty.

■ *Greet properly.* You should extend your hand to the interviewer and provide a firm handshake. Make sure your palm is dry. A remark such as "Hello" or "Good morning" or "Nice to meet you" is obviously appropriate.

■ *Enter confidently.* The initial glance by the interviewer(s) will automatically create a meaningful impression of you. Step into the room with your head and shoulders erect. Then pause for a second before stepping forward to greet the interviewer(s). This will help generate an impression of self-assuredness.

■ *Respond enthusiastically.* Your tone of voice and facial and hand mannerisms provide the interviewers with a message. It should be that you are glad to be there and are genuinely motivated to be selected as a resident at their program.

■ *Sit properly.* You should keep your torso straight. Avoid signs of nervousness by being fidgety, using your hands to play with some object, or touching your face. Appearing and acting self-confident will add presence to your appearance.

■ *Maintain eye contact.* This mannerism will suggest that you are being forthright and imply that you do not feel uncomfortable with the questions being asked. It is a recognized dimension of reassurance of the truthfulness of your convictions that the interviewer seeks to obtain.

■ *Depart gracefully.* At the conclusion of the interview, get up and shake hands with the interviewer(s), and thank them for having extended you the opportunity of the visit and for their time. You should offer to provide any additional information they may wish. Then leave in a cheerful manner.

Potential interview questions

Many of the questions you will be asked will most likely to be the standard ones commonly asked at residency interviews. Thus, preparing for them in advance can remove a heavy burden from you and help smooth your path toward a successful interview outcome.

The interviewers are seeking to ascertain if you feel strongly about your work as a medical student and to evaluate your communication skills. You need to realize that they seek to gain insight as to whether you think clearly when under pressure (a common situation for a resident). Bear in mind that many questions may not have a clear right or wrong answer. Finally, seek to respond in an organized and thoughtful manner to the questions raised during the course of interviews. If a question is unclear, ask the interviewer to repeat or to rephrase it. If uncertain as how to respond, pause momentarily to gather your thoughts before answering.

The following are twenty typical questions and suggestions as how to respond to them:

1. *Why did you choose this specialty?*
Your response should clearly be enthusiastic and consistent with your personal statement that you submitted along with your application. Your answer should be a substantive one; thus, for example, you might, if applicable, indicate that your choice of this specific field was due to the influence of your mentor or come from a very stimulating clerkship that had a profound influence upon you. In addition, you should indicate that there are certain characteristics of the specialty (e.g., procedures, major recent advances, etc.) that you find especially attractive and then enumerate them. Your interests may have been reinforced by conversations with attendings in the field and doing extra work to gain an in-depth familiarity with it. Give your answer the thought it deserves. This may probably be the most common question you will be asked. Nevertheless, although possibly repetative, make sure that your response to it sounds spontaneous.

2. *Where do you see yourself in 5 to 10 years?*
This question seeks to determine to what extent you have given thought to your professional career and your future plans. Before answering, bear in mind the

program that you are being considered for. Does it match up fully with your own career interests? Is securing subspecialty training a realistic option? Avoid leaving a rigid impression. Rather indicate that you are open to suggestion, when necessary, as time progresses.

3. *What are your strengths and weaknesses?*
You may be asked about either or both of these issues. The nature of your response may reflect a lot about yourself. It is important to avoid sounding uncertain while presenting your attributes in as positive a manner as possible without exaggeration. Identify one major, strong attribute and exemplify it. You may, for example, wish to demonstrate your sense of empathy by indicating your ability to establish a meaningful interpersonal relationship with a special patient whom you have dealt with during one of your clerkships. Where possible, exemplify with an experience that would be relevant to your future work as a resident.

As to weaknesses, your goal is to describe one that in reality will not make you look bad. You may wish to indicate that by nature you are very diligent about your work and need, at times, to 'put your foot on the brakes' to avoid becoming over-worked. Emphasize that you usually set realistic goals and then seek to complete them in a timely, thorough, and careful manner. Indicate that, when necessary, you stay beyond official hours, usually until your responsibilities are satisfactorily completed. This will make you look good, inspite of a potential weakness.

4. *Why did you apply to our program?*
You should be familiar enough with the strengths of the department from reading the material you secured and conversations with others, to be able to respond to this question in a convincing manner. You should obviously select factors that are of primary importance when exemplifying the reasons for your interest.

5. *What happens if you do not Match?*
This challenging question is commonly asked of applicants for highly competitive specialty appointments. Do not conclude from this inquiry that the program is not really interested in you. Rather, information is being sought to see if you are realistic enough to make alternative plans. The program seeks to learn about the level of your commitment to its particular specialty. It behooves you to indicate that, even though you are confident of obtaining a residency appointment, if need be, you have an alternative plan. This may involve having also applied for a one-year transitional program or a preliminary medicine or surgery residency appointment. This step would allow you to reapply, if necessary, in the next year for a PGY-2 appointment to your specialty without losing time.

6. *Why are you a more attractive candidate than others?*
This question needs to be responded to tactfully. Indicate that you cannot judge others, but only your own abilities. You should then briefly outline your assets without sounding arrogant. Emphasize that you have an attractive (or credible)

academic record, are a team worker, are highly dependable, and have an intense desire to become a competent specialist in the field in question. You should certainly never say anything negative about other candidates (or programs or schools) when responding to this type of question.

7. *Where have you applied other than here?*
This is also a common question and should be answered honestly and forthrightly. They probably want to know if you have been realistic in the choices of programs that you have applied to, both in caliber and numbers. Also, the interviewer may use this inquiry as a possible means of securing information about the programs you visited (which you should provide without making any negative remarks about them).

8. *Could you tell me about an interesting case that you were involved in?*
This is another popular question, because it can provide a great deal of information about your medical knowledge, ability to think under pressure, attitude toward the healing profession, and sense of compassion. The answer will require careful preparation, for it involves providing details about a case that you were actively involved in (preferably one in or close to the specialty in question). Read up about the specific medical problem you may have to discuss and any impact it may have on other relevant body systems. This should enable you to respond to any follow-up questions that you may be asked.

Your response to such a question, if possible, should be fourfold: (a) initially relevant to the medical problem raised, (b) reflective of the limits that a physician has in achieving a goal, (c) relative to the patient's response to their illness, and finally (d) the effectiveness of the health care system in dealing with the issues that arose. You should try to have followed-up on or be aware of the patient's progress, in case you wish to discuss the case at great length. If the patient expired, secure, if possible, a copy of the autopsy report (if one was done). The goal is for you to have demonstrated genuine interest in your patient and a desire to expand the depth of your knowledge base.

9. *What kind of people do you have difficulty working with?*
The interviewer is seeking to determine if you are a compatible individual. This question can also reveal a great deal about you. To avoid any pitfalls, it may be safe to say that generally you get along well with people, but have a problem with those who do not carry their weight when it comes to meeting their responsibilities. Perhaps you can provide an example of being able to work things out even with such or other difficult types of individuals. Such an attitude will prove advantageous.

10. *How are you?*
This is a common lead-off question. It need not be assumed that it is a mere innocent courtesy inquiry, although this may be the case; it is quite possible that it is specifically designed to judge your personality. Specifically, the question may aim

to determine your response to any frustration and pressures that may be associated with current events, such as your interview. The interviewer may wish to ascertain your reaction to some possible unexpected difficulties or irritants, manifested by your tone of voice, resulting from your trip or from an unforeseen delay in meeting with the interviewer. Complaining about some relatively minor inconvenience during your trip may conceivably raise a red flag that you may by nature be a dissatisfied person, who will find even minor difficulties or inconveniences during a residency very unpleasant. This may suggest the possibility that you could respond negatively to the postgraduate training experience and consequently you may not contribute favorably to the working atmosphere. Thus it is best if your response is polite but perfunctory, such as "fine, thank you" and thereby avoid giving any potential opening that can lead to negative impressions.

11. *I would like to get to know you a little better, so please tell me about yourself.*
This well-known, open-ended question is very challenging and it can be troublesome. It has the potential for being a favorable opening, if you look upon this question as a special opportunity to sell yourself. Your response should be concise and to the point. You may wish to indicate that you have had a long-standing interest in medicine, are a diligent team player who is very anxious to learn, and have a genuine interest in the specialty you are seeking a residency in. Emphasize that you have found both the diagnostic and (in most cases) therapeutic aspects of the field very appealing. Also, for procedure-oriented specialties (e.g., surgery and related fields), indicate that you believe you have the manual dexterity needed. You can then inquire if the interviewer wishes you to go into greater detail in some of the attributes you enumerated. It is quite likely that the topic will be changed. If not, utilize the opportunity to proceed to elaborate briefly by perhaps indicating some important experiences that motivated you to choose to become a physician or to choose this specialty (if you haven't already done so).

12. *How do you spend your spare time?*
Strive to avoid using this as an opportunity to enter a long monologue. Rather, provide a straightforward but concise answer (e.g., I collect stamps and specialize in a specific location, or participate in some special sports activity). Avoid merely saying that because of time constraints you have no hobbies, as well may be the case. Preferably, indicate that your spare time is quite limited and that you use it to keep up with your family and social life. Be certain that whatever you say in response to this question is expressed with enthusiasm, by indicating, for example, how enjoyable it is to spend free time with family and friends.

13. *Looking ahead, what are your basic career plans?*
Your response to this question should reflect your conviction that the program's goals, as stipulated in their literature, are in harmony with your own future plans. However, given the uncertainty in the provision of health-care services that is taking place, your answer should certainly not be dogmatic. Rather, it needs to reflect your

openness to considering the available options of solo, partnership, or group practice or joining a health maintenance organization. Indicate that at an appropriate time you will seek advice from a variety of individuals.

14. *How well do you accept criticism?*

Naturally, you may wish to respond that you, like anyone, much prefer praise to negative criticism. Indicate, however, that you welcome constructive criticism, when offered as part of a learning experience, and that this is the way you enhance your knowledge. Suggest that you recognize that constructive criticism can serve to avoid future mistakes. Indicate that for a supervisor not to be critical when it is called for is in a sense being negligent. Point out as you move up the ranks, you will have the responsibility of providing both instruction and criticism to junior house officers. State that you hope to do so in a positive and meaningful manner.

15. *What motivated you to become a physician?*

You should refer to your premed application's AMCAS personal statement, if it is still available, when preparing for this question. In all likelihood you covered this issue in depth in this document. It would be advisable to add to your rationale that your medical school experience has convinced you that your decision *certainly* was the correct one and that you anticipate having a satisfying professional life. If requested, you should be prepared to substantiate this statement in light of your experiences as a medical student.

16. *What kind of people and/or patients have you had trouble with?*

This is a critical question, because it is designed to see if you may become a problem resident because of a weakness in interpersonal skills. The above question may be asked in various guises. It is important to emphasize strongly that you have found that you usually get along very well with most people. You may wish to point out that you do get irritated, however, when a member of a team does not carry their load. But you try to resolve such issues in a nonconfrontational, reasonable manner. This kind of response will also serve to enhance your own image. As to difficult patients, you should indicate that you recognize that patients located in a medical facility are in a stressful setting and thus you feel that you must be especially tolerant and professional in your dealings with them. Then note that you have found that this type of approach has proven to be successful in securing their cooperation and compliance with the needs of their situation.

17. *Your record indicates you had difficulty with* _____ [subject or rotation]. *Please, clarify what was the problem.*

This question, uncomfortable though it undoubtedly is, should be anticipated and faced head on. Avoid any attempt in your response to obfuscate the issue. If the reason is nonacademic (e.g., because of being overinvolved with your wedding arrangements), briefly explain the situation. However, if the issue was academic, seek to put the situation in the most favorable perspective possible. Thus, if the deficiency is true, you should at the outset point out that overall you have a very credible or even impressive record and that this was the only problem situation to have arisen. You may then consider indicating that your time management, when the problem arose, was unfortunately not optimal. By devoting an excess amount of study time to one course or rotation, in which you achieved a superior grade, you apparently lacked the needed time to study for the exams in the course of rotation in question. Finally, note that the lesson you learned from this unfortunate experience proved beneficial in the future as regards budgeting your time and efforts.

18. *Where else have you had an interview?*
This question is commonly asked of many prospective residents, so you should not get flustered by it. Respond frankly and in a forthright manner. You should be prepared to answer questions regarding some of the programs you visited. Your response may be valuable for the interviewer. This information is for the edification of the interviewer. Review your notes about the programs that you have gathered, so that you will be prepared to respond appropriately. Be certain, however, that you do not make any negative comments about another program you may have visited. It will not reflect favorably on your standing if you do so.

19. *Can you work well under stress?*
The interviewer needs to be assured that you unquestionably can function effectively under pressure. It is up to you to do this in a convincing manner. Initially you can point out that all residency programs generate stress, albeit at different levels. You can then note that you have discussed this issue with residents and attendings in the field in question. Indicate that you have a good perspective on many challenges you may face and are firmly convinced that you that you will be able handle the challenge of a stressful work environment that may arise. Emphasize that you obviously will call for help whenever the situation warrants. Finally, reinforce your response by exemplifying, if possible, a situation where you were placed under stress, how you handled it, and how it has given you confidence for the future.

20. *Do you truely feel that you merit a residency appointment on this field?*
Your reaction to this question should not be one of shock or panic. Also, do not read into the question a prediction of things to come. Rather, since it may well be asked regarding a highly competitive specialty, the question attempts to see if you are fully aware of the challenges in securing an appointment in the field. Your response should initially indicate a high level of self-confidence. You can affirm that you are optimistic about your chances of being matched, based on your strong academic record and the fact that you have been granted a substantial number of interviews. Nevertheless, you can point out that because you cannot foretell the future, you have (if true) applied to preliminary medical/surgical or transitional programs that will allow you to reapply, if necessary, for your specialty of choice at a later date. Such a statement will support your strong commitment to the field you have chosen to specialize in.

Illegal interview questions. There are a wide variety of questions that if asked, violate federal or state law relative to employment. These commonly relate to marriage and family plans. There are, however, some personal questions that can be asked if properly formulated (e.g., what is your corrected vision?). If a clearly illegal question is asked, you obviously do not wish to antagonize the interviewer by bluntly saying so. They might not even be aware that it is inappropriate. Under these circumstances there are two real options available. One is to deflect the question by asking "Will the response to this question impact my chances for getting a residency?" This may induce the interviewer to withdraw it. The other suitable option is to indicate that regarding any of your personal life decisions, the success of your residency will in most cases have the top priority. You may also choose to use the latter response, if the first option fails.

Becoming program savvy

You should recognize that your site visit provides an opportunity for securing critical information about the structure of the program, the nature of the faculty, and the existing working atmosphere. You can secure this vital information from two sources, namely, faculty and current residents.

Questions for faculty

1. *Does your program aim to train its residents for practice in major cities or in rural communities?*
You are seeking insight into the scope and aim of the program relative to your own future plans.

2. *Do your graduates serve primarily in private community offices or in academic centers?*
Here to you are trying to find out about the program's goals, which will have an impact on your future professional activities.

3. *Is the program accredited?*
If the answer is no, then the program is not for you, since you would be ineligible to get an appointment through the Match or to take the specialty board exams. What you should do under those circumstances is self-evident. The answer may also be a clear-cut yes, a provisional yes, or being on probation. In the latter two cases, careful investigation is essential as to prospects of the program receiving full accreditation.

4. *What success have program graduates had on the specialty board exams (both written and oral)?*
Passing specialty boards is very important, because it will impact the type of position you can secure. Tactfully try to ascertain how many passed after more

than one try. Also, inquire if the program offers any Board exam preparation support.

The nature of the responses you obtain during the course of your interview should indicate the amount of time that is devoted to enhancing knowledge of residents through teaching (both formal and informal), exam preparation, and self-education by reading. There is a correlation between the clinical demands on residents, which when high limits educational advancement, and Board performance. This question probes the essence of this important issue.

5. *Can one anticipate curriculum change in the very near future?*
This question should be asked of the program director and it will serve to reflect your genuine interest in the program. The response may indicate how up-to-date the program is in terms of responding to change in the clinical aspects of the specialty.

6. *Aside from clinical responsibilities, what other obligations do residents have?*
The valuable time of a resident needs to be expended as constructively as possible. Thus it is vital to know of any obligations beyond clinical service that are expected from a program's residents. These may include research or other activities. Should research be of special interest to you, then pursue this issue in greater detail. If it is mandated, find out how demanding any research obligations are.

7. *How is the performance of residents evaluated?*
It is essential for the psychological well-being of residents to be kept updated as to their performance. You should inquire what method the program uses to achieve this goal. To provide feedback, many programs use national in-service examinations developed by specialty boards to test knowledge of residents working at the same training level. Some programs may utilize standardized tests for this purpose.

8. *Does the program provide job placement assistance?*
Securing a good appointment after completing a postgraduate program is not necessarily easy, because of competition among a large pool of qualified applicants. Seek to find out if the program has any provisions that facilitate being placed and, if so, what services they offer and how successful these services have been.

9. *How demanding is the on-call schedule?*
You need to inquire if the on-call schedule generally will allow time for reading or, if desirable, research. The response to this question should be followed up by a request to see (or obtain) a current on-call schedule and then judge for yourself.

10. *What type of clinical exposure can I anticipate having?*
If you are interviewing for a procedure-oriented specialty, seek to determine what and when will be your exposure opportunities, to what extent, and at what level in your training. Obviously, gaining expertise in the standard procedures of a specialty through adequate hands-on exposure is absolutely essential to your professional success later on.

11. *Is your program structured pyramidally?*
This question is primarily applicable to surgery and surgical subspecialties, where many residents above the PGY-1 or PGY-2 level are dropped at the completion of their service contracts. If this is the case, then obviously competition among residents to remain in the program will be intense. If your plan is to seek a one- or two-year preliminary residency and obtain a categorical residence elsewhere, this situation should not be an issue. Otherwise, find out the extent of retention of residents beyond the initial stages.

Questions for residents. You should seek to obtain as much information as possible about the program from the perspective of the residents who are currently in it. You should use any free time or postinterview interlude to secure opinions from residents.

The last two questions in the preceding section can also be asked of residents. The answers then can be compared and judged accordingly. To obtain a more comprehensive view of the program, the following additional questions are worth asking.

1. *How reliable and effective is the supporting staff?*
It is important to be aware of how dependable the nursing and ancillary staff is. You should learn to what extent you will have to carry the 'scut work' load and if routine tasks can be reduced by assistance from allied health personnel.

2. *How dedicated are clinical faculty to training residents?*
The answer to this question will have a major impact on both your training and residency experience. You wish to know to what extent you can call on the faculty for their expertise and how actively they participate in didactic training of residents (e.g., by means of lectures, seminars, and rounds). Determine how much contact with faculty is provided in the varied clinical settings (e.g., E.R., O.R., wards, and clinics). In these situations, their knowledge base can be tapped with enriching consequences for residents. You need to ascertain the extent of availability of the faculty as educators, so that your residency can be a genuine source of creative learning and a meaningful training experience.

3. *What are the characteristics of the patient population in terms of numbers and disease processes?*
The two issues raised are obviously essential to a successful residency. Even if patient volume is adequate, not having a broad enough disease spectrum would be limiting to one's future practice.

4. *In what clinical settings are patients treated?*
To lower health care costs, patients are increasingly treated on an outpatient basis. Residents can provide you with an overview of the scope of their patient contact. To what extent residents see patients in clinics and outpatient surgical facilities and even in private physician offices, as compared with hospital ward service, is useful

information regarding the range of experience you may be exposed to during the course of your training.

5. *How demanding is the routine of a resident?*
You are actually inquiring to what extent service as a resident dominates your life. You should seek to know if daily service plus on-call time allows you respite for reading, relaxation, and meeting personal commitments. You need to avoid becoming dehumanized by a process that is so time-consuming as to allow very little leisure time.

6. *Have residents transferred out to other programs in the same specialty?*
You should be aware that most defections from programs occur for personal reasons (e.g., illness, change in specialty goals). What should be of interest to you is the number of residents who have recently left the program because of dissatisfaction with it and perhaps their reasons for doing so. This should be of special interest, because the same issues can conceivably have an impact on you. Discretely seek some clarification on this issue if you see a tactful way to do so.

7. *Are you aware of any prospective changes in the faculty?*
Residents may be aware of information on pending faculty changes. They also will be cognizant of overall faculty stability, the level of professional maturity of the faculty, and their own satisfaction with the program's operation. An unstable, inexperienced, or disgruntled faculty will not generate a sound teaching atmosphere. On the other hand, a satisfied faculty will meet their responsibilities with enthusiasm, which can be educationally most stimulating, thereby providing a positive experience.

8. *Do you feel that your selection of this program was a sound decision, and if so why?*
You should ask this important question of each of the residents you speak with. As a consequence, you will get a consensus as to their satisfaction and a meaningful assessment of the program's attributes. You can then judge how relevant their comments are for you and if you feel the program can provide you with a congenial treatment team and employment atmosphere and with the quality of training you seek.

9. *Have you found the faculty to be helpful?*
You want to ascertain from as many residents as possible their personal experience with the faculty in terms of their accessibility when needed and their commitment to teaching residents. This is crucial to your securing quality professional training.

10. *What is the level of cooperation among residents?*
It is important to ascertain the nature of the rapport among residents. Is it an atmosphere of competition or cooperation? You need to know if you can count on the possibility of a colleague replacing you in an emergency. Seek to find out if the more

senior residents treat those at a junior level with appropriate professional respect. The nature of the working relationship among residents contributes very significantly to the overall working atmosphere. Parenthetically, you can also inquire as to the nature of after-hour socializing among residents, for a clue to the state of their coexistence.

Note: Among the questions *not* to ask are salary, benefits, and vacation allowance. Such information should be secured from the institution's Graduate Education Office.

Postinterview activities

Assuming that you are still interested in the program after the interview, you can do several things to try to enhance your chances of being favorably ranked.

1. You should *promptly* send a typewritten letter (or e-mail message) to the program director (a) thanking them for providing you an opportunity to spend time on _____ relative to your application for a residency appointment, (b) expressing your favorable impression of the program, (c) confirming your continued interest in the program now that you have been there for a site visit (and if appropriate, mention something special that impressed you or give a particular reason for your special interest in their program), (d) indicating briefly some essential facts that you may have inadvertently overlooked during your interview, and (e) providing any information that may have been requested of you during the course of the visit (or note that it will be forthcoming shortly).

2. You can also benefit by sending a copy of your letter to the program director or a special personal note to others of the staff who interviewed you. If writing to an individual, you may wish to refer to something significant that came up during the interview that proved of special interest to you.

3. Conclude all correspondence with an indication that you hope that things will work out and that there will be a mutually profitable association with the program in the future.

4. If you are genuinely interested in the program, in the conclusion of your letter, you can give some indication to this fact with a remark such as that you would very favorably view being offered an opportunity to secure your specialty training with them.

The motto of your mission to secure a residency should be, "Prepare adequately, submit early, and follow-up regularly." These steps may prove to be the keys to your success.

Prioritizing your residency choices

At some point your scheduled interviews for a residency appointment will be set. Getting ready for them undoubtedly will involve proper and adequate preparation. This basically implies the need to be able to (a) leave as effective an impression as possible and (b) seek to determine if the residency program in question is suitable for you. Arriving at a judgment about any program involves securing information relative to the critical issues outlined below (in addition to many general facts that are of interest to you).

When speaking with program representatives, focus attention especially on answers to the following (in addition to those enumerated previously):

1. *What has been the success rate of your graduates on specialty board exams on their first try?*
This will provide an indication of the caliber of the residents and quality of their training.

2. *What are some innovative aspects of the program?*
To prepare you for anticipated changes in medicine in the years ahead, evidence of innovation in postgraduate training will provide reassurance that the program is not overly conservative and will not leave you unprepared for future challenges.

3. *What are your program's strengths?*
Getting a perspective on this question from several faculty members independently can provide you with a meaningful picture in this regard.

4. *Is input from the residents about the program sought by the administration?*
It is important to learn if, as a resident, your opinion will be sought and has value to those setting policy. You do not wish to be viewed merely as a postgraduate student, but to be considered as a colleague.

5. *When did the most recent program evaluation take place and what are the results?*
A successful program will be prepared to discuss this matter with you and comment on how they are addressing any reported deficiencies.

6. *What support services and family assistance services are provided or are available?*
This would be in the area of recreational facilities, housing, and employment opportunities for spouses.

When conversing with residents privately, focus special attention on the following questions.

1. *What are the program's weaknesses?*
With some good fortune you will get a candid view of the program's deficits. How this impacts your plans is a personal matter. You need to realize, however, that probably every program has some limitations. It is important to bear in mind whether the strengths of the program markedly outweigh its deficiencies. Also, note what is being done to improve any weaknesses or eliminate them.

2. *Does the program director provide the desired level of leadership to ensure the quality of training you seek?*

Determine how long the director has held his/her position. Inquire if the director seeks input from the residents and gives their views ample consideration. Residents know what defects in programs exist and that their voices should be heard.

3. *What is the quality of the conferences offered by the program?*

A well-organized program includes lectures by knowledgeable, well-prepared, and enthusiastic speakers. Residents can provide you with information as to whether the conferences have motivated them to explore the topics further and if the information provided complements knowledge secured through patient contact.

It is advisable to prioritize and perhaps even narrow down your potential programs in anticipation of preparing your Rank Order List (see Chapter 12). You should now have the necessary information to do so, based on your completed interview assessments (see Form 9.2) and the responses to questions you have sought answers to from both the program representatives and current residents (see above).

To facilitate your task, you can devise a form in which you evaluate the programs you have been interviewed at, in terms of issues that are of most importance. These include such items as program location, nature of patient population, faculty, curriculum, reimbursement benefits, and the community. For this purpose you may wish to use or modify Form 11.1.

Form 11.1 Comparative residency program evaluations

Evaluation rating criteria: Unacceptable = 0, Acceptable = 1, Superior = 2, Excellent = 3.

Note. Since the value of each of the categories varies and is clearly subjective, they have to be weighed differently. To do so, you should calculate the average for each category and then multiply it by a *value* of 1 to 5 to determine its true *worth*. (The values given in the table are only suggestions and can be changed). Then move on to the next category. The quantitative rating of each program will thus be the sum total of all individual weighed category totals.

Program names and locations

#1 _____

#2 _____

#3 _____

#4 _____

#5 _____

(Add on as many programs as necessary)

(continued)

Form 11.1 *(continued)*

Programs	#1	#2	#3	#4	#5
1. *Location*					
Region	_____	_____	_____	_____	_____
City size	_____	_____	_____	_____	_____
Type	_____	_____	_____	_____	_____
Average	_____	_____	_____	_____	_____
Value (2)x average	_____	_____	_____	_____	_____
2. *Clinical Training*					
Patient volume	_____	_____	_____	_____	_____
Staffing level	_____	_____	_____	_____	_____
Patient/staff ratio	_____	_____	_____	_____	_____
Exposure	_____	_____	_____	_____	_____
Hospital type	_____	_____	_____	_____	_____
Responsibilities	_____	_____	_____	_____	_____
On-call schedule	_____	_____	_____	_____	_____
Average	_____	_____	_____	_____	_____
Value (5)x average	_____	_____	_____	_____	_____
3. *Program*					
Reputation	_____	_____	_____	_____	_____
Faculty	_____	_____	_____	_____	_____
Curriculum	_____	_____	_____	_____	_____
Work atmosphere	_____	_____	_____	_____	_____
Research option	_____	_____	_____	_____	_____
Support services	_____	_____	_____	_____	_____
Average	_____	_____	_____	_____	_____
Value (4)x average	_____	_____	_____	_____	_____
4. *Facilities*					
Laboratory	_____	_____	_____	_____	_____
Library	_____	_____	_____	_____	_____
On-call	_____	_____	_____	_____	_____
Parking	_____	_____	_____	_____	_____
Security	_____	_____	_____	_____	_____
Value (2)x average	_____	_____	_____	_____	_____
5. *Personal benefits*	_____	_____	_____	_____	_____
Health	_____	_____	_____	_____	_____
Dental	_____	_____	_____	_____	_____
Prescriptions	_____	_____	_____	_____	_____
Liability insurance	_____	_____	_____	_____	_____
Vacation allowance	_____	_____	_____	_____	_____
Maternal leave	_____	_____	_____	_____	_____
Average	_____	_____	_____	_____	_____
Value (3)x average	_____	_____	_____	_____	_____
Grand total average	_____	_____	_____	_____	_____

Finally, you should note that in formulating your prioritized list, it should not be based exclusively on the quantitative data resulting from your calculation on Form 11.1. These data should serve as a meaningful guide and be considered along with your subjective impressions of your interview experiences. This should be taken together with a realistic estimate of your attractiveness as a candidate. Thus, by combining all three elements, quantitative data, subjective judgment, and personal potential, you should arrive at a sound prioritization of your residency programs for your Rank Order List.

12 | Facing the Match

Overview

The origin of the Match goes all the way back to 1951. It was introduced to overcome very serious problems associated with obtaining postgraduate training positions. Originally using a card-sorting system, the Match was computerized in the early 1970s. It provides the principal means of placing medical students in PGY-1 or advanced residency positions. Some fellowship appointments can also be secured by means of the Match.

The official name for the Match is the National Residency Matching Program (NRMP). The directors of this organization are responsible for establishing general policy for the program. There are representatives from various professional and student medical organizations on the board of directors.

Generally about 90% of senior medical students from U.S. schools secure first-year residency appointments by means of the NRMP. A substantial number of international medical graduates (IMGs), whether U.S. or non-U.S. citizens, also succeed in being matched through this route. Foreign medical graduates are eligible to participate in the Match if they pass the USMLE. Information about the Match can be secured from the NRMP, One American Plaza, Evanston, Illinois 60201. The NRMP produces three publications to facilitate using its placement services. These are the *Handbook for Students, Directory of Programs*, and *Handbook for Independent Applicants*.

The Match

The Match is based on an algorithm that is described in the NRMP *Handbook for Students*. This being a complex, structured process, medical students are well advised to follow instructions and procedures, as well as meeting the deadlines mandated by the NRMP, in order to be able to properly participate in the program. It is thus essential to comply carefully with the guidelines provided in the NRMP *Directory*. This source also has a list of the names and codes for each specific residency program. The NRMP *Directory* can be secured at the office of the dean of students at your medical school, as well as from the NRMP. Signing up with the NRMP means establishing a contractual commitment that firmly commits you and residency programs to the outcome of the process. Consequently, when you are matched to a program, you are fully obligated to accept the appointment offered. Although approximately 50,000 residency slots need to be filed, the actual number of positions open each year varies. It is influenced by budgetary, accreditation, and other considerations.

The Match will align up to 15 residency choices which you submit, whose preference is identified in your Rank Order List, with a ranked listing of interviewed candidates submitted to the NRMP by the residency programs. On average, 60%, 15%, and 10% match up with their first, second, and third choices, respectively.

Standard Match schedule

The Match operates on a firm timetable and you must meet the stipulated deadlines to achieve credible results. The general outline of this schedule is given in Table 12.1. Your residency appointment search should be fully activated in the latter part of the third year of medical school. By this time your desired specialty most likely has been chosen. Should you still be uncertain as to your future plans you can delay the process until the early part of your senior year.

Postgraduate training appointments

PGY-1 positions. There are two types of first-year postgraduate training positions. These are known as preliminary and categorical appointments.

Preliminary positions are short-term appointments (one or two years) providing broad-based clinical experience. Such appointments are common before undertaking another specialty or subspecialty. These appointments can be secured in

Table 12.1 Standard Match application schedule

Year/Month	Activity
Third year May–Nov.	Secure adequate information about residency programs. Obtain, complete, sign, and return the NRMP agreement for the Match.
July	Carefully prepare your resume and personal statement. Request letters of recommendations from attendings.
Aug.	Apply to suitable residency programs. Check if supporting material is complete in your school file at the Dean of Students.
Fourth year Sept.–Oct.	Check if your school documents were sent off to programs to which you have applied.
Oct.–Dec. Nov.–Jan.	Arrange for your residency interviews. Attend interviews.
Feb.	Prepare and submit a Rank Order List.
March	Match Day.

the field of internal medicine or general surgery or within transitional programs (see Chapter 1). This type of appointment can serve as a preparatory stage in one's postgraduate training.

Categorical positions are long-term appointments (three to six years) that result in acquiring specialty training and thus becoming eligible for Board certification. Many of these appointments do not require completing a preliminary appointment. Specialties offering such positions are internal medicine, general surgery, pediatrics, obstetrics/gynecology, pathology, family medicine, and emergency medicine. There are, however, subspecialty programs also offering categorical positions, but these require completion of an appropriate preliminary residency as a prerequisite (see below).

Advanced positions refer to appointments at the PGY-2 or higher level. Many of these positions are in specialties such as ophthalmology, otolaryngology, radiology, and neurosurgery. Applicants for appointments in these fields apply for a preliminary PGY-1 position through the NRMP and simultaneously for an advanced program appointment. This procedure will ensure having completed the required prerequisites prior to initiating advanced postgraduate training.

Fellowships in some specialties can also be acquired though the NRMP and other Match programs. To participate, one needs to have completed specialty training. The NRMP Specialties Matching Services offers opportunities to apply in a wide variety of fields.

Your Rank Order List

Your prioritized list of residency programs to which you are applying is called a *Rank Order List*. A similar ranked list of selected candidates is also prepared by the residency program for submission to the NRMP. Your list should be placed on a worksheet located in the back of any of the aforementioned three NRMP publications. It should be submitted to your school's dean of students' office for transmission via their computer terminal.

Those applying for a residency appointment will receive an *Applicant Code*, which is located on the preprinted NRMP Student Agreement. A *Rank Order List Confirmation* is printed out at the time the list is submitted. The security of your list is ensured by built-in protection arrangements.

Registering for the NRMP allows you, after payment of the registration fee, to list up to 15 programs on your Rank Order List. Beyond this number an additional charge results. For each program you assign a *Rank Order Number*, and also provide the name of the hospital, city, and state and the specialty and type of residency sought, as well as the NRMP program code that is listed in the *Directory*.

Those seeking to gain a place in an advanced program should list their choices on the initial Rank Order List and then on a Supplemental Rank Order List along with associated PGY-1 positions.

Two suggestions as to how to maximize your chances of getting the best results out of your Rank Order List are (1) that you list your top choice first and (2) that you list all other programs in order of *your* preferences. To seek to guess how anxious programs may be to have you is highly speculative. It is an irrational basis for formulating a Rank Order List.

How many. Regarding the number of programs to place on your list, this depends on how competitive it is to secure a residency in the specific specialty you have chosen. Obviously, the more challenging it is to obtain an appointment in the specialty, the more programs you should apply to. In any case, you should place on your list the names of all programs you have been interviewed at and where a Match would be acceptable, because these programs potentially can meet your professional needs.

Results. The results of the Match become available annually on an NRMP-designated day in mid-March, known as *Match Day* (see below). They are mailed to applicants provided that a match has been made. Results as to whether one has matched can be ascertained by looking for a confidential code number in *USA Today* on the morning of the day before Match Day. But this source does not provide the name of the residency site. That information becomes available only on Match Day.

Unmatched candidates. Unmatched candidates will be notified of their being unsuccessful in securing a match on the day before Match Day by the dean of students at their medical school. This information is implied by the absence of the code number in *USA Today*. At the same time, these candidates will receive a list of unmatched positions that are still open in their specialty. Unmatched individuals should *directly* contact appropriate program directors where such openings exist, to attempt to *promptly* arrange a telephone match. This requires retaining one's composure, in spite of a potential major personal setback, by acting quickly and decisively to possibly reverse the situation.

Starting at noon on Unmatched Day, those still seeking a residency appointment should prioritize their phone lists of available residency openings in their specialty. Next, *promptly* contact program directors sequentially by phone. After describing the highlights of one's credentials, and note the nature of the directors reaction. If it sounds affirmative, then determine the extent of their interest by inquiring if you should fax the appropriate credentials to the program for an immediate decision. If the program director procrastinates or responds in the negative, proceed *at once* to contact the next program on the phone list, until success is achieved or all the possible opportunities have been eliminated. One should feel encouraged in this challenging effort, by the fact that statistics show that by that at end of Unmatched Day most candidates still seeking positions usually are placed by this approach.

Match Day. This decisive date, for the overwhelming majority of medical students, occurs the day after Unmatched Day. Soon-to-graduate students (and their families) usually assemble at their schools and at noon each receives an envelope that contains the name of the hospital or medical center where they will initiate their postgraduate training. This marks the high point of an extended and very trying interlude lasting many months.

It merits noting once again that having been offered an appointment through the Match, the applicant cannot refuse to accept it, because of the contractual commitment made with the NRMP at the time one signed up for the Match. The only possible exceptions are, if one accepts a position with the military or in the event that the candidate has decided not to undertake any PGY-1 position during the coming year.

It is in your best interest, soon after being advised of the favorable outcome to your quest for a residency, to contact the program director and inform them of how delighted you are with the turn of events. You may wish to express that you are looking forward joining their team. This will serve to initiate your professional association in a positive manner. You might take this opportunity to inquire if anything is still missing from your file and if so, arrange to provide it.

Other matches

In addition to the standard PGY-1 individual Match, there are several others. These matches are as follows:

Early Matches. Many specialties have separate matches for advanced (PGY-2 or higher) appointments. These take place earlier than the standard NRMP PGY-1 Match. They include matches for positions in neurology, neurosurgery, ophthalmology, otolaryngology, plastic surgery, radiation oncology, and urology. The results of these matches are provided to candidates weeks prior to the NRMP's mid-March deadline.

Most of the specialties that use separate matches are sponsored by their academic societies. The advanced positions are usually filled one or two years in advance by those who are planning to undertake preliminary or transitional positions at the outset of their postgraduate training.

Information and applications regarding advanced matches can be secured by contacting _____ (Name of specialty) Match Program, P.O. Box 7999, San Francisco, CA.

For urology, material can be secured from the American Urological Association Residency Matching Program, 6750 West Loop South, Bellaire, TX 77401.

Late Match. Dermatology is the only specialty to have a late Match announcement date, as determined by the NRMP.

Couples Match. Medical senior student couples are not an uncommon phenomenon. To reduce the possibility of serious marital hardship by placement in diverse locations, NRMP instituted the Couples Match Program to obviate such possibilities. This Match can facilitate couples being placed in geographically compatible locations relative to their training sites.

The Couples Match is different from the standard one. At the outset, each member needs to apply to the Match as an independent individual. However, when they submit their Rank Order Lists, these should be coordinated to meet the needs of the couple. Thus, if each member of a couple applies to programs in two common cities, they thereby enhance the probability of securing a mutually suitable match. The required applications consist of a special worksheet for couples and instructions, both of which are found in the NRMP publications. Naturally, the dual Rank Order Lists formulated by the couple will be the result of their determining the most appropriate common locations for both of them, based on their individual interview experiences and evaluations of program sites. The final list submitted therefore represents the merger, by consensus, of their individual choices for residency locations.

Shared Match. This match involves a pair of individuals who are linked by virtue of their seeking a common scheduled residency appointment to be shared on a part-time basis. It provides an opportunity for those who, for personal reasons (e.g., wishing to care for a family) or special obligations desire to extend their training over a longer period of time. It should be recognized, however, that only a limited number of specialties have programs that offer shared positions. These include family practice, internal medicine, and psychiatry. The NRMP *Directory* has a listing of such programs. Applying for such a match requires submission of a special form found in the NRMP manuals. By late October, the pair of applicants are assigned a single number for their application. They will apply using a single hyphenated name. In contrast to the Couples Match, only one Rank Order List is submitted, to secure a shared residency appointment. It is a major challenge to secure such a position and thus considerable thought should be given prior to initiating such a process.

Osteopathic Matching Program. Osteopathic medical students match through an intern matching program executed by the National Matching Services. This service sends out to eligible students a single application packet. All match participants also receive a listing of all osteopathic residency programs, but only those that are funded need to be considered. In October, the matching service sends registered candidates a personalized Rank Order List form on which to submit their selections. The National Matching Service is located at 595 Bay Street, Toronto, Ontario, Canada.

Canadian Resident Matching Service. This program announces its match results prior to those of the NRMP. A Match applicant is eligible to apply to both U.S. and Canadian programs should they so desire. If they do so, they should rank the Canadian programs first. In the event they match up through the Canadian service, the NRMP will remove their name from its lists, making applicants ineligible for a U.S.-based appointment.

Your contract

In due course you will receive a contract from your program. Below is a checklist of the things you should look for:

_____ Length of your appointment

_____ Annual salary (on a year-by-year basis)

_____ Nature of your responsibilities

_____ Working hours

_____ Maximum on-call service and days off

_____ Other benefits (stipend for meals, uniforms, laundry, pagers, etc.)

_____ Insurance coverage for disability, health (including family), etc.

_____ Personal leave policy (disability, illness, for family needs, etc.)

_____ Professional leave policy (to attend conferences, meetings, etc.)

_____ Vacation policy

_____ Policy relative to grievance and disciplinary procedures

_____ Policy relative to contract termination and appeal procedures

_____ Policy relative to transferring

_____ Policy relative to program termination

In the event that you are uncertain about an issue that is important to you, contact the program secretary or, if necessary, the director for clarification. If you question the validity of an issue, you can contact the Committee of Interns and Residents at the institution.

PART THREE

SURVIVING A RESIDENCY

T HERE IS A STRONG SENSE OF SATISFACTION AND RELIEF WHEN YOU DEFINITIVELY select a specialty for your professional career goal. For some, the decision-making process is quite simple, straightforward, and almost preordained. For others it involves many inquiries, much investigation, and considerable agonizing thought. With this decision behind you, the next task is facing the challenging process of securing the most appropriate site where you can obtain your postgraduate training. This is a difficult, demanding, and time-consuming process. This is the reason for the well-deserved celebration by medical student seniors and their families that takes place each year on Match Day. Being matched is another major professional milestone in your life.

With the issues of selecting and securing a residency resolved, the next major hurdle is faced from the very onset of postgraduate training. This involves coping with the rigorous demands of your prospective training program. These are usually both physically and emotionally highly stressful. Overcoming the daily challenges, advancing your knowledge and skills, and developing self-confidence are essential components of residency survival.

The impact of residency training on each individual depends on the demands of the specific specialty as well as on the nature of the individual program. Some residents can take the training process in stride. They may get fatigued and stressed out at times by the intense demands of their daily activities. However, they become rejuvenated after a good night's (or day's) rest. On the other hand, for many others, there are deep ups and downs in their personal state of being, depending on the events that transpire and the extent and nature of the workload placed upon them. Physical fatigue and emotional stress can often make the training process very challenging. For a very small number of individuals, residency can, unfortunately, wreak havoc with their personal lives. In some cases the pressure of residency may even induce substance abuse, as well as such personal problems as depression of varying degrees, marital difficulties, divorcing one's spouse, and tragically, in rare instances, even suicide.

This section of the book is designed to help prepare you to cope with what may lie ahead during the lengthy physician-in-training interlude, which is so crucial to molding your professional attitude and skills.

This third part of the book begins with an orientation chapter that puts into context your position as a PGY-1 trainee in the scheme of things and how best to manage some of your personal affairs. Next follows a discussion of ways of meeting your professional responsibilities. The third chapter provides suggestions on managing personal issues to help ensure your survival. Advice is then given regarding how best to function while protecting your well-being in the face of the demanding tasks you may confront. The following two chapters in this section deal with the professional and personal challenges you can expect to face during residency. As to the former, your position as a resident will be viewed from several professional perspectives. In the subsequent chapter, the challenges facing special groups of residents will be addressed. Finally, the last chapter summarizes the best means of not only surviving during your residency, but thriving as well. To achieve this goal you need to seek not only to properly manage your activities, but to enjoy this challenging interval in your life so that you can later look upon it with some degree of fondness.

13 | Becoming Oriented

Overview

The start of your PGY-1 or internship year is a time of considerable excitement. Undoubtedly you have been looking forward to obtaining advanced clinical training in your chosen specialty. This period of professional growth is unique by virtue of the especially intense demands and responsibilities that are placed on each individual. It is important that you start off well on this vital new adventure. To do so, you need to make a smooth transition from (medical) student to doctor (albeit one who is in training).

To facilitate this transition in your status, it is essential at the outset to be familiar with (a) a resident's professional goals, (b) the position of the various members of the treatment team, (c) your relationship with the ancillary staff, (d) how best to resolve professional conflicts that may arise during training, (e) the benefits of time management, (f) responsibilities relative to covering for other doctors, (g) issues concerning securing personal time off, and (h) the question of moonlighting. These eight important topics will be discussed in this chapter. Together with the next one, it should help you be better prepared for the challenges that lie ahead.

Residency goals

There are a number of goals that a resident should bear in mind as their training proceeds. These goals can be placed into two categories.

1. The resident as an apprentice. In this capacity you should seek to

■ Always have the best interests of your patients in mind as your highest priority.

■ Strive intently to master essential diagnostic skills by gaining expertise in the art of performing a work-up, to facilitate arriving at a meaningful preliminary diagnosis.

■ Seek to enhance your skills in carrying out the basic routine procedures called for in the specialty you are working in.

■ Aim to improve any deficiencies in your interpersonal abilities for dealing with patients, colleagues, and ancillary staff.

■ Observe closely the clinical styles of your attendings, to see what best suits your own approach and philosophy of patient care.

■ Find practitioners as role models who are dedicated and empathetic and practice medicine in a superior manner.

■ Endeavor to maintain your emotional equilibrium even in the face of the intense pressures and trials that you may likely experience.

■ To avoid errors and potential problems, recognize your limitations and do not exceed the boundaries of your knowledge and skills when treating patients.

■ Be firmly committed to carrying your share of the workload as a responsible member of the treatment team.

2. The resident as a teacher. As you move up the ranks in the course of your residency, your level of responsibility for teaching junior colleagues will increase. This obligation can start even in your PGY-1 year, when you may be involved in supervising medical students. Your general approach to teaching should be to

■ Provide orientation to residents medical students at each training level in order to smooth their transition.

■ Be available, when possible, to personally provide guidance to appropriate personnel, so that their assignment is properly executed.

■ Respond promptly to being paged and then determine the degree of urgency.

- Tactfully provide meaningful feedback on a resident's performance when warranted.

- Correct resident's errors patiently, without causing them embarrassment.

- Provide instruction calmly and pleasantly to make learning enjoyable.

- Offer practical and useful advice that can be applied directly to patient care.

- Give individualized instruction, when appropriate, to improve its effectiveness.

- Strive to treat all colleagues equally, to avoid jealousy on the treatment team.

- Willingly accept constructive comments and suggestions from subordinates.

- Delegate responsibilities, when appropriate, to enhance learning opportunities.

- Demonstrate an empathetic attitude toward patients and their families.

- Help generate a tension-free environment, so that work proceeds efficiently.

- Seek to know the assets and liabilities of subordinates in order to be able to evaluate them is objectively as possible.

The treatment team

Upon admission to a hospital service, the patient will receive medical care provided under the supervision of an attending physician and his/her supporting house staff treatment team. It is thus important to be cognizant of the role that each member of the team plays in caring for patients' needs. The treatment team commonly consists of a chief senior resident, a junior resident, one or two interns, and possibly one or two medical students. The status and basic responsibilities of the individual members of the team are distinct and will now be briefly summarized.

Attending physician. This individual carries ultimate clinical responsibility for patient management. The attending is the one who is obligated to (a) definitively decide on a treatment option choice, (b) determine patient treatment protocols, and, (c) help to amicably resolve crucial issues which team members face. In addition, the attending is responsible for supervising training of team members and thus for sharing their knowledge and skills collectively or individually.

Attendings are also expected to write evaluations and recommendations for residents at various levels whom they have supervised. This is critical in applying for a fellowship, subspecialty, or categorical appointment.

Attending physicians should serve as master teachers during rounds and conferences. Physicians vary as to the extent of their clinical knowledge and skills, as well as teaching abilities. Most are anxious to interact effectively with their team members, but some may tend to be remote. Usually there is a congenial working relationship between attendings and residents of their team, which enhances the working atmosphere.

In some cases, unfortunately, difficulties with attendings may arise because of occassional lapses in professional behavior on their part (or on the part of other superiors). It is helpful to recognize evidence of errant activity. This may be manifested as

■ Subjecting a resident to embarrassment and painful criticism in the presence of colleagues.

■ Generating excessive anxiety among residents in the course of providing supervision.

■ Antagonizing residents by personally deprecating and offensive remarks.

■ Failure to provide constructive criticism that would enhance professional growth.

■ Creating an atmosphere where residents feel that the attending can never be satisfied.

■ Writing what are perceived as grossly unfair evaluations of resident performance.

■ Generating an impression of being omnipotent, by discouraging dialogue.

Obviously it is a major challenge to cope with an attending physician manifesting such forms of behavior. Some possible approaches to dealing with this difficult problem are as follows:

■ Absolutely avoid responding to any abusive rebuke in a retaliatory manner. It is essential to retain your composure and act responsibly, especially under trying circumstances. This will ensure against compromising your own delicate position as a resident in good standing and reflect favorably on your professionalism.

■ Document in writing any unprofessional behavior by an attending (or other supervisor), recording the date, place, circumstances, nature of the offense, and any possible witnesses.

■ Privately and respectfully express your concerns regarding the issue(s) at hand to the attending physician. This should be done only if you feel emotionally comfortable doing so without worsening the situation. Seek to attain a satisfactory resolution of the existing difficulties and try to create a basis for a more satisfactory relationship for future professional interaction.

■ Should you not wish or be unable to resolve your concerns directly with the attending, you may seek to secure the assistance of the senior resident, the program director, or an attending who is both your friend and a friend of your supervisor to mediate the dispute. This step should be taken only if very serious difficulties have arisen.

■ As a last resort, higher officials in the administration can be contacted. Alternatively, the legal counsel of the residents' union at your institution may be able to provide assistance.

■ Refrain from signing an evaluation that you genuinely believe to be unquestionably inaccurate. Determine established institutional policy in order to be able to consider an appeal from such a report.

Chief resident. This resident is in charge of and responsible for the routine daily activities of the entire team. In addition to supervising basic patient care, chief residents have a significant role to play in observing and teaching other members of their teams and should be reasonably available for consultation by them. Customarily, when conducting rounds and discussing medical issues relevant to patient care, a senior resident may frequently call upon the juniormost member of the team and then move up from there.

When you are an incoming PGY-1 appointee, the chief resident should introduce you to the traditions and practices in your new setting. When necessary, the chief resident can serve as your representative. He/she will, over time, usually gain a good perception of the quality of your performance. This person can help resolve any issues that may arise in the course of working with other senior and junior residents and the ancillary staff. The chief resident can, in the event of an unexpected need for a resident to be absent, make adjustments to your on-call schedule to fill the gap. They can also serve as your liaison with attendings as well as the program administrator.

Junior resident. The move up to this level from that of PGY-1 or the internship year marks a major increase in your professional responsibility for patient care. Where necessary, junior residents report directly to the attending physician. They have the obligation of teaching the medical students assigned to the team. Another significant role of the junior resident is supervision of new interns, whose activities must be more closely monitored, especially during the early phase of PGY-1, when they need reassurance and guidance, as they make the transition into the postgraduate training program.

Intern. Having received a medical degree, the intern is now considered to be in a position to assume direct responsibility for patient care. Naturally, this will be carried out under the supervision of a junior resident or when appropriate, a senior resident. Responsibilities at the PGY-1 level include initial patient work-up, routine care decisions, and arranging for tests or providing treatment based on the determined protocol. The first several months of the program can be especially stressful, because they involve functioning under new circumstances. This is due also to understandable insecurity in decision-making and the pressure inevitably generated by your new, important responsibilities. Long hours of work, possible assignment to the intensive care unit or the E. R., and other demanding duties are especially challenging. One should gracefully accept the imposition that some routine or non-intellectually-stimulating activities (scut work) impose. Avoid demonstrating frustration even though your time is limited. This type of work includes starting IVs, removing sutures, and removing casts.

Fellow. Although no longer a member of the treatment team, having completed residency training, this physician, who may be engaged in research or advanced training, can be a very useful source of valuable information and advice. This would be based on their own recent postgraduate training experience. They may be able to assist you in making decisions when issues are not clearly black or white. If such an individual is available, seek them out and see if you can establish a personal relationship that can prove rewarding and enhance your educational experience.

The dysfunctional treatment team. A treatment team consists of people with a variety of personalities and operational styles. Establishing a cohesive, constructively functional unit therefore presents a major challenge. This difficult situation is further compounded when a member of the team is impaired (see also *The Impaired Resident*, Chapter 14). Team dysfunction generated by an impaired resident may not be readily evident. Such individuals tend to be able to mask their serious imperfections from others and, consequently, they may provide a seeming appearance of professional competence.

The intense pressure of postgraduate training can, however, produce such a high level of stress among house staff as to result in some individuals becoming impaired. Although the presence of an impaired resident usually goes undetected, because of their active coverup, it is also due to the fact that the supervising attending has very limited opportunities to become aware of the situation. In addition, the other residents are too intensively involved in their own activities to do anything about such a situation if they become aware of it. Consequently, a dysfunctional team can result in compromised patient care and increased anxiety among team members.

It is thus important to be alert to signs of dysfunctional difficulties associated with a resident. These may be manifested by

- Frequent disputes over insignificant issues in the course of routine activities.

- Persistent lateness or time off for sickness beyond what is reasonable.

- Expressing low morale and a high level of anxiety when conversing.

- Increased use of sarcastic or angry responses when communicating.

- Frequent passing on of blame for personal errors to others on the team.

- Increased assertion of status during conflicts, rather than applying reasoning.

In light of the above, two issues need to be touched upon, namely, (1) how to deal with team dysfunction when it exists and (2) how to avoid its developing.

1. In terms of dealing with the problem of team dysfunction, the following three suggestions may prove helpful.

• At group sessions, seek to uncover troubling issues and ventilate them, so that they do not remain barriers to effective patient care and postgraduate training.

• In any group discussion, avoid finger pointing. The focus should be an improving collegiality in team function and generating and/or enhancing group morale.

• Should a group meeting be unable to resolve troubling situations, seek to involve the attending physician to defuse and ameliorate existing problems.

2. To reduce the potential for the occurrence of team dysfunction, the following three suggestions may prove helpful.

• Residents should provide each other with genuine support, especially during stressful events (an all-too-common hospital phenomenon).

• Residents should be encouraged to participate in periodic group sessions that allow discussion and resolution of potentially troublesome issues.

• Team members should participate in social gatherings, away from the hospital, to help foster better interpersonal relationships between them and their families.

The ancillary staff

One critical factor in determining your success as a resident will be your relationship with the ancillary staff. This group includes such professionals as nurses, physician assistants, health care therapists, technicians, and social workers. The importance of establishing and maintaining good relations with the ancillary staff is reflected by the fact that residents have intensive contact with staff during the course of their activities. Moreover, to significant extent, residents are dependent upon the goodwill of such personnel. While recognizing that a PGY-1 resident is still "green" in terms of practical experience, one need not feel threatened when dealing with an experienced ancillary professional. Also, because there are a large number of female physicians, one should not behave in a superior manner toward women who are members of the support staff. Always remember that they also are part of the patients' treatment team and serve to facilitate their well-being and a physicians activities.

To develop good relations with support personnel, the following suggestions should be borne in mind.

■ Upon initiating your service, introduce yourself to the support staff present. Find out if they customarily call residents by their first names. If so, tell them yours and make a point of getting to know theirs.

■ Learn and accept the standard protocol and routines relevant to patient care (e.g., scheduling of tests and writing orders, etc.).

■ When in doubt, do not hesitate to ask an experienced ancillary professional for a suggestion or opinion on a subject or technique that he/she has substantial experience with.

■ Be prepared to admit to errors on your part, explaining that they are a component of a normal resident's learning process.

■ When it is necessary to rebuke a support staff member for a mistake, first be certain that you are correct. When circumstances clearly require you to do so, handle the matter tactfully and aim to educate the individual, not merely to criticize.

■ Make a special effort to obtain the friendship of the head nurse on your assigned floor. She is probably a repository of much information and can ensure that her staff readily provide you with essential support and assistance when needed.

■ When you are discussing a medical issue with an ancillary staff member and you are uncertain of the correct response, do not try to obfuscate. Rather, indicate that you will provide a definitive answer as soon as possible, and do not fail to do so.

■ If challenged by support personnel, do not bully your way through by pulling rank. Clarify the rationale for your proposed action and indicate that you will fully assume the responsibility for any possible consequences.

■ When requesting assistance, be polite, and express your genuine appreciation for any help provided.

■ When being humorous, do so in a tactful manner, so that no one is personally offended.

■ Be certain that any disagreements focus on patient welfare and not become personal disputes.

Conflict resolution

In the course of meeting your professional responsibilities you will have contact with a wide variety of individuals, including practicing physicians-in-training, medical students, administrators, and support staff. Differences of opinion might arise. Obviously, these should best be resolved in the most amicable manner possible, because this will allow the maintenance of future productive relationships. When a conflict cannot be readily settled and it involves patient care management, it is best to refer it to the more senior house staff for resolution. When challenged by a member of the nursing staff, one should recognize that many of them have a great deal of practical experience. Thus pulling rank should not be the approach used; rather, clarifying the problem and determining what is in the patient's best interest is essential. It is obviously wise to seek to eliminate opportunities for disagreement at as early a stage as possible. But it is absolutely critical that discussion of differences be resolved privately and certainly not in the presence of patients or their families.

The following guidelines in the area of conflict resolution should be considered:

■ Utilize direct private discussion with the other person as a first step. This obviously should be done prior to requesting that others intervene on your behalf.

■ When satisfactory resolution is not attainable by direct discussion, seek assistance up the house staff ladder of responsibility.

■ Documenting your complaint will significantly strengthen your arguments, especially if the disagreement is a serious one.

■ As a last resort, you can consider obtaining the help of the program director, but only if the problem merits going to the top, because a disagreement also reflects upon your status as a team player.

Time management

Proper expenditure of a resident's time is a very high-priority item and proper management is a key element in ensuring success. To use your time efficiently, you need to budget it in an appropriate manner. Difficulties in time management arise from (a) underestimating the amount of time that scheduled activities will take, (b) scheduling an excessive number of activities to the point of becoming overextended, and (c) not allowing enough free time for unforeseen circumstances.

The very nature of the residency experience involves being intensely preoccupied with requests for information, judgments, and decisions. This activity requires prioritizing your responses. How well you succeed at this task largely determines your overall effectiveness. You can categorize requests on your professional time into three groupings: (a) urgent, (b) important, and (c) not important. Although some tasks will be completed earlier than others, it is essential that in due course you should respond to *all* of them.

Specific guidelines that facilitate time management to meet the demands for your services are as follows:

■ *Be flexible*. Although, you should have a structured plan for each day's activities, it is essential to avoid being rigid, for this can prove to be counterproductive. Realize that in medicine the unexpected is commonplace and you need to respond to sudden changes in circumstances by using good judgment, bearing in mind relevant issues and possible consequences.

■ *Promptly answer pages*. Because you cannot be certain of the degree of urgency of a page, it is in your best interest to respond without delay to all calls for your assistance.

■ *Avoid delaying decisions*. When you feel qualified to act, based on your knowledge, experience, and level of responsibility, do not procrastinate unjustifiably; rather, act decisively. If you have valid reason for holding off, seek advice and guidance from your superior as soon as possible and then respond.

■ *Update your knowledge.* Where you note some deficiency in your grasp of a clinical problem or subject, seek to close the gap promptly by reviewing the appropriate sources. This can prove valuable in improving the quality of your patients' care and further your base of clinical knowledge.

Covering for others

It is quite common that you will periodically have to cover for other physicians who are off. This occurs not only on days but also on nights or weekends. It may result from residents being unavailable due to sick leave, vacation, personal leave, or days off. Your performance in replacing another resident during such times is critical for patient welfare as well as for maintaining your own professional standing in the department.

Your guidelines on dealing with this issue should be as follows:

■ *Secure a sick patient roster.* Be certain to find out the names and room numbers of all patients whom you must cover who are in an unstable or serious medical condition. These individuals may need to be seen more frequently. They may well require special monitoring of their status while you are covering the service.

■ *Stay current.* Keep your list of patient problems up-to-date to facilitate work of the treatment team by being able to report on existing conditions.

■ *Determine assignments.* Formulate a list of all the laboratory and other test reports as well as x-rays that must be checked during the time interlude you are covering.

■ *New admissions.* It is essential to work-up assigned new admissions to your service to facilitate the patient care that will be provided by the regular team that will subsequently assume responsibility for these patients.

■ *Resuscitation status.* Be familiar with the appropriate response to terminally ill patients in regard to resuscitation instructions that may be in force for each individual.

■ *Transfer responsibility.* When your tour of duty is over, alert the on-call team as to the status of any unstable patients. They will then be able to better respond, when necessary, after they take over. The information you provide the team should be concise and precise, because they will be receiving reports concerning a host of patients and thus their time is limited.

Personal time off

Vacation and time-off policies vary among institutions. Your contractual agreement with the residency program will stipulate the specifics in your individual case.

The following guidelines will facilitate your retaining in good standing with your program with regard to the issue of personal time off.

■ Notify your program director as far in advance as possible and in writing of your need for time off, briefly specifying the reason and identifying the time interval. If necessary, outline in greater detail the reasons behind this request. This approach will allow a replacement to be conveniently obtained for your scheduled absence if it is other than the standard vacation. Obviously the earlier the director can be informed the better it is, because it facilitates scheduling of a replacement.

■ Make arrangements with another resident to cover your clinic patients during any absence that you are granted. A lapse in coverage will reflect negatively on your sense of responsibility and is unfair to the patients in question.

■ Provide your program director's secretary and hospital switchboard with a phone number where, if essential, you can be reached during your off time.

■ If you must depart from the hospital on very short notice to meet a personal emergency, it is incumbent upon you to arrange for coverage of your patients. Should this prove impossible for you to do, secure the assistance of the chief resident in making the necessary arrangements.

■ Whenever possible, seek to arrange time off for personal needs in advance. This facilitates scheduling of personnel in your department with the least disruption of scheduled activities.

Moonlighting

Supplementary employment, known as moonlighting, can be defined as work performed by residents during off hours at medical facilities other than their own. It is a relatively common practice and can serve as a meaningful source of enhanced income. After paying off monthly loan payments, it is estimated that not very much remains from a resident's modest salary for essential living expenses such as food and rent. Thus for many residents there is strong pressure for an additional source of income, and moonlighting provides such an avenue.

Many residents thus depend on moonlighting to earn extra income, whereas some also do so to gain additional medical training. The latter group obviously strongly prefers that their work be in their specialty, which frequently cannot be arranged.

Those residents moonlighting primarily to increase their income will seek to obtain the most lucrative positions available. The most common site of service for moonlighting physicians is in the hospital emergency room. Putting in a robust number of hours over a weekend moonlighting can earn a resident up to $2,000.

Moonlighting, however, does have a potential negative impact on a resident. The hospital environment, already stressful, becomes even more challenging when a sleep-deprived, moonlighting resident has to resume responsibilities at their hospital training site. Residents readily admit that sleep deprivation poses dangers both to themselves and to their patients. They also admit that under these special circumstances, residents may be less careful, thorough, and compassionate than is desirable. Many residents, however, argue that hospitals resist work-hour reform in their resident schedule. This, they claim, is because the present situation provides far lower reimbursement costs than engaging additional personnel to cover for a shortened work program.

Moonlighting may also negatively affect a resident's learning experience by interrupting continuity of care after a short interlude. This is a consequence of restriction of the possibility for long-term relationships between patient and physician, a major element of postgraduate training. As a compromise, many programs offer in-house moonlighting opportunities, which provide control over the extent of the resident's extracurricular activities. This also allows supervision over the nature of the services, thus mitigating, to an extent, some objections to moonlighting that have been raised. For many medical educators this is an acceptable means to solve the problem, financially helping meet legitimate needs of physicians-in-training and yet monitoring the nature of the activity.

Major changes in the provision of health care have been going on for quite some time. Irrespective of which direction health care reform takes, moonlighting will most likely remain as a potential funding source for residents. It will help some of them cope fiscally during a very difficult phase of their professional growth.

In summary, moonlighting should be considered only if the additional money is absolutely essential to maintain at least a modest, but adequate, standard of life. It is certainly ill-advised for residents who, because of intense professional demands, are having difficulty meeting their current responsibilities. By moonlighting they risk overextending themselves as a result of placing additional demands on their limited free time and energy. It is obvious that under such circumstances, their performance of medical services can be impeded, which would impact on their postgraduate training careers negatively. For this reason, residents should very carefully weigh their options before undertaking supplementary work obligations.

14 | Meeting Responsibilities

Overview

Upon initiating service as a resident you should recognize that your position requires you to simultaneously wear three hats, namely, medical apprentice, hospital employee, and committed physician. As a consequence, you have obligations toward your treatment team colleagues, the department chairperson who represents the institution that hired you, and the patients who have been placed in your care. All of these obligations put heavy demands on you, which in turn may generate tension and anxiety that can lead to stress. Obviously this can impact a resident's professional performance negatively. The overall issue of functioning effectively under the pressure of multiple obligations will therefore be the main topic of discussion in this chapter.

Keys to patient care

The extent of a resident's clinical responsibilities obviously depends on his/her stage of postgraduate training. It also is governed by the status of the patients namely, whether they are classified as private or public. In the former case, a resident's responsibilities toward the patient will be limited. For public patients, residents have greater supervisory responsibilities and thus can establish a more in-depth relationship with them. In either case, it is essential that you develop strong communication skills, which will improve your interpersonal relationships with individual patients, who undoubtedly will come from a wide variety of backgrounds.

To enhance your interaction with patients. The following suggestions should prove helpful:

■ Always seek to practice good medicine. Although your time is very limited, be sure to take an adequate history and perform a reliable physical exam. Shortcuts may jeopardize the accuracy of your findings and preliminary diagnosis.

■ Being able to communicate well with the patient will facilitate building trust. Thus, the patient will be more likely to confide in you, which improves your chances of securing essential information and cooperation for testing and treatment.

■ To be objective in your approach, treat all patients equally irrespective of their social class. Make the patients and their families feel comfortable in your presence. The feeling can in part be generated by minimizing the use of highly technical terms.

■ Focus your full attention on the patient, so that you really listen to what they are trying to say. By this means you will gain the most from your interpersonal contacts and can better provide the needed help. Thus, it is important, when conversing with patients, to read between the lines to ascertain the true facts behind their complaints.

■ Demonstrate concern toward your patients by spending at least a brief amount of time at their bedside, preferably sitting a moment at each visit. This will suggest that your concern is genuine. This small display of empathy can leave a strong impact.

■ Maximize the use of your time by working efficiently. This means carrying out your duties in an organized and methodical manner. Even when pressed for time, stick with this approach.

■ When carrying out your physical examination, do so in a well-lit room. Neutral light is better than the florescent type, because, for example, it reduces the risk of overlooking a jaundiced or cyanotic appearance. The examination room also needs to be absolutely quiet if you wish to pick up symptomatic heart sounds, such as a murmur or gallop.

■ Like all professions, physicians have essential "tools of the trade," which in reality are extensions of yourself. Thus, be certain to carry all appropriate instruments and use them effectively. This can provide you with maximal clinical information so vital to your mission.

■ When interviewing patients, it is important that you ask the right questions. Your questions should stem from your placing the observed signs and reported symptoms in a pathophysiological context. This will allow you to explore the nature of the patient's condition in greater depth. This way of utilizing your knowledge can lead you to arrive at a possible diagnosis.

■ When examining a patient, you should approach the subject with an open mind. It is essential to be unprejudiced and formulate your own unbiased personal opinion concerning the nature of their illness. Thus, you should initially examine the patient, and only then look into the chart. Then consider the case in the light of all the available evidence and information.

■ Remember that the ultimate source of information is the patient, not the textbook or the chart. The examination and test results are the best road map to a definitive understanding of the problem and its possible resolution.

■ If a patient's room is closed, be sure to knock before entering, because many are uncomfortable with a surprise visit, even from a physician.

■ Identify yourself by name and if necessary repeat it on the next visit, until the patient gets to know it. This will help better personalize your relationship and facilitate interaction.

■ Determine what the patient prefers you to call them (i.e., using their first name or Mr./Mrs./Miss./Ms.). This will effectively indicate your respect for their individuality.

■ After entering the patient's room, make a brief effort at small talk, so that your entrance is more in the nature of a visit than merely a brief clinical inspection.

■ Give each of your patients a human face. Identify them in your mind by some special feature that can serve to characterize each of them as a distinct entity, rather than only by room and bed number.

■ Allow your patients to briefly express their emotions. Even though this can be somewhat time-consuming for the doctor, it can be therapeutically valuable by serving to relieve some of the psychological strain that the patient is under.

■ Respectfully entertain a patient's suggestion regarding utilizing an alternative healing approach. Consider such a request seriously, especially if it presents no risks to a patient's health and can complement conventional therapy. You may suggest they initiate this approach upon returning home. If the request is inappropriate, do not dismiss it in a light-hearted or offensive manner. Rather, be tactful when responding in a negatively.

■ Avoid getting upset when confronting compliance failure on the part of a patient. Seek to discover the underlying reasons for this behavior. Try to determine if it is due to misunderstanding, fear, or ignorance. Attempt to educate the patient, in a constructive and conciliatory manner, as to establish how essential their cooperation is to achieve therapeutic success.

■ Try, when possible, to become acquainted with a patient's family. Allow them time to consult with you. This will enhance your chances of securing the patient's future cooperation and thus facilitate compliance.

■ If you personally have had an episode of serious illness in the past that required hospitalization, recall this experience in the context of providing patient care. It will serve to strengthen your sense of empathy for those whose future is your responsibility.

■ Determine if patients of a specific type, age, race, or background, for some reason, elicit strong negative emotions on your part. Self-awareness of this bias may possibly allow you to better control your feelings in such cases and help you respond in an objective manner toward such patients.

■ When dealing with a patient who is *justifiably* angry, agreeing with them will put you on their side and may serve to defuse the situation.

■ When you are applying a newly learned procedure, anxiety on your part can reasonably be anticipated. It is best to focus your attention on the patient's reaction to your executing the procedure more than on your own performance. This will help you get through the process with greater ease.

■ Recognize that the response of patients to pain, illness, and fear of the unknown varies widely. It depends on their personality, gender, and cultural and religious background. Thus brave individuals should be commended and fearful ones be appropriately reassured. Both groups, naturally, should otherwise be treated equally.

■ When imparting information to patients, explain yourself in a brief but clear manner. Inquire if you were fully understood; if not, present your thoughts once again from a different perspective. Get a family member involved, if necessary, to ensure clarity and facilitate compliance.

■ Make a strong effort to maintain good eye contact with the patient while conversing. This serves to establish a bond that facilitates better communication.

■ In presenting a treatment plan, respond, when possible, to a patient's reluctance or opposition by negotiation. This will facilitate chances for greater compliance and ultimately thus secure better results. Just saying "trust me" may not necessarily achieve your goal. Rather, allowing the patient a reasonable degree of input can prove to be a useful device for acceptance of your recommendations.

■ Upon discharge, provide patients, where appropriate, with sources for self-help, so that they can better adjust to nonhospital life. This is especially important after a lengthy hospitalization.

■ Seek to enhance your learning experience and its impact on your patient by providing continuity of care. You should seek to maintain this in both inpatient and outpatient venues.

Retaining empathy

Service as a resident is an intensely demanding experience. It can generate psychological pressures, physical fatigue, and emotional discomfort, which collectively can have a very negative impact on the nature of one's response to patient suffering. In some cases, residents unfortunately react by becoming immunized to a patients' ordeal. Psychological buffering is a mechanism utilized subconsciously by such residents to reduce emotional stress that has been generated in the course of their professional activities. Such individuals can continue to meet the technical demands of their responsibilities. However, regrettably, they may not fulfill the holistic needs of patient care. Those who permanently develop such an emotion-numbing trait will, because of this handicap, find it difficult to resist the employment pressure of high-volume processing, when working for for-profit managed care organizations, and of moonlighting. They may be prone to be transformed into technician-like practitioners.

Another negative feature of becoming unsympathetic to pain is that it can serve as a major barrier to achieving career satisfaction. Moreover, it has been found that such impaired physicians have difficulty establishing a private practice and are prone to have more negligence lawsuits. This situation can also generate difficulties in the family lives of such physicians. Thus, loss of empathy potentially can have devastating consequences for a health care professional.

It is common that residents treat a population that contains a broad spectrum of individuals. These people range from congenial and cooperative to demanding and argumentative. Some may be seriously ill or even moribund. Clearly, providing health care is a major emotional challenge, given all the work-related pressure in a hospital environment. Dealing with a diverse population obviously can add to the challenge of an existing situation and make it even more demanding.

One major means of combating psychological fatigue that induces diminished empathy, is to recognize its onset and/or evidence of its symptoms. These include experiencing a composite of *several* manifestations from among those listed below:

■ Developing an unprofessional attitude toward patients, reflected in making disparaging remarks about them or direct impoliteness. Such negativity suggests an existing underlying anger toward those, one is called upon to serve.

■ Executing perfunctory histories and physical examinations, including failure to secure vital patient information, all of which, obviously, can impede formulating an accurate diagnosis.

■ Exhibiting impassive emotional responses to tragedy, in spite of the expectation of a positive outcome. Some sympathy under such circumstances, even from a hardened physician, would be likely, and even more so from a physician-in-training.

■ Referring to patients by room number, nature of their disease, or body component that is in disrepair.

■ Denying the existence of a patient's illness, irrespective of unquestionable medical evidence to the contrary.

- Fantasizing a disliked patient's disappearance or death, thus theoretically eliminating the problem from one's agenda as a recipient of one's medical care.

- Having excessive emotional involvement with a patient's problems (both medical and personal). Sound professional behavior requires maintaining a healthy distance from a patient.

- Consciously avoiding of professional contact with specific patients whom one is responsible for.

- Being overeager to refer patients to other specialists to avoid the challenges of personal treatment.

- Becoming increasingly dictatorial in attitude, seeking to force patients to conform to one's wishes, instead of having a reasonable dialogue to facilitate patient cooperation and compliance.

Coping with stress

The inherent character and demands of the postgraduate training process clearly lend themselves to generating a stressful lifestyle. Thus, a major element in succeeding as a resident is learning how to cope with stress.

The ability to cope with stress is dependent upon your personality as well as your prior life experiences. Some people can withstand very intense stress before they feel pressure, whereas others have a lower stress tolerance threshold.

Mastering the art of coping with stress is also essential in helping you maintain your physical and mental health. Under stress, your breathing becomes shallow and uneven, your pulse may speed up, and your senses sharpen. Consequently, a stressful day frequently results in a feeling of tiredness. Prolonged stress has been demonstrated to contribute to headaches, skin rashes, and even more serious illnesses such as ulcers and asthma.

If you have any problem coping with stress, you should seek information about deep breathing, stretching, or regular aerobic exercises that can help you control the troubling feelings generated by pressure. Consulting your advisor/mentor or even a psychiatrist can also prove useful. In severely stressful situations, medication may be indicated.

At the very outset, it should be clearly recognized that, if you are capable of graduating from medical school, you have already proven that you can cope effectively with stress induced by intense educational and training demands. A successful medical education involves obtaining attractive grades, especially in relevant clerkships, as well as performing well on the USMLE Step I. These achievements should strongly reinforce your sense of confidence in being able to cope with stress while serving as a resident.

The goal in coping with stress should be twofold: (1) to limit the extent of your exposure to stressful situations and (2) to learn how to respond to stress.

The following seven suggestions may be useful in coping with stress:

1. Maintain your physical health as optimally as possible. This includes following an appropriate diet and a suitable exercise regimen and obtaining adequate sleep.

2. Try to meet pending responsibilities without becoming overwhelmed. Thus, tasks and problems should be prioritized and addressed accordingly. When possible, subdivide large problems into small, more manageable tasks, which in turn should also be solved in a prioritized manner.

3. Utilize your time efficiently. This means budgeting time in an appropriate and efficient manner. Don't overextend yourself with an excessive number of scheduled activities or underestimate the time they may require. Be flexible in making changes in planned activities when circumstances require it.

4. Realize and accept the fact that some stressful situations are completely unavoidable. These include scheduled rounds, challenging new procedures, and presenting cases. Because you cannot exercise control over potential stress-inducing events, try to prepare for them as adequately as possible and then accept them and the results calmly and matter-of-factly.

5. Find satisfying and wholesome outlets for dissipating stress and frustrations. This can include participation in some exercise or sports activities, or seeking a close friend to whom you can confidentially ventilate your feelings and fears.

6. When possible, avoid situations that you know in advance will be stressful. Thus, for example, last-minute preparation for executing a new procedure can obviously generate stress. Schedule study time so that you are fully prepared in advance of hospital activities and therefore can avoid cramming. Similarly, if getting to the hospital is an erratic experience timewise, schedule your departure to work to be able to avoid the frustration and stress created by the fear of arriving late.

7. When possible, allow for several periods of relaxation, however brief, during the day. These can be taken during mealtimes and during night call. More extended rest periods should be standard parts of weekends. Occasional vacations, even limited ones, can help you to recover from long spells of intense activity. Such changes in environment are very conductive to maintaining one's mental well-being.

Coping with stress will also be facilitated by recognizing certain common realities. Namely, in making the transition from medical student to resident, you can expect

1. Being somewhat disoriented at the outset by your new status.

2. Feeling frighteningly unprepared for your new challenging responsibilities.

3. Finding that procedures that seem simple and straightforward actually complex and confusing in the inexperienced hands of a novice.

4. Hospital staff tend to assume you to know much more than you actually do.

5. Facing the difficult task of extracting essential information from seriously ill or even hostile patients can be quite challenging.

6. Possibly being embarrassed by being reprimanded by an attending or more senior house officer's in front of others, even for minor mistakes or for lacking knowledge on some specific issue.

7. Not being the first person doing a work-up on a patient. Hence, some sense of competition with others may arise.

8. Having the obligation to meet patient responsibilities that mandate a change in your plans to attend rounds, a conference, or lecture.

On the positive side, you also should recognize that many of these troublesome issues will, over time, gradually become resolved as you gain more experience and self-confidence. Moreover, you will feel increasingly fulfilled as you mature as a resident and find the satisfaction that practicing medicine has to offer.

Finally, you should realize that during your postgraduate training, in addition to clinical proficiency, characteristics such as personality, diligence, reliability, respectfulness, honesty, flexibility, and cooperation will also be judged by attendings and senior house staff. These personal attributes may carry as much weight as your medical knowledge base. Remember that competence is important, but decency, dedication, and compassion also count for a great deal.

The impaired resident

It is widely recognized that an impaired resident can jeopardize patient welfare and lead to treatment team dysfunction. Dealing with such individuals is difficult because it generates a inner conflict within an individual who is cognizant of the situation. The cognizant resident is caught in a dilemma by their desire to assist one of their colleagues, while at the same time ethically doing the right thing and protecting patients. Of paramount importance in this type of situation is the need to confirm the existence of genuine impairment, rather than a transitory reaction to excessive fatigue due to stress generated by the demands of one's activities and responsibilities. Making this distinction will now be discussed.

Evidence suggesting that a resident suffers from burnout is reflected by observing multiple signs and symptoms, such as the following:

■ Repeated unjustifiable lateness or absences over a meaningful period of time.

■ An obvious attitude of apathy and indifference toward one's professional responsibilities.

■ Carelessness in patient care as reflected in an increased frequency of unjustifiable mistakes.

■ Manifesting evidence of serious emotional disturbance reflected by symptoms associated with depression and paranoia.

■ Being involved in an increased number of professional and personal conflicts with colleagues.

■ Disappearance, while on duty, to a secluded area of the hospital without justification.

■ Convincing evidence of substance abuse involving alcohol, drugs, or chain smoking.

■ Demonstrating inappropriate behavior toward patients, as reflected by serious complaints from them.

■ Showing a persistent marked decline in personal appearance unbecoming a professional.

■ Demonstrating, over an extended period, wide mood swings over short periods of time.

Assuming that the impaired resident does *not* present an *immediate* risk to his/her patients or themselves, the problem of responding to this type of situation can be approached by

■ Having a close colleague of the impaired resident privately and tactfully express their serious concern about the situation. Identify the multiple ways it is evident. This should be coupled by a forceful suggestion that it is essential that help be sought *promptly*, so that the situation does not get worse. Intimate a readiness, if necessary, to take the matter up with higher authorities in order to protect patients from being harmed. Explain your great reluctance to avoid this unpleasant course of action on your part, if at all possible.

■ Indicating that not only you, but others, are aware that something is seriously amiss and that erratic behavior has been observed on his/her part has also alarmed them.

■ Listening to the individual's response. If it is denial and/or defiance, point out that continuing without securing help will unquestionably very seriously jeopardize the individual's career. Emphasize that promptly seeking assistance can minimize dislocation of their professional and personal life. Indicate that what is at stake is the basic well-being of a competent physician like yourself and prompt action is absolutely essential.

■ Following up by providing sources of confidential professional help at the hospital or local mental health agency. Indicate that you fully expect the person to inform you very shortly of what action has been taken regarding seeking help.

■ Indicating that if you fail to be updated on steps being taken (which should be confirmed as being valid), or if the help sought is inappropriate, or if the nature of the situation deteriorates, you have no choice but to take the matter up with the residency program director.

When a situation is *critical* and there is a clear danger to patients or to the resident (e.g., intoxication while on service), immediate action is called for. This should be done by notifying the psychiatrist on duty or escorting the individual to the E.R.

If possible, offer to fill in for the impaired resident until the immediate crisis is resolved.

Maintaining efficiency

It is common knowledge that residents are overworked by their multiple and demanding responsibilities. To maintain one's well-being under such circumstances, it is essential to find the time to retain a reasonable semblance of your personal life. To achieve this goal it is important to do your work efficiently so that you have some time available for your private needs. Therefore, avoiding the unproductive use of time, provides an important source of flexibility to pursue nonprofessional activities.

There are a number of ways that efficiency can be improved, each of which will be briefly discussed below:

Set goals. You should be clearly aware of the goal before you start a task. You will then be able to focus your efforts and thus save time. To maximize your chances for attaining goals, it is best to categorize them into short- or long-term groups. In doing so, there is a need to be flexible, to allow for delays.

To measure progress you may write down your goals. Noting your achievements, you will keep your sense of momentum going. Such an event, for example, takes place when you chart a patient's daily activities from admission to discharge. A clear goal and the progress record can be followed within a projected time frame.

Set priorities. To maximize efficiency and thus best utilize your time, it is imperative to prioritize. This means determining which are the most important items that require your attention and alloting them more time. There are various approaches to prioritization. The simplest is to establish "must- do" and "should do" lists. The latter contain items that can be deferred, but deserve not to be neglected. By checking off items on such lists as they are completed, you get gratification from a sense of accomplishment. A more complex scheme requires subdividing items into four categories, namely, urgent and important, can wait and should wait. The use of an electronic organizer is a very convenient way to record and prioritize your commitments (as well as recording important reference data).

Delegate responsibility. There is a natural tendency among physicians to do all tasks themselves. Nevertheless, it is more productive if routine tasks are delegated to ancillary staff who are equally or frequently even better qualified to carry them out. Similarly, when possible, delegate responsibility to junior house staff, or even medical students. It is important that you impart a clear idea of what you wish to have done and transmit your instructions in an understandable and decisive manner. It is also essential that equipment be available to carry out assigned tasks before they are begun. Clarification regarding instruction given should be sought from a superior, when necessary, to avoid any misunderstandings.

Time-saving approaches. Aside from the use of electronic organizers, another useful device is a miniature dictating machine. This allows you to make verbal notes of vital information and tasks that need to be done. This approach takes getting used to, but it can prove advantageous in carrying out the details of a demanding schedule.

Responding to pages. Interruptions in your routine activities are commonly expected as part of the hospital routine. They come from various sources such as other physicians and nurses. By evaluating the importance and urgency of issues raised by their call, you can determine how urgent the problems are and how much time you need to devote in responses to them. This also can help maximize efficiency.

Avoid procrastination. One may readily rationalize delaying performance of certain tasks. One consequence of doing so unjustifiably may result in feelings of personal frustration and anxiety later on. To overcome such behavior, requires gaining an understanding of underlying causes of such behavior. This issue obviously requires some elaboration at this point.

To help modify this behavior it is important to note when, where, and under what conditions the desire to procrastinate arises. One of the common factors generating this behavior is a desire for perfection. This unfortunately can be self-defeating, because it raises standards to unrealistic heights. The goal should be to aim for optimal results by doing your very best and be satisfied if you attain or come close to your goal. A second factor inducing procrastination is a lack of self-discipline. When full recognition is given to the importance of facing up to challenging tasks promptly, because it increases the chance for success, a change in attitudes may come about. Two other factors involved in procrastination are a fear of failure or conversely a fear of success. In the former case it should be recognized that one learns to be successful from failures and that they need not be equated with futility. To overcome a sense of doom and gloom, it may be desirable if possible, to divide a project into several natural components. Accomplishing each task individually will then motivate you to move on to the next one until the entire project is completed.

Fear of success, if it occurs, is more likely to take place among women. They may regard success in their professional life as presenting a worrisome challenge to achieving a successful family life. They may be concerned that one cannot maintain a proper balance between what they conceive as two opposing commitments. Consequently, they may tend to procrastinate and delay professional success. By realizing that this concept is inaccurate and finding role models that exemplify a well-balanced personal and professional life, one can overcome this impediment to success.

Thirty steps to success

Although experience usually proves to be the best teacher, the following guidelines should help to facilitate your success as a resident:

■ *Provide good medicine.* Don't let the demands on your time so overwhelm you as to deflect your performing a thorough history and physical exam. Although this is a time-consuming task, you owe it to yourself and your patient. It will pay dividends in mastering the art of patient care.

■ *Be tolerant.* Your patients will come from all walks of life as well as social and economic strata. Make the patient (and their family) feel comfortable irrespective of the impression they leave with you.

■ *Listen well.* Pay careful attention to what the patient and family tell you both during the formal interview and in informal conversations. The clues they may provide can prove invaluable in formulating the correct diagnosis of the patient's illness.

■ *Evaluate carefully.* It is often essential to read between the lines of comments and symptoms described by patients. There may be a purposeful or subtle desire on the part of the patient to mask the real problem that exists. Clarification can sometimes be elicited from a spouse or other family member as to what the underlying problem really is. Do not hesitate to seek their help when necessary and possible.

■ *Inquire appropriately.* It is essential during the course of a history and physical to ask the right questions. These should not be focused exclusively on signs and symptoms. Such questions, although useful in indicating the possible underlying disease, need to be reinforced by an understanding of the possible pathophysiology that may be involved. This kind of knowledge will stimulate further questions that in turn may facilitate uncovering the nature of the heretofore elusive ailment.

■ *Demonstrate concern.* Although you may be pressed for time, avoid reflecting a sense of haste to your patient. Even sitting down *briefly* at a patient's bedside will demonstrate compassion and empathy, which are qualities sought by patients in their physicians. Such an expression of interest, albeit minor, will help cement the doctor–patient relationship and further your patients' treatment and recovery.

■ *Act with humility.* Although wearing a white coat confers higher status, it should not be reflected in arrogant behavior. Recognize the complexity of the human condition and the ultimate limitation of every physician's powers in the healing process. This awareness should be reflected in one's speech, behavior, and actions.

■ *Be prepared.* Carry essential professional diagnostic equipment with you. You can't do your job and get the information you need without it. When proceeding to a patient's room to carry out a procedure, think of all essential items that you will need, to avoid delaying or interrupting the procedure due to the absence of essential components.

■ *Focus on the patient.* Managing patient care requires maintaining an accurate record of the patient's status on a day-to-day basis. Certainly the chart contains vital information that is an asset for patient evaluation and care. However, the physician needs to recognize that the final arbiter is the patient's condition. Both in treating the patient and in learning about medicine, it is essential to recognize that the health status of the patient is the ultimate source of information, for each patient is a living textbook.

■ *Don't be overconfident.* Make it your policy to call for help when you need it. Don't even think of proceeding unsupervised beyond your level of competence. If you do, you may regret it, if you run into an unforeseen difficulty and then need help.

■ *Proceed promptly.* Respond immediately if called about a patient who is in an intensive care unit. See them even if their vital signs are reported to be stable if something else is or seems amiss. For other patients, visit them as soon as possible. Try to avoid medical management by phone, because it presents too many risks of overlooking important clinical signals and signs.

■ *Ascertain the facts.* When you receive an on-call message, secure the patient's full name, exact location, attending physician's name, diagnosis, and current therapy and a clear brief description of the immediate problem. This information can provide a basis for considering further action, even as you proceed to the patient's bedside.

■ *Speak carefully.* Be discrete in your discussion of patients' cases in areas where privacy is lacking. You may be overheard by a family member or stranger who may misconstrue your remarks as disparaging, or you may inadvertently reveal medical information that may turn out to be unnecessarily alarming. Any such comments can reflect badly on you and your attending physician.

■ *Be courteous.* This policy is applicable under all circumstances (e.g., in the emergency or operating room as well as in a patient's room or on rounds). Courtesy is obviously mandated in your dealing with attendings and fellow house staff physicians, as well as with all patients and supporting personnel (e.g., nurses, technicians). This is true even under very trying or seemingly justifiable circumstances, such as when being deliberately provoked. Courtesy is an essential part of professional behavior and it will enhance your status at the institutions.

■ *Avoid arrogance.* Although you, as a resident, certainly rank higher than a nurse or technician, their fund of practical knowledge obtained from extensive experience may be superior to yours in specific areas. Take advantage of any input they provide and act upon it appropriately, in the context of your own medical knowledge.

■ *Start early.* When possible, arrange to see patients early in the day, so that you can formulate suggestions for treatment plans. Later you can compare your judgment with that of the attendings as well as offering thoughtful comments on rounds. This approach can prove to be an educationally meaningful exercise and can improve your clinical judgment as well as self-confidence.

■ *Access data efficiently.* Successfully managing patients' illnesses requires, among other things, securing data regarding relevant laboratory and diagnostic tests. Obtaining this information by computer can save much time and effort, which can be expended on other worthwhile tasks. It is important to make sure the data are as up-to-date and as complete as possible.

■ *Set a routine.* When possible, schedule routine activities at fixed intervals (e.g., securing lab reports at convenient regular times). This will make overly long "must do" lists unnecessary. Moreover, even if you can't achieve the task at its set time, you will better remember that this element of your routine is incomplete. Also, try to schedule all activities on the same floor for completion when you are there, so that you aren't moving unnecessarily back and forth between floors.

■ *Get sleep when possible.* Whenever time allows, try to take an undisturbed catnap. This is especially desirable if you will be on-call at night, when you may not always have a chance to nap when you would like.

■ *Exercise whenever possible.* Use even short free time intervals as opportunities to exercise moderately. Exercise can lower your level of stress and fatigue and allow you to get through the day (or night) better.

■ *Use discretion.* Respond to patient questions about medical progress, biopsy results, discharge date, or disease diagnosis with the suggestion that it would be best for the individual or family member to obtain such information from their attending physician. This may make you feel uncomfortable, but it is better than being admonished or contradicted by an attending physician or a senior house staff member and thereby losing face in the eyes of the patient or their family.

■ *Act with consideration.* If special circumstances (e.g., an acute illness, an important family affair) necessitate your early departure from the hospital, don't leave without appropriate notification. Make sure that your essential responsibilities are met and that a senior house staff member knows your plans, so that all your patients will be covered. You can generally expect a sympathetic response from your colleagues and superiors under such special circumstances.

■ *Communicate.* Discuss your activities with fellow residents. It may turn out that they have a more efficient way to carry out tasks, or you may be of help to some of them. In any case, it strengthens the bond of fellowship and cooperation within the treatment team by sharing ideas and experiences.

■ *Obtain feedback.* Try to discreetly ascertain from attendings and senior house staff how well you are doing. Soliciting constructive input will indicate how sincere you are in wanting to enhance your knowledge and skills. Positive comments will also encourage you when things are difficult. Any negative comments should induce you to work harder, ascertain your deficiencies, and thus improve your performance.

■ *Eat appropriately.* Treat your body with respect. Eat healthful and wholesome food. Coffee and junk food are not substitutes for meals. Mealtime may also be an ideal opportunity for taking a break and socializing with others. Avoid talking shop whenever possible when taking time out.

■ *Join a support group.* Your long days and nights will not only be physically stressful, but emotionally trying as well. In the course of your activities, things may go badly at times; you may make some mistakes; patients may be troublesome; senior staff may come down hard on you. Expressing your feelings in the context of a compassionate and discreet support group may go a long way to relieve the tension that tends to build up under trying working conditions.

■ *Remain in touch.* Remember that beyond your job there are people with whom you have to stay in contact for your own social survival, for example, your husband/wife, children, parents, and close friends. Use free time to place the calls that help maintain relationships. You will feel much better after doing so.

■ *Educate appropriately.* When at home, give your family the full benefit of your presence. Try to save some of your reading, although important, for the nights. Also, change your hospital uniform (e.g., scrubs) so that you don't bring the job atmosphere home with you.

■ *Be organized.* This key piece of advice should be the hallmark of your activities. Use a prioritized "must do" list, preferably made up each night, as your guide. However, be flexible when circumstances require. This will help keep your head above water even at times when the demands are most intense.

■ *Learning is the key.* Medical students come from an educational background where the emphasis is placed on grades and academic achievement in order to advance one's career. This approach to gaining knowledge can become an ingrained habit. For those planning to treat patients, the critical factor is achieving the depth of knowledge that comes from genuine learning. This will make a vital difference when it comes to saving lives. Patients will never ask for your transcript, Board scores, or evaluations. They will judge you by the work you do how you go about doing it and the quality of the help you provide them.

15 | Protecting Your Assets

Overview

Residency places heavy demands on physicians-in-training, not only intellectually but also physically and emotionally. The work schedule is usually very lengthy and interruptions in the daily routine are frequent. Sleep-deprived nights are quite common. Consequently, it is essential to advise residents, in spite of the fact that they are physicians, to pay careful attention to both their physical and emotional well-being. This should be done both out of self-interest and out of concern for the welfare of their patients. Consequently, this chapter will discuss the various issues relevant to maintaining one's good health during the lengthy rigors of postgraduate training. Consciously training yourself to guard your health will prove to be a constructive habit. Moreover, it may carry over into your later years when you are in practice and thus may prove a rewarding adopted trait to facilitate maintaining your well-being throughout your life.

Guarding and maintaining your physical health

There are many elements that will help protect your physical health, namely, proper nutrition, adequate sleep, adequate exercise, infection precautions, safety precautions, and illness precautions. Each of these factors will be discussed separately.

Nutrition. There are a number of reasons that residents are prone to be subjected to poor nutrition. These include (a) lack of sleep and stress (factors that suppress the appetite), (b) the tendency to eat junk food, (c) dissatisfaction with hospital menus, and (d) the frequent inability to find time to eat three wholesome meals daily.

A number of reasonable suggestions have been made that facilitate active individuals obtaining the essential nutrition that will provide a good energy level and avoid drastic weight alterations. The suggestions for sound nutrition include the following:

■ Focus your eating habits on maintaining a balanced diet consisting of 35% carbohydrate, no more than 30% fat, and about 35% protein.

■ Arrange for an adequate intake of complex carbohydrates (e.g., rice, potatoes, cereals), while reducing intake of simple carbohydrates.

■ Diminish usage of caffeine, alcohol, and fatty foods as much as possible.

■ Eat an adequate amount of food with a high fiber content to maintain regularity.

■ Supplement your diet with fruits and vegetables and vitamins when appropriate (e.g., when meals are skipped).

■ Drink adequate amounts of fluids at varying times during the day to avoid dehydration.

■ It may be helpful in securing proper nourishment to switch to eating multiple small meals each day, rather than three large ones.

■ Make use of healthful snacks between meals, such as dried fruits, nuts, and graham crackers, as well as fruits and vegetables.

Sleep. Unquestionably, the major factor generating stress and fatigue among residents is sleep deprivation. This is due to the requirement for on-call service that mandates being duty-bound for 36 consecutive hours at regular intervals (usually every second or third day). Sleep during such intervals is usually limited and frequently interrupted by requests to provide medical assistance for assigned patients.

The need for adequate amounts of sleep to perform responsibly on the job, has been established for many professionals holding demanding positions (e.g., airline pilots). To maintain essential cognitive and motor skills, a minimum of five hours of sleep is absolutely essential. Evidence suggests that residents lacking adequate sleep and suffering from fatigue manifest a variety of symptoms, such as irritability, inability to concentrate, reduced fine motor skills, and a decline in accuracy. The impact of such deficiencies on residents, even if only transient, and the concomitant increase in danger to patients are quite obvious.

In spite of these facts, residents are still exposed to a prolonged, exceedingly demanding training system that makes them susceptible to becoming impaired. The reason for the existing situation is that medical institutions view the current state of affairs as being in their economic self-interest and also because it is a long-standing tradition of postgraduate training. However, it is possible that if residents were routinely granted more humane working hours, their efficiency would be higher and consequently their productivity improved. Such an enlightened situation would be fiscally advantageous for hospitals as well as of great benefit to patients and residents alike.

The fact is, however, that many, if not most, postgraduate training programs have an excessively demanding schedule. Thus, it is in your own best interest to take reasonable measures that will facilitate maximizing your opportunities for sleep when you are on-call. This is important because it has been shown that a significant number of beeper pages of residents are unnecessary. (Moreover, responding to some of these night calls may inadvertently result in waking up other patients in the room and may be counterproductive, an unfortunate side effect of hospital life.)

The following *general* suggestions can facilitate a resident's opportunity to meet their responsibilities when being on-call at night, while at the same time facilitate securing needed rest:

■ Where possible, try to obtain the privacy of your own room, with access to a phone and bathroom.

■ Seek to arrange, if possible, with the head nurse to screen all after-hours pages, prior to your being contacted. This request should not be considered as an imposition, but rather a request for cooperation in order to more effectively utilizing your time and efforts.

■ Secure the help of the ancillary staff to do as much of the 'scut work' as is appropriate during the day. This will lessen the burden on the resident during the night when support staff are usually not available.

■ Try to arrange, where possible, for split shift coverage with another resident. As a result you will be on-call only part of the night and thus you may be able to get at least a minimum of uninterrupted sleep during a 36-hour on-call shift.

■ See if you can arrange to be paired with another on-call resident, with each of you handling a specific set of chores. This will make the demands on you less burdensome. With this arrangement, you will be spared responsibility for multiple major activities that may arise simultaneously during one time frame.

There are some *specific* suggestions on how most effectively to handle on-call requests for your services:

■ Secure a well-written manual providing step-by-step on-call management procedures.

■ Provide yourself with reliable pocket manuals for differential diagnosis and treatment.

■ Be certain that your pager is operational; to do so, check its status periodically.

■ Become fully cognizant of any special problems associated with specific patients by comments made at evening rounds prior to sign-out time. This will help prepare you for potential difficulties you might anticipate during the night.

■ Be certain that you understand the instructions given to you by the senior resident at sign-out time. If not, seek clarification before they depart for the evening.

■ Prioritize your list of the sickest patients on your service, so that if called on their behalf, you might anticipate what to expect.

■ Make a list of scut work assignments that await your attention. These should be carried out in a prioritized and efficient manner. It may prove worthwhile to do all your work on the same floor and then move on to the next floor.

■ Establish an understanding with your supervising resident as to under what circumstances you should call for advice and how best to contact them.

■ When contacted by a nurse, ask if they feel that the patient should be seen. If in doubt, whenever possible, do so, to avoid any regrets later.

■ When called to a patient's bedside, use the opportunity, after resolving the existing problem, to inquire if he/she has any other serious patient problems, thus possibly avoiding the need for a return visit.

■ Write a brief note in the chart for every patient seen, for both medical and legal reasons. Indicate any issues the patient may have raised that need attention, but could not be taken care of during the night, so that follow-up care can take place during the daytime. If especially important, also report verbally during the change in shift on the need for action on a specific patient problem, so that it is not overlooked.

■ When you become aware of a potentially serious medical situation, take care of it promptly whenever possible. Such preventive activity is obviously far more effective and preferable to treatment later on.

■ After seeing a patient, advise the nurse precisely what, if anything else, needs to be done and under what circumstances you wish to be contacted again.

■ If provided with an accompanying medical student, utilize their presence to assist you with your work, while at the same time providing some useful instruction to such individuals to enhance their learning experiences.

■ Systematically organize your essential activities for the night, so that, if possible, you meet the needs of your assigned patients as well as processing all lab reports and x-rays in a sequential manner.

■ To be better prepared to handle a challenging situation into which you have been called, review the steps you anticipate taking in your mind on the way to the patient's room. You will then be better ready to apply them, should you confirm that a situation exists that warrants its application.

■ In admitting patients via the E.R., it is desirable, if time permits, to do the work-up there as well as writing orders, some of which may be carried out from that facility.

■ If you see a patient admitted via the E.R., do not rely on the admitting officer's work-up and tentative diagnosis, but do your own. This is because you may have to justify your recommendations regarding patient management at the morning report.

▪ Keep concise, accurate notes of the important events of the night (e.g., new admissions, critical patients, transfers) so that those can be reported in the morning.

▪ Be prepared to fully report all major events to the incoming treatment team in a concise fashion prior to signing out.

Exercise. The time limitations of residents and the fact they frequently suffer from fatigue does not usually permit them to set intervals for exercise during their busy daily schedule. Nevertheless, it should be possible to incorporate in your schedule this vital activity, even if only to a limited extent. To this end, spending about half an hour several times a week doing exercise can counter the effects of stress and anxiety, as well as enhancing one's well-being physically and emotionally in a number of other ways.

There are a variety of ways to obtain adequate exercise that residents find useful. These include walking or running to work or not using elevators and favoring stairs (except when time is critical). These activities can be supplemented by working out with an exercise bicycle or treadmill. Some find it possible to utilize a swimming pool where they live or even at the hospital where they work. Others will try to manage to periodically visit a gym for a workout.

To supplement standard exercise activities, for which opportunities may not always exist, one should secure information regarding one or more of a variety of breathing exercises, some of which can be quite simple. These can assist in reducing the tensions that daily activity of a resident traditionally entails.

Infection precautions. While working in a hospital, residents are exposed to a variety of viral and bacterial agents, as well as other hazards. These can be quite dangerous to your health, and thus appropriate precautions must be taken to guard against unforeseen contamination.

These precautions fall into the categories of both active and passive.

ACTIVE PRECAUTIONS. This involves making sure that you have had all the required vaccinations, including the following:

▪ Diphtheria and tetanus (DDT) booster. If more than a 10-year gap exists, you need revaccination.

▪ Polio, measles, and rubella. This is necessary if you have not been previously vaccinated or have had exposure to the disease.

▪ Influenza vaccination. This is advised for those with special health risks.

▪ Mumps vaccination. This is recommended for those who were never protected from or exposed to the disease.

▪ Hepatitis B specifically, but hepatitis A vaccination is also desirable.

The following two tests should be done when appropriate:

- For tuberculosis status, using the tuberculin skin test.
- For susceptibility to rubella, for female residents.

PASSIVE PRECAUTIONS

- In dealing with blood and most body fluids, the universal precaution of wearing gloves and thorough hand-washing is *essential*.

- When possibly subject to radiation exposure, maintain an adequate distance from x-ray equipment, both fixed and portable. Wearing a radiation meter will serve to alert you to any dangers.

- When required to do heavy lifting (e.g., patients, equipment), ask for help and be sure to lift properly to protect your back.

- When using equipment, be certain that it is in good working order and is being maintained properly.

- Check to be certain that equipment that should be disinfected or sterilized before use has been properly cared for.

- Be especially careful when using needles. Never recap them, because this may cause stick injuries. Dispose of all used needles (and other sharp objects such as scalpel blades) in a container designated for such items.

- If a needle stick inadvertently happens, then allow bleeding to take place. Wash the injured body part with soap and water, disinfect with alcohol, and promptly seek follow-up treatment at the appropriate hospital site.

- If it is necessary to attach scalpel blades, do so with the aid of an instrument.

- Where infection of a patient, bacterial or viral, is suspected, appropriate isolation and hand-washing procedures should be stringently observed.

Safety precautions. The occurrence of violence at a hospital unfortunately is commonplace. Your work environment can unexpectedly become dangerous to patients and staff alike. What becomes public knowledge is only headline-grabbing committed acts, not threats of harm. In response to this situation, safety programs have been introduced at health care institutions and facilities and security precautions have been significantly enhanced. This proactive stance has markedly helped improve the safety situation at many hospitals. To this end, the number of security personnel at hospitals has considerably increased, metal detectors have been installed at strategic locations, and personnel, including physicians, have been instructed on how to deal with the possibility of violence. These measures have been supplemented by the use of TV monitors and electronic identification cards. The key element in enhancing personal security, however, is to learn how to anticipate dangerous situations and recognize and where possible avoid poor safety locations.

Obviously, there are no guaranties of absolute safety anywhere. Thus you should not assume that you are immune to the dangers of workplace violence at your own facility. There are some distinct steps you can take to make yourself less vulnerable. These are as follows:

■ Recognize that wearing a stethoscope (or necklace) around your neck, or having hair tied in a ponytail, provides aggressors with a readily available place to grab you.

■ Similarly, carrying exposed scissors or wearing a tie can be risky, especially in a high-crime setting. Thus, borrowing scissors when needed and utilizing a clip-on tie may be advisable, for circumstances that warrant such precautionary measures.

■ Seek to carry out patient physical examinations in a well-lit setting. Proceed to do so in a nonprovocative manner and, if you are suspicious, that the patient has any hidden, dangerous items in their possession, always have someone with you at such times.

■ When involved in a blood-related procedure on an agitated patient, obtain the assistance of another individual to prevent complications, should the patient became unruly. Apply physical restraint if necessary, but be aware of hospital rules regarding this procedure.

■ When in doubt as to the stability of a patient's state of mind, call for a staff member's assistance and, when appropriate, advise security personnel.

■ If an unstable situation develops, seek to avoid escalating it into a major incident.

■ Tactfully sidestep provoking a patient, since you cannot foresee their reaction. This means not being condescending or expressing your frustration with them, even when you have the right to feel that way.

■ Do not touch or point at an angry patient, since this may possibly ellicit an unexpected angry response that can accelerate a minor issue into a full-blown conflict.

■ When a dangerous situation appears imminent, promptly discontinue an interview or physical exam in progress and leave the area and/or signal for help.

■ Be knowledgeable about security code protocols and the location of alarm buzzers and video cameras.

■ When genuinely concerned about the state of affairs securitywise, position yourself closer to an exit than your patient, so that you can make a quick retreat before the situation becomes more dangerous.

Illness precautions. As noted above, bring yourself up to date as regards vaccinations. This is important for both your and your patients' well-being. The other vital factors, such as proper nutrition, adequate sleep, and exercise, discussed earlier, will similarly contribute significantly to maintaining your health while you are serving as a resident.

It is also important for you to seek appropriate medical attention at the first sign of any significant illness. This will thus avoid more serious complications that could result in disruption of your personal and teamwork schedule, as well as possibly jeopardizing the welfare of colleagues and patients. The latter obviously are especially susceptible to illness because of their potentially weakened condition.

It is also essential to guard against the impact of stress and fatigue on your physical health. The excessive burden of professional pressures can be reflected by an increased amount of smoking and greater usage of alcohol and even experimenting with drugs. The impact of such behavior on one's physical and emotional well-being is obvious. It will clearly impact one's physical health, both in the short and long term, and also one's capacity to function intellectually at an optimal level.

In light of the serious detrimental effect's of substance abuse, it is critical to recognize the warning signs of such behavior. Some of these are as follows:

■ Excessive alcohol consumption on days off, when one feels liberated.

■ The tendency to deny overuse of alcohol or drugs, when it is certain.

■ Secretive use of addictive substances, so that others do not become suspicious.

■ Increased radical mood swings or personality changes over short intervals.

■ Greater frequency of unjustified interpersonal conflicts with colleagues, patients and family.

■ Experiencing physical discomfort characteristic of overuse of alcohol or drugs.

■ Repeated failure to curtail or terminate usage of alcohol or drugs, in spite of genuine attempts to do so.

■ Seeking to rationalize the abuse of substances as being only an essential short-term expedient.

■ Developing an evident inability to control one's negative behavior habits.

■ Increased unsatisfactory performance at work, such as excessive lateness and absences.

■ Excessive frequency of unquestionable or poor judgment as reflected in errors in one's personal and professional activities.

Guarding your mental health

The intense demands of the residency experience on an individual's physical and mental health have been emphasized repeatedly. Having discussed ways to protect your physical health in the preceding segments, we can now focus on doing the same for your mental health.

Stress and fatigue are major factors challenging your well-being during the course of a residency. You can anticipate having to carry increasingly weighty responsibilities as, over time, you move up the ladder to a higher status and need, at times, to make major if not critical medical decisions. Among the most difficult emotional situations that occur is when one needs you to transmit bad news to patients or their families or to respond to the death of a patient. They are commonplace events in a hospital setting. These are emotionally very trying situations for all concerned. For private patients, the attending physician usually is responsible for carrying the burden in such situations. For public patients, residents will be the principals involved in facing such emotionally difficult challenges as communicating bad news and losing a patient who is under your care, two issues that will now be discussed in greater detail.

Communicating bad news. When you are delegated or required to deliver bad medical news to a patient, the following guidelines should prove helpful. Bad news may take many forms. It may involve a lengthy period of hospitalization, the necessity for major surgery, a need for a drastic change in life-style or career activity, or the existence of an incurable disease.

■ Prepare yourself before any such meeting. Clearly know what you wish to say and how to phrase your remarks. Think of any questions you may be asked by the patient, and how you might respond to them.

■ Make sure you have adequate time in your schedule to spend with the patient when imparting bad news. Avoid giving the impression that you are pressed for time or wish to be through with this unpleasant chore.

■ Sit down to talk with the patient in comfortable, private surroundings.

■ Before breaking the news, prepare the patient somewhat by indicating that your task is to carry a distressing message with to regard his/her medical condition.

■ Be straightforward when presenting the bad news, but avoid being blunt or procrastinating in your remarks by an extended preface before you get to the point.

■ Used lay person's language to explain the situation and to clarify any medical terms that must be used, and make certain that they are understood by the patient.

■ Observe the patient as to the nature of their reaction and response to your comments.

■ Allow the patient to express themselves fully, both emotionally and verbally.

■ Respond to all questions honestly and for those that do not have definite answers, say so. For questions that require you to secure a response from another source, advise the patient that you will get back to them with an answer as soon as possible.

■ Advise the patient that they can feel free to be contact you if they wish to do so, and that you plan to see them again quite soon.

■ Do not leave the patient alone if they appear agitated or distraught. Call someone in to stay with them if you must leave for some urgent task.

■ Ask the nursing staff to give extra attention to the patient for the balance of their stay.

■ Keep all your commitments to and reactions about the patient confidential, even if you have been rotated onto a different service.

Losing a patient. The second special emotionally draining issue is the loss of a patient who was on your service and while you were on duty. To reduce the psychological impact on yourself, after confirming the patient's demise, you are well advised to do the following:

■ Pause for a few moments to meditate on the limitation of every physician's capacity to heal and the ultimate fragility of human beings as living entities.

■ Express genuine condolences to any family member who may be present.

■ Be sensitive to any religious or cultural customs applicable under the circumstances.

■ If family members are absent, determine from the nursing staff if they know how to contact them.

■ Contact the supervising attending physician, advise them of what occurred, and inquire as to their preference as to who should contact the family.

■ If you are elected to speak with a family member, identify yourself and seek to speak to the next of kin. Indicate the extent of your prior contact with the patient and inform them of what has transpired and when. Point out that you believe all the appropriate medical care that could be provided was indeed given and express regret that the patient could not be saved.

■ Inquire if the next of kin will be coming in and advise the nursing staff accordingly.

■ Make sure to record in the patient's chart the date and time you confirmed the patient's passing and your clinical findings. Find out who will be responsible for completing the death certificate.

■ Take a short but adequate break, before you resume your routine activities. If you feel distressed, you may wish to be alone or to talk to your mentor, a colleague, or a member of the clergy about your recent sad experience.

Maintaining your mental health

From the above, it is clear that the routine activities of a resident can be emotionally very demanding. For some, the stress may be intense enough to generate a sense of emotional unease. This may be reflected by feeling distraught or overwhelmed.

Stress, fatigue, heavy responsibilities, lack of sleep, facing trying emotional situations, and making challenging decisions, as well as possible clinical failures and mistakes, may over time take their toll. To combat such a negative situation requires utilization of one or more of three approaches: (a) reduce sources of stress, (b) seek support services, and (c) strengthen family and social contacts. Each of these avenues of assistance will be discussed individually.

Reduce sources of stress. The following suggestions on possible ways to reduce stress are applicable even for those who do not feel distressed, but certainly for those who do.

■ Find a personal residence as close as possible to the hospital you are affiliated with. This will minimize travel time, ensure your availability at special times of need, reduce lateness, and facilitate getting home quickly after a hard day or night's work. Such an arrangement allows you to maximize your chances for eating properly and securing adequate sleep, key factors in diffusing stress.

■ Seek, if possible, schedule a long weekend that incorporates a statutory holiday. If this is done well in advance. Chances are that you are likely to get the time off. This will give you something to look forward to. It can serve to reduce the tension generated by a long spell of uninterrupted activity as a resident.

■ If you have the option, seek your program director's cooperation, as early as possible, in scheduling your rotations so that they will alternate between strenuous and less challenging ones.

■ Where a choice of services is possible, get input on attendings and chief residents as to which prospective and pedagogically attractive supervisors to work under. Try to be assigned to their services. Working under them is likely to place you in a less stressful environment.

■ Where feasible and appropriate, consider undertaking an elective or special project that particularly appeals to you. The challenge and novelty will likely raise your spirits and serve to counteract stress stimulated on other services. Make the necessary arrangements with your program director and confirm them in writing.

■ Prioritize your tasks and problems and address them in due course accordingly. You should feel a sense of accomplishment when they have been completed.

■ When possible, subdivide large problems into smaller more manageable tasks. These then should also be solved in a prioritized manner.

■ Utilize your time as efficiently as possible by budgeting it appropriately.

■ Don't overextend yourself with an excessive number of scheduled activities or underestimate the time each of them may require and thus become overwhelmed.

■ Be flexible in meeting needed changes in planned activities due to unexpected altered circumstances.

■ Recognize that some stressful situations are beyond your control and are thus unavoidable. Under these circumstances it is best to accept such unfortunate circumstances in a calm fashion, realizing that they are of a transitory nature.

■ Actively avoid, when possible, stressful situations that you may be aware of in advance (e.g., the need to cram for exams, last-minute preparation of case presentations).

■ Accept positive rotation evaluations of your performance as meaningful evidence confirming your ability and progress in the program. Any negative evaluation should serve to stimulate your efforts to improve and should not be viewed as an inherent professional weakness on your part.

■ Become familiar with the residents' union contract. Carefully reading a copy will allow you to become aware of the prerogatives you are entitled to. This knowledge may improve your attitudes regarding your rights and responsibilities.

■ When especially frustrated, be good to yourself by indulging in some meaningful source of pleasure (e.g., a favorite meal, a long-distance call to a friend with whom you haven't spoken in a while, or a swim at a pool). This type of self-indulgent activity may serve to lighten your spirits.

■ Plot forthcoming major events in your life on a one-year calendar. These should include both personal events (e.g., birthdays of important people, vacation days) and professional events (e.g., rotation changes, exam dates). Crossing off each day will make you feel you are nearing each event step by step and that the end of the road is not so far away, after all.

■ Remember that you are entitled to days off due to illness. If the pressures are too intense, you may wish to take a day off for rest and relaxation. You should, however, bear in mind its impact on the schedules of your colleagues who would have to fill in for you. Thus, try to schedule such time off appropriately and judiciously.

■ Should you genuinely feel that you need more extensive free time to regain your mental and emotional equilibrium, check if your program has any provisions for a leave of absence. If this is essential, discuss such a possibility with your program director.

■ If you are disillusioned with your residency program to the point where you wish to opt out of it, seek the guidance of your mentor. If they concur with your judgment, see if you can identify a suitable vacancy elsewhere. If so, try to see if a transfer can be arranged with a minimum of inconvenience for all concerned.

Seek support services. In times of difficulty, keeping to yourself when you believe you are in physical and emotional turmoil can compound the situation. It will make it more difficult to handle and resolve the problem in an objective manner. This is because the distressed individual may be too self-centered to be capable of making the most objective decision or choosing the best course of action. Thus, input and advice from relevant professionals can be most helpful in putting the real troubling issues into proper perspective and in providing useful guidance on how to remedy them.

Residents who are aware of and acknowledge the existence of serious personal problems, can seek assistance from a variety of individuals and even some organizations. Some of these sources of help will be discussed briefly.

Advisor/mentor. While in medical school, you undoubtedly had contact with an advisor/mentor. If your choice was appropriate, and relationship congenial, then you undoubtedly benefited from the relationship. The same can be equally true for the role of an advisor/mentor during your residency. You may be assigned one or need to find such a person yourself. If the latter is the case, ask the program director or chief resident for suggestions of possible suitable individuals. The following criteria will help define the person you should seek:

■ Someone whose clinical interests are similar to yours and whom you feel especially comfortable with.

■ Someone who has the credentials, experience, and desire to serve in this capacity.

■ Someone who can serve as a role model and is patient, flexible, and nonjudgmental in attitude.

■ Someone who has the time to provide you with guidance that you may seek during your residency, and would be sympathetic to your state of being.

■ Someone who has the connections to facilitate your securing a subspecialty or fellowship, should you so desire. Thus he/she can stimulate you.

Personal physician. It is valuable for a resident to have a personal physician and establish a meaningful relationship with them. By this means you may have a medical professional with whom you will feel at ease in terms of discussing your serious personal concerns. To rely on hospital staff may limit the extent to which you can communicate about issues that are very intimate. A suitable personal physician can make an initial assessment of your situation and then make valuable suggestions as to how best to resolve any difficult situation.

Clergy. It will serve your long-term interests to establish a relationship with a member of the hospital's affiliated clergy of your faith. In the care of critically ill patients, ethical as well as nonmedical issues frequently arise. These can have an impact on one's emotional state. Such circumstances may arise from the possible occurrence of medical errors or the need to communicate bad news to patients or after confirming a patient's death. Having periodic discussions with knowledgeable clergy can help reduce stress and provide guidance in areas of ethical concern. Such a person can also prove helpful when you feel emotionally distressed, by serving as a sounding board as well as an ethical lighthouse.

Resident support group. A support group can help diffuse some of the tension associated with being in a residency program. The fact that others share your own trials and tribulations can be a strong source of consolation. Moreover, this group can be a means of establishing friendships with like-minded individuals. There is a need for openness, to discard the sense of competition and feelings of omnipotence that are common among residents. A support group of sympathetic residents can serve as an ideal forum to discuss issues of self-doubt, feelings of lack of adequacy, and inner signs of anxiety. An open exchange of views will provide an opportunity for ventilating your thoughts and emotions. You may find that you are not alone and perhaps may secure some sound advice as how to cope with your problems as well as how to put them into proper perspective. The effectiveness of such support groups depends in part on senior residents acting as role models for their junior colleagues. They can also serve to generate an atmosphere where other residents feel comfortable in discussing common experiences and in expressing their concerns and feelings. Such group meetings can also provide practical opportunities to arrange to cover for others when circumstances warrant and to reciprocate in turn. Such meetings also allow planning social activities that are of common interest. Groups of varied makeup, such as an all-women groups, and spouses' groups are also useful means of retaining a sense of community.

Strengthening family and social contacts. Family and social contacts are another pillar of importance in maintaining one's mental health during residency. A resident's unique work environment can serve to establish an invisible barrier to their prior relatively normal life. By focusing primarily on gaining knowledge and experience in the context of caring for the sick, one can unfortunately lose sight of other vital elements of life. This is compounded by being disconnected at regular intervals from home and society, especially when on night call. Given these circumstances, it is imperative to maximize the use of available time to strengthen one's interpersonal contacts. This will serve not only to help maintain a healthy perspective, but also to secure emotional support and moral encouragement.

The impact of the disruption of normal social life caused by the demands of residency in large measure depends on one's marital status. It will thus be briefly discussed from this perspective.

Unmarried residents. The effect on single residents of their intense professional life-style, places them at greater risk of stress-related problems. This is the result of a higher degree of social isolation than for married individuals. Limited free time and the need to maximize rest, as well as being responsible solely for maintaining one's household, obviously contribute to the problem. All of these obligations limit the extent of a single resident's social contacts. Because residents have left their home base in medical school after four years, for a new environment and possibly also a new city, their available social contacts are initially limited.

Some possibly helpful suggestions to enhance the situation follow:

■ Maintain maximum contact with the outside world. This can be facilitated by means of an answering machine and beeper.

■ Seek to expose yourself to the society that you are in a position to meet. Thus, participate in hospital social events and join special interest groups (even if you can't participate fully).

■ Keep up your family ties in person, by phone, and by e-mail. Do not procrastinate in responding to outside communications.

■ Consider sharing an apartment with a compatible person who can accommodate your special professional needs and who is willing to share the burden of maintaining the facility in a comfortable, livable condition.

■ Schedule your potential free time to coincide with that of friends whom you can join for social activities.

Married residents. Being a resident has a profound effect on the life of a couple. It has the potential to produce serious strains in the relationship. There are numerous factors contributing to this situation. These include frequent absence, fatigue when present, uncertainty as to the future, substantial debt, and being located in a strange place. This situation is obviously compounded significantly when a resident is distressed by their activities, thereby lowering their compatibility threshold.

Another complicating factor is that many spouses of residents are themselves working, thus scheduling quality time to share is difficult to arrange. Unfortunately, the nature of their work and pressures on residents may generate temporary personality changes that can contribute to the deterioration of a relationship. Finally, the demanding chore of running a household and raising children can be a major source of tension and conflict.

Some suggestions on reducing difficulties among married couples are as follows:

■ Arrange to go out socially on a regular basis and seek to share other pleasurable activities together.

■ In a one-physician household, discuss your activities in lay person's terms, but only as a component of other shared conversations.

■ Lay out your schedule in full, to the best of your knowledge, in advance, so that your mate knows when to expect you. Call your home if an issue arises and you can't meet a commitment.

■ Schedule chores as equitably as possible, bearing in mind your mutual schedules.

■ Come home promptly when you have signed out from the hospital.

■ Minimize calling the hospital when off duty. Do so only when it is essential. In other words, don't bring your work home with you.

■ When possible, stay in contact with your mate during the day over the phone.

■ Try to share dinner at your worksite together during on-call nights. This can somewhat compensate for your absence.

■ When returning home from a difficult and tiring day, acknowledge your experience and physical/emotional state to your mate, so that he/she may be more understanding.

■ Arrange for periodic discussion with your mate of existing problems, concerns, and upcoming short- and long-term plans that you both can look forward to.

■ Strongly encourage mutual continuation of prior family and social contacts of both spouses.

16 | Professional Challenges Facing Residents

Overview

Although patient care is the principal focus of residency activities, it simultaneously entails expanding the depth of your education and gradually assuming greater professional responsibilities. This chapter will therefore discuss how to maximize learning and how to meet teaching obligations as you move up the house staff ranks. While carrying out their duties, residents frequently must face up to ethical and legal challenges that can impact their performance and themselves. These topics will also be considered in this chapter. Finally, considerations relative to gender, religious views, and life-style and their impact on residency will be discussed.

The resident as a student

Medical school serves to provide prospective interns primarily with the fundamentals of the basic sciences and an introduction to the clinical sciences. In-depth education and training in a specialty, however, are provided only during the course of a residency. Whereas in medical school learning takes place in the classroom and hospital wards, during residency it occurs in hospital wards and in outpatient clinics.

Your clinical experience during the course of a residency will focus on four aspects:

■ *Learning by observation and participation.* This takes place during rounds when diagnoses, treatment plans, patient progress, and prognoses are discussed.

■ *Learning by performing tasks.* This involves carrying out, frequently under supervision, procedures usually relevant to the specialty.

■ *Learning by listening.* This occurs during the course of conferences when medical topics are discussed in depth by attending physicians, visiting specialists, and house staff.

■ *Learning by self-education.* This involves the use of a wide range of resources: texts, journals, audiotapes, videotapes, online Web sites, abstract services, etc.

The last learning approach mentioned is of special importance, for it is the key to continuing education, a most essential element in keeping a physician's knowledge up-to-date. Moreover, each resident is aware of areas of knowledge which they believe need reinforcement. They can call upon the resources enumerated to provide them with the information sought. Finally, residents themselves are called upon to make presentations on selected topics and therefore must utilize reference material to satisfactorily achieve this goal.

To enhance your learning, the following suggestions may prove useful:

■ If during the course of rounds useful knowledge is offered, make a note of it so that the information is available for future reference.

■ Become a subscriber to at least one major journal in your field of specialization.

■ When scanning journals, pay particular attention to recent review articles. These will be a sound source for obtaining in-depth, current, and comprehensive information on relevant topics.

■ When possible, read up on the topic to be discussed prior to a lecture or conference. The information presented will likely then be more meaningful.

■ Utilize appropriate pocket manuals to obtain on-the-spot information while on duty.

■ Use the occasion of leading a grand rounds presentation to focus on a topic that would be both of general interest to the audience and of special interest to yourself.

■ Utilize synopses of comprehensive texts to obtain relative quick reviews of a subject.

■ Seek to learn by asking questions at rounds. Showing interest in gaining knowledge will also leave a favorable impression on your supervisors.

In the course of your residency, you will need to take exams. Some advice in preparing for these challenges is as follows:

- Secure early on a schedule of written and oral exams from the departmental office.

- Set aside a specific time for study and whenever possible, try to stick to that schedule.

- Inquire from senior residents as to the nature of the examinations given previously. This will help familiarize you with what to expect.

- If it fits into your learning style, join a study group, which may facilitate your learning.

- Begin studying with the relevant topics you are most knowledgeable about or most comfortable with. Productive learning reinforces your self-confidence and encourages moving on to more difficult topics.

- Try to master a subject in its logical framework, rather than as distinct blocks of knowledge and/or data. By this means your retention of information should be better.

- Make use of study techniques that have worked for you on previous exams that are similar to those you anticipate taking.

- Allow some study time for review of the basic sciences that are relevant to your specialty.

- Incorporate into your study plan reading about specific common cases as well as some rare ones.

- Be aware that the patients you care for on your service may be chosen as case presentations on exams. Carrying out a thorough work-up, followed by some relevant reading, will help prepare you for such eventualities.

- Bear in mind a resident's limited time and that you will tend to be fatigued by day's end. You should, therefore, pace study activities to be consistent with your physical and mental state. Efficient study is productive, facilitating both absorption and retention of information.

- Focus your efforts on problem-solving, rather than memorization. This should enhance your exam performance.

- Seek to comprehend the subject at hand before trying to commit it to memory.

- Remember that knowledge associated with concepts or principles is retained more readily than isolated facts.

- After a solid study session, get a good night's sleep. Your chances for retention of the material are thereby increased.

- A major aspect of retention is repetition. Short reviews of the material will enhance achieving this goal.

■ Avoid cramming for exams. This feeling of inadequacy of knowledge can induce pretest anxiety.

The resident as a teacher

The postgraduate medical education system is predicated on a policy of sharing knowledge, with the more senior members teaching the more junior ones. The chain starts with the attending physician and goes down to the intern instructing medical students.

Teaching of residents takes place in a wide variety of settings. These include the bedsides of patients, rounds, and conferences. The ability to teach well is itself an art. Residents tend to imitate their favorite teachers. Some programs offer guidance on approaches to teaching. It is, therefore, appropriate at this point to offer suggestions as to how to be more effective as a resident-teacher in various settings. The advice will be offered under three headings, namely, (a) bedside teaching, (b) case presentation, and (c) conference teaching.

Bedside teaching advice. The relevance of the suggestions listed below depends on the resident's level.

■ Respect a patient's wishes regarding being presented at rounds. You can expect that some may demur.

■ Take care to respect the patient's sense of privacy, so that they are not made to feel uncomfortable during the course of teaching.

■ Indicate to the patient that you intend to make the visit as brief as possible.

■ At the end of the presentation, express your gratitude to the patient for helping facilitate the teaching program.

■ Introduce the accompanying team members to the patient at the outset.

■ Prepare team members in advance to focus on the body area to be discussed and examined. This should be done with appropriate dispatch and discretion.

■ Upon completion, seek an appropriate setting to review the case in a confidential manner. Be certain that no visitors are within earshot of these discussions.

■ Encourage an exchange of views among team members. These should be carried out in a congenial, collegial manner.

■ Foster a desire to ask questions, and avoid anyone feeling put down because of their comments.

■ Make sure, when appropriate, to be complimentary to those who merit it.

■ Present suggestions for further reading and study about the subject(s) raised. Offer to provide reference sources that will contain additional information.

Case presentation advice. As a resident assigned to a service, you can anticipate that your day will be filled with a wide variety of activities. These will include routine tasks such as ordering lab test and x-rays, removing stitches, and attending rounds and conferences, as well as case presentation.

Case presentation involves making a clear, concise report of a patient's illness to your audience. Your remarks should be presented in the form of an organized, flowing medical report of the events connected with the patient's present illness. The goal of your presentation is to guide the group in formulating a differential diagnosis. You need to facilitate this effort by selecting both positive and negative elements of the patient's history, physical examination, and available medical data. This information should be placed, in the context of the patient's story about its impact on the disease process. Your approach is akin to designing an outline of a puzzle with only a limited number of key pieces available. It is indeed difficult, but certainly doable.

It is common practice for residents at some point to be required to make a case presentation during rounds, to the members of their treatment teams or perhaps even to larger groups. It is therefore important to be familiar with the protocol associated with this method of clinical education. It is highly desirable to make a favorable impression on your peers, especially because it will affect your evaluation as a resident.

The following guidelines should facilitate a favorable presentation:

- Dress professionally for the occasion to present a positive image.

- Focus your efforts on making a brief presentation of up to about 10 minutes.

- To attain brevity, be organized and provide only the information that is essential.

- Consider yourself to be comparable to a prosecuting attorney. Aim to weave the facts regarding the patient and their medical status so that your colleagues arrive at the same conclusion that you will be advocating.

- Be ready to discuss the details of the case after your presentation is completed.

- Do not view questions asked of you as reflecting negatively on the quality of your remarks. They are a natural follow-up during which the depth of your knowledge and the validity of your diagnosis are being challenged.

- When multiple medical issues are found to be present, the typical situation in the case of elderly patients, present each condition separately, beginning with the most significant one.

- When dealing with a complex systemic disease, initially discuss the most important condition and its implications and then move on to secondary ones.

- Seek to account for any significant abnormal symptoms, physical findings, and anomalous radiographic or lab reports in the context of your diagnosis.

- For long-standing patients, you need to recognize that your diagnosis should be considered tentative. It is quite possible that over the course of time, misleading findings may disappear and a clearer picture will emerge, leading to a more definitive diagnosis.

■ Make a special effort to speak clearly, at an unhurried pace, and loudly enough to be properly heard by all present. In other words, adjust your voice to your audience and room size.

■ It can be beneficial for you to prepare your presentation by means of a timed taped rehearsal. This will facilitate your giving a more polished performance in person. If necessary, you may refer to notes, but avoid using a script.

■ The following protocol will serve to guide you on how much time to devote to the various parts of your presentation:

History: 3–4 minutes

Physical examination findings: 2–3 minutes

Laboratory findings: 1–2 minutes

Summary: 1 minute

Total: 7–10 minutes

Each of these four components will now be discussed in greater detail.

HISTORY. Concentrate on the patient's complaints that can serve to catch the listeners' attention. Provide the initial reason that resulted in the patient's being admitted to the hospital. It is important to note how reliable the source of the history is, since there may have been language or other communication problems. The history is a key element in formulating a diagnosis; thus knowing the extent of its veracity is very important. Information about the patient's social history can be deferred until later and then presented, if relevant.

When presenting the major complaint, be sure to include the following:

■ Information about the nature of the onset of the symptoms (acute or insidious).

■ The level of intensity (mild or severe).

■ If the symptoms are increasing or diminishing.

■ Any factors influencing the level of pain.

■ If the progress of the illness has been steady, rapid, or slow.

■ Describe the nature of any disability directly resulting from the illness.

Next, briefly outline any related symptoms and clarify their relationship to the main symptoms. If the patient has been treated, you should note what was done and its impact, if any, on the medical condition.

Finally, present the differential diagnosis and your own conclusion. You should offer in support of your diagnosis evidence from the history, the etiological factors, and the presence or absence of diseases commonly associated with the major complaint.

PHYSICAL EXAMINATION. The results of the physical examination should be presented in an abbreviated fashion. Describe the patient's appearance and mental state. Findings regarding nonrelated systems can be defined in terms of being normal. If relevant, the neurological exam findings also can be characterized similarly.

Regarding the body area that is under consideration, you can devote a little time to noting additional relevant findings, whether negative or normal. This may provide a clearer picture of issues related to the illness.

LABORATORY FINDINGS. In this component, information about the hemogram, urinalysis, blood chemistry, and, when relevant, x-rays, EKG, and any special tests are presented. For hospitalized patients, relevant lab findings following therapy, if helpful, may also be mentioned.

SUMMARY. Make a short statement wrapping up your case, incorporating the differential diagnosis. At the conclusion, you should be prepared for probing questions. Seek to be knowledgeable about the disease processes relevant to the presumed illness, including etiology, pathogenesis, and manifestations.

Conference teaching advice. An occasion may present itself when you will be called upon to make a presentation before an expanded audience. This is a more formal presentation before a larger group than just your treatment team. Some guidelines as how to make an effective conference presentation follow:

■ Be punctual in your presentation by starting and finishing on schedule. Remember that members of your audience have their own commitments.

■ Arrive at the lecture site early so that you can test the microphone and familiarize yourself with the audiovisual (AV) equipment and room lighting system.

■ Feel free to use slides, x-rays, scans, and photographs to more effectively present your information.

■ Avoid overwhelming your audience with excessive AV material. Just use what is necessary to present relevant evidence that helps clarify the medical problems.

■ Carefully arrange your AV material in a proper sequence in advance so that your talk will proceed smoothly.

■ If you present figures or graphs, make them straightforward, so that they are easily grasped by your audience.

■ Try to avoid a formal lecture style approach; rather, seek to be case-focused in your presentation.

■ When the presentation is complete, summarize the key points you wish to get across.

■ Allow adequate time at the end of your talk for questions from the audience.

■ If feasible, provide your listeners with a handout presenting your conclusions. It should include relevant references.

The resident as an ethical caregiver

Most residents have quite limited knowledge regarding ethical issues associated with the practice of medicine. Some may gain limited exposure during a course in ethics as medical school undergraduates, whereas others have an opportunity to acquire some ethical insights as part of some formal lectures, if offered by their residency program. This common situation of a limited background in medical ethics may serve to complicate a resident's clinical decision-making. Thus, when dealing with ethical issues, residents, by virtue of their personality, prior background, and limited experience, may come into conflict with both patients and their superiors.

The following guidelines regarding medical ethical issues can prove helpful.

■ Seek exposure, as your time permits, to ethically challenging cases by attending grand rounds, conferences, and lectures to observe what judgments are made by other physicians in such situations.

■ When faced with an ethical dilemma, seek guidance from your hospital's ethicist or another appropriate individual (e.g., attending physician, chief resident, hospital chaplain).

■ Attempt to gain insight into ethical perspectives from your mentor, attending physicians, and senior residents.

■ Encourage discussion of ethical issues at resident gatherings such as rounds and case presentations.

■ When your personal ethical concerns are aroused, do not dismiss them. Discuss them with an associate to see if they are legitimate. If so, seek proper guidance to avoid adding to your stress level by developing guilt feelings.

■ Try to secure guidance from appropriate medical ethics texts and/or by attending a suitable workshop or seminar on the subject.

Several major ethical issues facing residents will now be briefly discussed.

Patient cooperation. Given the diversity of the current patient population, one may anticipate being assigned patients of varying backgrounds and cultures. Their views on the nature of their illness and the best method for treatment for it will probably diverge widely from your own professional judgment. The temptation to react in an authoritarian manner under these conditions is understandable, but it should be strongly resisted and repressed. There is an obligation, however, for you to provide your best professional advice, even when a patient wishes to exercise their self-determination, which in your opinion may not be in their own best interest. It is essential to allow the patient to fully express their views and for you to seek to be understanding. Nevertheless, your ethical obligation is to try to be persuasive about the benefits of your recommendations, perhaps trying to facilitate matters with the aid of a family member. If unsuccessful in your efforts, document the situation on the patient's chart and turn the case over to your attending physician for further action or for guidance.

Patient incompetence. Individuals who, because of their mental state, are unable to arrive at decisions regarding their health care can be considered incompetent. Being incapable of understanding the facts regarding their illness, such patients lack the ability to make choices as to potential treatment protocol options that may be available to them. Incompetence usually is the result of some neurological condition brought on by the aging process, a psychiatric disorder, or a traumatic event. The legal requirement for declaring a patient incompetent varies among different states. In competence can be certified in some states by a licensed physician, but others require a psychiatrist's authorization. The hospital's social services department will be familiar with the required procedures. A mental status exam is normally mandated in such situations.

Where informed consent (see below) is not possible because of the patient's incompetence, the resident and a social worker will be responsible for initiating the establishment of guardianship. A proxy will need to be appointed whose function is to judge what the patient would have wished, were they able to make a choice. Commonly a spouse or sibling will serve in this capacity, hopefully in the patient's best interest.

Informed consent. Patients for the most part are lay people with limited knowledge of medical issues. Although currently there is significantly greater interest in managing one's own health, the legal concept of informed consent exists to protect patients' interests. Three elements are associated with the concept of informed consent, namely, (a) information, (b) competence, and (c) authorization. Each of these issues will be elaborated on briefly.

Information. When the resident recommends a procedure or therapy, the patient must at the same time be provided with the rationale behind the recommendation, with its potential benefits and possible risks and anticipated outcome. Although a resident may encourage a patient to take their advice as being in the patient's own best interest, this should not be done by withholding any essential information. Thus the patient is not denied an opportunity to arrive at a judgment based on all relevant facts.

Competence. It is important to ascertain that the patient is capable of comprehending the nature of their illness and the treatment being recommended, with all of its ramifications. This includes evaluating options and making responsible, independent judgments.

Authorization. Upon entering a hospital, a patient is required to sign a consent form agreeing to *general* medical care at the institution. This authorization does not, however, cover specific procedures (e.g., surgical) or therapies (e.g., radiation) provided subsequently during one's stay. For these procedures, approval has to be given separately for each new procedure or therapy undertaken. The patient needs to give permission to proceed with any medical care that entails a genuine health risk. This should be administered to the patient only, voluntarily, and not under any pressure. Although a resident can express, even with conviction, a strong preference for a preferred course of action, the patient should not feel intimidated by their physician's opinion and they should be allowed to arrive at their own decision as independently as possible.

Managing the terminally ill. It is an unfortunate fact that in the course of residency training, it becomes necessary to make very difficult decisions regarding treating terminally ill patients. This situation raises three challenging issues, namely, (a) what to tell the patients about their poor prognosis, (b) when to discontinue proactive treatment, and (c) when to recommend promulgating a "do not resuscitate" (DNR) order.

Each of these three difficult bioethical issues will now be discussed briefly.

CONVEYING DIRE NEWS. In the past, it was common practice on the part of physicians to be quite discreet in conveying grim prognoses. It was felt that this was not in the patient's best interest. Over the course of time, withholding information from patients, and passing it on only to close family, has largely been rejected. The current consensus favors adopting a "right to know" policy and dealing with the consequences of doing so. It is thought that this approach is both ethically and legally appropriate, provided that it is done in a sympathetic manner. The issue of the manner to be used in presenting bad news was discussed earlier (see p. 216).

CHANGING GOALS. The second aspect of managing terminally ill patients is the major problem of discontinuing active therapeutic treatment in favor of palliative care. The determination of the incurability of a medical condition should obviously be definitively confirmed by the use of appropriate clinical procedures relevant to the disease in question. When in doubt, appropriate specialty opinions should be sought. If confirmed with certainty, the information can then be acted upon in an appropriate manner. In many cases, hospice care may be the most desirable option to be considered by all concerned and the resident (or attending physician) can advise the family accordingly.

DNR ORDERS. The third issue is that of nonresuscitation instructions. In this regard, one needs to determine if the patient's condition is *unquestionably* irreversible and how long they can live if intervention does not occur and to convey the implications of assigning a DNR designation. The competency of the patient with regard to this question also needs to be evaluated. If they are found to be incompetent, an appropriate family member needs to be consulted. Finally, the DNR decision needs to be approved by the patient's attending physician and a second physician (or clinical medical ethicist). The DNR instruction should be unequivocally noted in the patient's chart, so that all those on duty are aware of this instruction.

Confidentiality. Information about a patient should not be released without approval or authorization. If it is granted, this fact should be noted in the patient's chart. It is prudent to seek the patient's permission to discuss their condition even with members of their own family (and also note the response in the chart). Caution needs to be exercised with regard to communicating patient information to fellow professionals. The best approach is to make judgments on divulging information on an "as needed" basis. Moreover, care should be exhibited as to where such a discussion is held, so that its contents are not overheard by inappropriate individuals. Obviously, there are certain situations where privacy privileges are superseded by legal requirements (e.g., court orders for records, subpoenas for evidence, reporting criminally suspicious medical findings, or reporting the possibility of danger to a patient's life or that of others).

Resident legal guidelines

Residents who perform their duties conscientiously, bearing in mind the need to communicate effectively with patients (and where necessary their families) as well as to maintain high ethical standards, will not likely be involved in legal difficulties, such as malpractice suits. Nevertheless, there are a number of specific suggestions that, if followed, can further reduce the risk of legal complications. These are as follows:

■ Seek to establish good relationships with your patients. They will be less likely to undertake action against you, even if things don't work out well.

■ Listen carefully to patient complaints and do something about those that are legitimate as soon as possible.

■ Always leave the impression that you are genuinely concerned with the patient's best interests. Be sensitive to cultural nuances relevant to the patient's background.

■ If a conflict arises with a patient, make every effort to resolve it amicably, so that the patient does not retain a grudge against you.

■ When suggesting a procedure or therapy, avoid either exaggerating its benefits, minimizing its risks, or pressuring the patient to acquiesce in your recommendation.

■ Make sure that you carry out a comprehensive work-up when obliged to do so. Clearly identify any allergies to drugs the patient (or their family) is aware of.

■ When unsure about managing a patient's care, whether based on an uncertain diagnosis or questionable treatment protocol, consult with an appropriate superior and clearly note the determination made in the patient's chart.

■ When discharging patients, be certain that they are fully aware of their responsibilities for maintaining proper care of themselves and that the chart contains documentation of the advice given them.

■ Be certain that an order to discharge is, under the circumstances, not premature.

■ Be meticulous in securing written consent from a patient prior to carrying out a significant procedure or treatment.

■ If you make an error, discuss it promptly with your superiors and seek their advice on how best to handle the situation.

■ Be certain that instructions you give to the ancillary staff are clearly understood and are sufficiently detailed to be accurately carried out.

■ When countersigning orders written by junior staff members, be sure to read them very carefully and thoroughly to ensure their appropriateness and accuracy. Your written approval transfers the burden of legal and ethical responsibility over to you.

■ When performing a gender-sensitive procedure, do so in the presence of an appropriate witness. The same is true when it is necessary to carry out procedures that entail risk. The presence of witnesses will ensure that what was done was carried out using proper medical and ethical standards.

■ When you are required to treat a (legal) minor, seek to have them contact their parents or do so yourself. When needing to perform a risky procedure on a minor, try to gain the concurrence of a consultant and then insist on obtaining written parental consent.

■ Make a maximum effort to keep your charting up to date, and use appropriate detail when doing so.

■ Document, by date and time, in the patient's chart all your visits, orders, and activities on their behalf. Inquire from your attending how frequently documentation is required for patients suffering from extended illnesses.

■ Be certain that any equipment to be utilized is in proper working condition to properly provide the service sought.

■ Determine the extent of discretionary authority your attending wishes you to exercise in managing the care of their patients.

■ Be sure to document all transfers of care, whether service rotation or postshift. This documentation is to ensure adequate coverage during transition of responsibility intervals.

■ Avoid releasing information to inappropriate sources without authorization by the patient, when necessary, or the hospital's legal department.

■ Carefully prepare all prescriptions, being sure that your writing is legible. To this end it is best to print drug names accurately with the exact dose and frequency of usage. Oral orders should be avoided. Bear in mind any possible drug-to-drug interactions relevant to the patient's medications.

■ Be alert to the possibility of injury due to spousal abuse, child maltreatment, or other crime-associated issues or dangers. These need to be accurately documented and, when necessary, reported to appropriate authorities.

■ Determine if your malpractice insurance is adequate and if it extends for the length of time that your medical services as a resident are subject to the statute of limitations. Also clarify what insurance protection you have if and when moonlighting. Make certain that it is adequate.

17 | Personal Challenges Facing Residents

Overview

The composition of the resident population has undergone dramatic change over the past several decades. This is the result of the alteration in the makeup of medical school classes, which obviously directly influences the nature of the resident pool.

For well over a century medical school classes in the United States consisted, with few exceptions, almost entirely of white males. Acceptance of women into medical school was relatively meager until 1970, when a sustained increase in their numbers ensued. The road for women gaining admission to medical school has been long and difficult. The first woman medical student was Elizabeth Blackwell, who graduated from the then existing Geneva Medical College in 1849. She was followed by a handful of other women. The educational opportunities for women improved somewhat when a school exclusively for women, Medical College of Pennsylvania, opened up in 1850 in Philadelphia, sponsored by the Quakers. Nevertheless, even in the 1880s women still went overseas, to such places as Paris and Zurich, to secure a medical degree. Neither the introduction of medical coeducation by Johns Hopkins University nor the advent of World War I, with its reduction in available male students, significantly changed the gender imbalance in medical schools. Clearly, discrimination against women as physicians had deep roots.

Compounding the problem for training women was their long-standing inability to be allowed to secure clinical training. As late as the 1920s more than

90% of U.S. hospitals did not accept women as members of their house staff (residents). The situation eased somewhat during World War II (1941–45), but it took another 25 years for the situation to change significantly. Thus by the onset of the 21st century about equal numbers of women and men were being accepted into medical school. Consequently the ranks of women residents have been growing very significantly over the past decades.

Currently underrepresented minority student groups in medicine recognized by the AAMC are black Americans; Native Americans, which includes American Indians, Alaskan natives, and Native Hawaiians; and Mexican Americans (Chicanos) and mainland Puerto Ricans. More than even in the case of women, minority applicants had very limited access to medical education for a long time. The academic community, which controls medical school admissions, has in recent decades responded in a very positive manner to provide greater opportunities to minority group members to secure places in freshman classes.

By World War II, one-third of U.S. medical schools were still exclusively white. As late as 1960, black Americans were not on the student rosters of 12 schools. Three medical schools, Howard (Washington, DC), Meharry (Nashville, TN), and Morehouse (Atlanta, GA), continue to play a major role in training primarily minority medical students. Their current enrollment remains predominantly black.

Currently there also are three medical schools serving mainland Puerto Ricans. These are the University of Puerto Rico (San Juan), the Universidad Central del Caribe (Bayanon), and the Ponce School of Medicine (Ponce). These schools also accept some nonmainland students.

It has been estimated that the total minority representation went up from 5% to about 12% over the last two decades of the 20th century. The positive consequences of the increase in minority school admissions for the number of comparable residency appointments are obvious. With the enlarged pool of minority medical students continuing each year, a steady stream of minority residents can be anticipated for the foreseeable future.

Finally it should be noted that with the more tolerant social and academic atmosphere, not only women and minority group members have benefited, but also so have prospective medical students with strong religious values, as well as those with disabilities. More of such individuals are entering undergraduate and postgraduate medical education. Thus information relative to all four groups will be discussed in this chapter.

Women residents

The gender gap as related to salaries and occupational presence has narrowed during three periods of American history: namely, the industrial revolution (1820–1850), the later interlude of a dramatic increase in white collar jobs (1900–1930), and recent decades (1970 to the present). The most current trend involves women in very significant numbers entering higher paying jobs and professions, such as business, law, and medicine. Furthermore, there are many indications that this trend will continue into the foreseeable future.

There are at least three major reasons for the dramatic increase of women in the general work force. First, there are more jobs available than capable men to fill them. Second, the expectations of women have been elevated by their ability to more readily secure advanced education. Third, discrimination against women has decreased, although it is still prevalent. The last reason is the major one that impelled the opening of doors for women into the medical profession during the last quarter of the 20th century.

That the barriers to equality have not completely fallen is reflected in the wide range of percentages of women who make up entering medical school classes. This extends among schools from 10 to 60%. Interestingly, the proportion of women in Southern and North Central medical schools has been consistently lower than in those in other sections of the country. It is unclear whether this difference is due to women's attitudes regarding medicine as a career or an existing bias on the part of the admissions committees in those regions.

In any case, with women now making up about 50% of medical school enrollees nationwide and filling a large percentage of existing residencies, it is not surprising that it is estimated that they currently represent about one-third of practitioners in the United States. Obviously, this percentage will increase overtime.

The significant influx of women into the medical profession has resulted in a change in attitude regarding the intellectual abilities of women. There were some who assumed that thinking and reasoning are gender-specific attributes. Moreover, men have generally been viewed as assertive, dominant, worldly, tough, and unemotional. On the other hand, women are perceived by many as gullible, weak, and emotionally fragile. The fact is that thinking and reasoning are at most gender-related, not gender-specific. Crossover between gender attributes is now being recognized as not only possible but common.

Women have a unique position in the medical establishment. This will be considered from several perspectives, namely, in terms of residency choices, gender bias, establishing a family, status advancement, influential personalities, and leadership potential.

Residency choices. Traditionally women tended to select primary care specialties, namely, internal medicine, pediatrics, obstetrics–gynecology, family practice, and psychiatry. With the doors to medical school wide open to women, they have, to varying degrees, moved out of the traditional fields noted above into many specialty areas. The distribution of women among the different fields shows that they can be divided into six groups, which are categorized in terms of percentage of all residencies.

1. Above 50%: Pediatrics, geriatric medicine, dermatology, obstestrics–gynecology.

2. 40–50%: Preventive medicine, psychiatry.

3. 30–40%: Family practice, internal medicine, pathology, pediatric subspecialties.

4. 20–30%: Anesthesiology, emergency medicine, internal medicine subspecialties, diagnostic radiology.

5. 10–20%: Surgery and its subspecialties.

6. Below 10%: Orthopedic surgery and urology.

Gender bias. Over the past decade, several medical journals have published the results of surveys among female medical students and residents regarding bias based on gender. The results indicated that between 50 and 75% experienced some form of gender discrimination. The offensive behavior took a wide variety of forms. These included malicious gossip, sexual slurs, denied professional opportunities, and even sexual advances. Surprisingly, harassment varied with different specialty fields, being most prevalent in general surgery and least in pediatrics. Medical students were reportedly harassed by both faculty and residents. The hierarchical nature of the medical power structure, with men in the upper echelons, is thought to be a contributing factor in harassment of women.

Gender bias obviously impacts women negatively, both directly and indirectly. It may slow their professional advancement, thereby keeping them at a relatively lower salary scale. It may also be psychologically damaging, enough to lower self-confidence and sometimes affect work performance. The choice of a specialty by women may even be strongly impacted as a result of gender bias incidents.

Ongoing efforts are being made within the medical education profession to curtail harassment. These include periodic publication and distribution by medical schools and hospitals of their official policy statements against such activities, presenting "gender-neutral awards" to faculty who are especially sensitive to bias issues, establishing workshops where the relationship between genders is discussed, sponsoring and publishing antibias newsletters, and encouraging support groups that are involved with this issue.

Establishing a family. The issue of childbirth during medical education and residency is not new. However, with the substantial increase in women entering medical training, pregnancy has become an acute problem confronting the medical educational establishment. It is estimated that more than 20% of the female members of recent medical school graduating classes already have one or more children. Unfortunately, although the problem has been recognized, little has been done to address it in a serious, structured, and comprehensive manner. For example, school curricula have not been made more flexible and few schools have a written policy regarding maternity leave. Nor does a uniform policy regarding this important issue exist for residency programs.

Female medical students have received conflicting advice as to the best time to start a family. Many residency programs do not have pregnancy leave policies and those that do exist vary as to their detail. Generally a six-week leave of absence is provided. This should be scheduled well in advance with the administration, to allow adequate coverage during one's absence.

It is very important that a female resident gain full cooperation of her spouse in planning for a pregnancy. Appropriate child-care arrangements need to be worked out together. It should be noted that a study showed that no male, but 44% of female physicians said they had changed their career plans to be able to meet family responsibilities. In another study it was found that women specifically sought positions with shorter, regular hours to meet family needs. Although it is true that children need mothers, it is not true that the nurturing role must be assumed exclusively by women. It is thus reassuring to note that many if not most women somehow have the ability to find their own way to satisfactorily combine motherhood and a medical career.

Status advancement. The advances in the status of women are the result not only of a changed attitude on the part of the medical establishment, but also because of increased resources available to support their interests. Thus, for example, there are women liaison officers (WLOs) at all medical schools who are affiliated with the Office of Women's Programs of the AAMC. These officers receive information about seminars, as well as background material concerning women's issues, which assists them in publishing newsletters and organizing workshops. WLOs have also had a positive impact on the issues of maternity leave and sexual harassment.

An air of optimism abounds as women increasingly choose the time-honored profession of medicine and join their male colleagues on the road to becoming physicians. The overall climate has improved as women add their skills and brainpower to the pool of medical talent. Prospects for women in medicine will continue to improve with time, as old attitudes change and new ways of practicing evolve. Continued success depends on the degree of success women have in reaching positions of power and influence in the medical establishment and hierarchy.

In spite of significant advances, women still have a way to go. Nevertheless, they are assuming a larger role in academic medicine. They have increased in number in both the basic and clinical science faculties, especially in the departments of family practice, obstetrics/gynecology, pediatrics, physical medicine and rehabilitation, psychiatry, and public health. These advances are comparable to their specialty interests. Nevertheless, women are still behind in obtaining recognition for their work by advancement in academic rank and remuneration. Regarding medical practice, recent studies have shown that young male and female physicians with similar characteristics are compensated equally. This, however, is not true among older physicians, especially in certain specialties.

Influential personalities. For a very long time during the first half of the 20th century, it was commonplace that when little girls and young women expressed thoughts about a medical career; these thoughts and ideas were dismissed by adult listeners as fantasies. However, if little boys or young men expressed similar ideas, these were considered to be dreams. Thus, for young females, the concept of becoming a physician was considered a capricious image, but for young males, such thoughts were viewed as a conceivable possibility. Unfortunately, the negative reaction to the thoughts of young girls regarding a medical career may have stymied the potential of some of them to achieve such a lofty goal.

As noted, the thought of a woman becoming a successful physician changes from a fantasy to a dream, when gender stereotyping disappears. The influence of different types of individuals impact the human developmental process. Therefore, this issue is being discussed as it relates to women choosing medicine as a career.

Three types of people play a role in the destiny of youth, namely, molders, role models, and mentors. The shaping of people is initiated by individuals who are characterized as molders. This shaping process begins at birth and is greatly influenced by parents and others with whom the child has constant contact. General social molding of the child depends a great deal on gender stereotypes. This situation is, unfortunately, still widespread and deeply ingrained in society. It is regrettable, because such stereotyping is a vehicle for discrimination against women and can restrict their personal fulfillment.

Role models are a second type of influencing figure. This phrase generally refers to individuals who have traits or skills that are missing in others and from whom one can learn by observation and comparison. It is essential for female physicians to have role models who lead both successful professional and personal lives. Attaining this ideal goal of many females can then be seen as being realistically possible.

The third influencing individual is a mentor. Mentors are generally older, more experienced professionals who encourage, sponsor, and support young members in their career advancement. It is beneficial for female physicians to have female mentors. A mentor's academic or administrative rank is the major component in successfully sponsoring the advancement of female physicians. Because the number of female physicians who can serve as mentors is still quite limited, it behooves members of the male physician population to serve in this capacity until the pool of appropriate females is adequate. In due course, as their numbers increase, female physicians will undoubtedly assume a greater role as mentors for male medical students and residents.

Leadership potential. With the substantial influx of women into the medical profession, it is not surprising that their numbers are increasing, albeit slowly, in positions of leadership as well. Women have already demonstrated that they can serve as effective leaders in medium-sized organizations. The first female executives copied the male style of management, which they felt ensured success. The new generation of female leaders are following a different and gentler path than the command-and-control pattern utilized by their male counterparts and, nevertheless, they are succeeding.

Women holding supervisory responsibilities characterize their style as transformational leadership. Namely, they view their goal as getting subordinates to transform their own self-interest into that of the group, through concern for a broader goal. Moreover, they ascribe their power to personal characteristics such as charisma and interpersonal skills, rather than the power emanating from organizational status.

Successful female leaders have sought the following:

- To enhance other people's sense of self-worth and to energize their subordinates.
- To make people feel good about themselves and the work that they are doing.
- To create situations that contribute to the individual's personal contentment.
- To make people feel that they are an integral part of the operations of the group.
- To use a conversational style that emits signals inviting people to get involved.
- To use an interactive approach that has worked in the past to promote their goals.

The following suggestions may prove helpful for advancing the career of women medical students and residents:

- Secure for yourself a mentor who can provide meaningful guidance (see p. 105).
- Establish positive relationships with women attendings who have proven to be capable of being successful professionals as well as spouses and mothers.
- Consider the presence of a meaningful number of women residents in a residency program as a plus when evaluating it as a site for postgraduate training.
- Join or help form a women's support group at your institution to serve as a site to exchange views and ventilate frustrations.
- Be aware that there are groups such as the American Medical Women's Organization that have a strong interest in women's concerns relative to their professional life.
- Seek to secure information from various sources, including the Internet, regarding the advancement of female physicians.

Minority group residents

As indicated earlier in this chapter, members of a variety of minority groups in increasing numbers have belatedly succeeded in entering medical schools and residency programs. Getting accepted into medical school is not the end of the difficulties that may arise for minority group members. This is because at some residency sites, preferential treatment may be extended to some individuals because of their ethnic background. This may generate resentment on the part of other residents.

An additional potential source of frustration is that the increased income received by minority residents, although by itself not high, may place them at socioeconomic levels superior to other members of their families. At the same time, their situation may still keep them below the status of their white peers. This sometimes places the minority residents in an awkward position, being between two societal strata, namely, above their families but below their fellow residents.

The following suggestions may prove beneficial to minority residents.

■ Seek to gain acceptance into a residency program that, in addition to meeting your educational needs, also has other minority group residents who feel comfortable there.

■ If possible, see if you can secure a mentor who is known to be sympathetic to your special needs and can facilitate your adjustment to the residency process.

■ React calmly to indications of negative bias regarding any issue. View your task as educating individuals to judge someone by their professional performance rather than by nationality or shade of skin.

■ Consider forming or joining a support group of individuals of similar background or point of view so that you can share your experiences with others.

■ Seek to secure community representatives to enlighten the staff on the mores of culturally diverse groups that are represented in the patient population. This can sensitize individuals to the special needs of such patients and to the concept of multiculturalism.

■ Although you should perform at maximum efficiency, do not feel obliged to overcompensate and extend your efforts beyond what is reasonable because of having minority status.

■ Seek to obtain information from outside support sources, such as national medical groups, that can prove helpful to adjusting to the demands of a residency.

Religious residents

It was noted earlier that in the course of treating patients, various ethical questions arise (see Chapter 16). Such issues impact residents, whether religious or not, and they frequently present challenging moral dilemmas.

When residents are devout members of religious denominations, their convictions may be severely tested when they are faced with responsibilities that are in direct conflict with the principles of their faith. Such dilemmas may arise, for example, relative to abortion and contraception. When confronted with medical responsibilities in this regard, some religious residents may face intense inner conflict resulting from ethical issues that arise.

The following suggestions may prove helpful to residents with strong religious convictions:

■ Seek to secure a mentor who either shares or is sympathetic to your religious convictions. Such a person may provide you with meaningful guidance on how to face challenging issues that may arise.

■ Determine if any residents in the program have religious convictions comparable to yours or if there is a diversity of religious opinions that would suggest an atmosphere of tolerance being present at the training site.

■ Make the acquaintance of the hospital chaplain or ethicist to secure advice on how to relate to patients and colleagues on issues relevant to your religious convictions.

■ When relevant issues arise, seek to educate others about your views so that they become knowledgeable and more understanding of your convictions.

■ Help form or join support groups that serve to enlighten residents about diverse religious perspectives. This may contribute to a tolerant atmosphere.

■ Emphasize the importance of faith to individuals involved in the stress-related activities of medicine. Point out that faith can provide strength and fortitude, especially at times of emotional distress, as are common in a hospital setting.

Residents with disabilities

In the case of many physical impairments, barriers have been lowered and relaxed for disabled prospective medical students. It has been estimated that as a consequence of this development, there currently are upward of 1000 physicians-in-training with physical or learning disabilities, as well as chronic illnesses.

The goal of disabled students is to gain admission on their own merit and to secure reasonable accommodations from the school in order to facilitate their attendance. Residents with disabilities expect a comparable response as defined by an appropriate interpretation of the Americans with Disabilities Act (ADA).

Disabled residents fall into two categories: those with chronic illnesses and those with physical or learning disabilities. In the former group are individuals who suffer from such illnesses as asthma or diabetes. These and other chronic conditions can be exacerbated under the stress generated by the demands of a residency. Therefore, such residents should have their medical conditions regularly monitored by their local physicians to ensure that their health is not impaired by their professional activities.

Residents with obvious handicaps must establish appropriate working relations with colleagues, who usually seek to be helpful. In addition, it is essential for these individuals to establish suitable rapport with patients, which obviously can be challenging.

The following suggestion can prove helpful for residents with disabilities.

■ Have your personal physician speak with your program director indicating the extent and nature of your handicap or chronic illness. The contact established may be needed if complications develop in the future.

■ Discuss your handicap frankly with your program director and chief resident. Seek their advice on ways to overcome specific limitations, to enable you to maximize your service.

■ Make an accurate assessment of your prospective special needs in terms of providing you with mobility, elevator service, access to certain areas, parking, etc.

■ Establish favorable contacts with nurses, aides, orderlies, and porters. They are most likely to be glad to be of assistance and facilitate your meeting professional responsibilities.

■ If you suffer from a chronic illness, don't persist when overwhelmed by your own medical problem. It places both you and your patients at risk.

■ Accept the fact that you have a disability and do not seek to overcompensate because of it. Just be the best doctor you can under the existing circumstances by meeting your obligations to the fullest extent that you can.

18 | Surviving Yet Thriving

Overview

Having received your residency appointment on Match Day and your M.D. degree at graduation, you probably will have a short interlude of several weeks before you are back working as an intern at a hospital. Once there, you will be assigned to a treatment team consisting of an attending physician, other physicians-in-training, and medical students (see Chapter 13). Starting with PGY-2, you will be directly involved in managing the medical care of patients. You will be expected to know the clinical backgrounds of all patients supervised by your team and be assigned to do 'scut work' and write up medical notes regarding them. You may probably wear a longer white coat and will have the authority to order diagnostic tests (and need to follow them up) as well as prescribe medications (which may require being countersigned). Nurses and medical students will now respond to your instructions and everyone will usually address you with the title "doctor."

From the outset of your residency, you can anticipate that your workweek will be 60 to 100 hours long. Every third or fourth day, you will be required to arrive at the hospital for the usual early morning shift, meet all your daily responsibilities, be on-call throughout the entire night, and then leave work the following morning. At that time you will report the night's events to the incoming day team. Under these demanding employment conditions, you will nevertheless hopefully seek to maintain your personal life and your physical and mental well-being to the fullest extent possible.

As a new resident, your goal should be not only to survive this experience, but also to try to thrive under it educationally and emotionally. This introductory chapter will provide some strategies that can facilitate this goal and maximize the benefits of the unique experience that you will be involved in for a good number of years.

Adjusting

The fourth year of medical school may be a less stressful educational interlude than the preceding ones. By then you are familiar with the layout of the hospital that you have been working at and have learned the basic hospital routine. Once your subinternship is out of the way, you most probably will have some interesting electives as well as graduation to look forward to.

Moving on into your internship year is a great leap forward. Although clearly demanding a great deal of hard work, it is much more than that. The PGY-1 year places you in a new position in which you will be looked upon differently by staff and patients. As a medical student you always had somebody above you, to whom you could say, "What do I do and how do I do it?" As a resident, while still being subject to supervision, you nevertheless have direct responsibility for patient care. This puts you in an entirely different situation than you were in during your student days.

To prepare for your new role and its obligations, you should bear in mind the following three axioms that can help you get through.

■ Count on help from the people around you, residents who have gone through this rite of passage and the support staff who have assisted others in your predicament.

■ Realize that as far as patient care is concerned, you do not bear full responsibility but only a limited share. Your supervisors carry the largest portion.

■ Recognize that at the outset of residency no one knows everything and no one expects you to know everything.

With these three concepts in mind, your burden, at least psychologically, should be lessened.

Making it work

There is considerable and understandable concern among new residents regarding their lack of skill in the essential clinical techniques associated with their field of specialization. This apprehension, advanced residents will testify, will be ameliorated with the experience gained through repetition. Such concerns, while natural for the newly initiated intern, usually prove to be unwarranted as time goes on.

To facilitate your transition during your internship, it is advisable to keep the following eight *specific* suggestions in mind:

Get a head start. It can be helpful to start initiating residency-type experiences during your fourth year of medical school. Focus on mastering technical skills such as advanced cardiac life support (ACLS), learn how to manage an airway, volunteer for on-call service to see what it is like, and get a sense of what takes place during a code call. Since your internship will probably take place at a hospital other than where you were during your student days, knowledge of such basic techniques and exposure to common medical experiences will make it easier for you to focus on other issues relative to adjusting to your new surroundings and responsibilities.

Learn to prioritize. During a typical day you can anticipate being involved in multi-tasking responsibilities, with some conflicting demands on your time. These might, for example, include caring for routine inpatient medical needs, planning to attend an in-house conference, monitoring the state of a critically ill patient, and having to provide your services at an outpatient health center. Prioritization of your obligations may require you to skip the conference or to come late to the outpatient clinic. What is reassuring to know is that prioritization will become easier as you gain experience and become comfortable making thoughtful judgments.

Listen carefully. There is a natural and understandable temptation to define patients in terms of illnesses described in textbooks. However, it usually doesn't work out that way. Rather one may often hear an attending say: "I had a strange case that presented the following symptoms that are certainly not classical for the specific disease in question." It is clearly beneficial to keep your ears open and learn from experiences such as these. They will better prepare you for diagnostic challenges that lie ahead.

Other learning opportunities will surely also arise, including monthly, weekly, and occasionally even daily lectures and meetings, both formal and informal. Take advantage of them whenever possible, even if they are not mandatory. They can provide meaningful information that may be beneficial at some point in your training or later in your career.

Allow patients time. It has been reported that the bulk of a resident's time is spent in ordering and evaluating lab reports and x-rays and also in discussing patient management with other members of their treatment team. Only a relatively small portion of a resident's time may be devoted to direct patient contact. This is an unfortunate fact generated by the demands of a resident's many activities. It is certainly worthwhile to consciously make a periodic effort to slow down somewhat, whenever possible, and make time to get to know your patients personally, even if it is only a little better. It can prove to be a mutually rewarding experience.

Write it down. Your white coat has pockets and there is a reason for this. It is to your advantage to make full use of them. They may be larger than those of the white short coat worn as a medical student. The pockets can serve to hold handheld computers, manuals, index cards, pens of varying kinds, and small diagnostic instruments. Your computer can be used to access the *Physician's Desk Reference* or the *Merck Manual*. A different computer can be utilized for taking down notes that are of value. Index cards provide a useful patient database. It is easy to add or take out cards when new inpatients arrive or are discharged from your service.

Be a team player. Having acquired significant authority by your appointment as a resident, make sure not to abuse it. Show appropriate respect to your colleagues and members of the support staff. You need their cooperation and they can help you succeed. Some individuals may be difficult to get along with, but that needs be accepted, since it is a situation that is often part of any workplace.

Be creative. Although the overwhelming majority of residents follow their program's established educational track, this need not always be the case. You may at some point, be inspired by a meaningful novel idea that has scientific merit. To test it may require securing some time off from your duties to carry out your project. This project, for example, may involve writing an article or developing a research proposal. You may feel free, at an appropriate stage in your training, to inquire from your program director as to the feasibility of your request. The response you receive may come as a pleasant surprise and, if affirmative, will add a meaningful experience to your postgraduate training.

Ask questions. It is important not to lose sight of the fact that as a physician-in-training you are still a student seeking to learn the art of medicine. One of the best ways to do this, in addition to observing and doing, is by asking questions. These should be addressed not only to attendings or residents who are senior to you, but also experienced nurses, who, based on many years of service, can provide sound advice on patient care. That residency is a major learning endeavor will become increasingly apparent over the course of your postgraduate training, as you become cognizant of how your knowledge base enlarges over time. Asking questions and securing answers will undoubtedly contribute to an enhanced state of proficiency.

The human element

There is a general consensus that the actual details of the practice of medicine are the most manageable component of the residency process. It is the other elements, namely, the schedule, workload, and real and self-imposed expectations, that result in anxiety, stress, and on rare occasions even depression. Such are the genuine problems of residency experience. The negative impact of such issues, if felt by the intern, usually occurs about half a year into the program. Then they may experience a sense of being overwhelmed and bone-tired. Here are four important suggestions as how to combat this state of affairs, if it occurs.

Focus on each day. A sense of despair usually comes from the cumulative impact of a burdensome, intense, lengthy period of responsibility. If one concentrates only on each individual day's activities as an entity unto itself, the load and pressures will seem to diminish significantly. One should make a strong effort to devote attention to the positive aspects and accomplishments of each day's activities, to avoid acquiring a deeply negative view of events that may lead to a psychological morass.

When off duty, disconnect. Residents do get days off and they should make full use of them in a constructive manner. It is most important to disassociate yourself *completely* from all your routine hospital activities during your time off. These have been turned over to others, who presumably are equally qualified to handle them. Avoid wearing a scrub suit at home, which reminds you of your job. There is also no need to call the hospital to inquire how a favorite patient is doing. This free time should be used to strengthen personal ties to others, to become recharged physically and emotionally, and to meet essential chores and obligations, including, if necessary, studying for exams. It is essential that you maintain some semblance of a normal life during the periodic breaks that your schedule allows. These can be used for entertainment, socializing, or just relaxing with a good book or watching an interesting movie.

Indulge yourself. Residents have limited incomes; nevertheless, there is a need to keep one's spirits up during the long, trying residency period. To this end, it is advisable to invest in items that will impact favorably on your life-style and thus improve your frame of mind. Depending on your available financial resources, this may be tickets to a sports event or shows, a good-quality home entertainment center, or even a car. Some people may opt for a short, but elaborate weekend vacation to get away from it all. In any case, let the source of prospective enjoyment be one that you will look forward to having. This will make your demanding daily chores more acceptable. Take note of your next time off, so that you can foresee pleasure lying not too far ahead.

Seek help. There may occasionally come a time when, as a result of the intense pressures placed upon you, a sense of being overwhelmed occurs. This certainly is a most appropriate time for you to seek help. Many programs have support groups, where residents have the opportunity to ventilate their feelings. It certainly is preferable to join such a group early on, which may help you adjust to the challenges of residency, as well as possibly mitigating problems from getting out of hand and possibly impacting negatively on one's professional activities.

Should efforts to gain help via a support group not prove productive or should no such group exist, then seeking assistance from a chief resident is appropriate. Undoubtedly, the experience that they have, should be such as to put them in a position to provide useful advice or suggestions as to available sources of assistance. If the problem is severe, see the discussion in Chapter 15.

Mastering the art

The residency interval represents the ideal time for one to develop and enhance one's diagnostic skills to become adequately proficient as a physician. A key element is observation at the patient's bedside, which can be decisive in establishing an accurate diagnosis of an illness, which is the prerequisite for appropriate treatment.

The art of bedside examination is a most demanding component of the practice of medicine. As with any art, there is a sense of accomplishment in achieving and integrating knowledge, more than merely acquiring a collected body of facts. Conducting such an exam is a creative process. Its results are usually meaningful and broadly useful. The process is comparable to detective work, which is initiated by simple but careful inspection. Observation of a patient's appearance, dress, language, and behavior by a physician is especially instructive, for it may indicate where to look further and what exactly to look for. What is revealed by observation is the connections between all of the elements that reflect a person's sense of self, along with specific clues about the current illness and the patient's history. The goal is to recognize the physiological reality behind the patient's outward appearance and symptom manifestations. This can at times be achieved without the need of technology, but involves appropriate interaction between two individuals, physician and patient.

Clinical instructors can offer facts that can be memorized or teach how to operate diagnostic tools. They can even motivate and unlock a student's intellectual potential, but making the most of observable facts requires the artistic talent of making the intuitive leap from clues to hypothesis. Gaining the creative sensitivity to bridge this gap comes from learning how to properly conduct a bedside exam. This requires a strong commitment to achieving this goal during one's residency. The rewards for such an effort can be profound.

There is a strong impression that the art of bedside observation is dying out. Many perceive the decline in physicians' clinical skills to have begun decades ago. Exactly what constitutes a physician's bedside exam is difficult to define precisely. As practiced in the 1930s it involved obtaining the history of the patient's current illness and of the family's health, conducting a head-to-toe exam of a disrobed patient, listening to the heart and lungs, and performing a mini-neurological exam (looking into the eyes and striking the extremities with the patient's eyes closed). Early diagnosticians could tell much about a patient at the bedside, but how accurate they were is unclear, because records are not available. Physician training gradually increased in sophistication. Eventually, technology began to play a larger role in the diagnostic process. Starting in the 1970s, there was intense pressure to spend less time with patients, at the instigation of third-party payers to achieve more income. This drive was initiated as technology became more sophisticated, leading to a greater dependence on laboratory test results. In the 1980s the process of deemphasizing the bedside exam was accelerated, and no questions were raised as to what was replacing it. As a result many clinicians, regrettably, have lost the skill of observing their patients. Apparently, it is no longer an aspect of medical practice that many physicians depend on as an essential diagnostic tool and it may unfortunately become lost by lack of practice.

Like anyone else, physicians are good at what they do repetitively; however, not enough time is spent with patients at bedside teaching, where a great deal of information can be secured. Instead, time is devoted to arranging for tests and then to checking and calculating the results. In addition, there is the issue of the rapid discharge of patients from the hospital. This also limits the extent of time for bedside interaction available to residents to devote to their patients.

Although medical students and residents are very impressed when a clinician comes up with a bedside diagnosis, based on observation, not too many are willing to take the time and commit themselves to developing this art. This is apparently because we live in a highly technological age and individuals feel more comfortable relying on machines than on their own powers of observation. When one has strong observational diagnostic skills, tests will have value to confirm judgments, and thus may not contribute decisively to the ultimate decision as to the course of treatment.

The basic source of the problem of the decline in bedside emphasis on diagnosis lies in the current approach to medical education and training. The reality is that it takes years to acquire the skill of meaningfully listening to a heart with a stethoscope or auscultating a chest and interpreting the meaning of its sounds. For this reason, young doctors often are satisfied with a cursory physical examination followed by a technological evaluation. This is appealing, because it takes only months to acquire the skill to obtain an echocardiogram or to learn how to use an endoscope. Consequently the focus of medical preparation has placed much greater emphasis on technology than on facing the challenge of mastering the basics of observation, physical examination, history-taking, and bedside diagnostic skills.

It has been well established that meaningful diagnostic information can be gleaned by interviewing patients. This means that physicians need to be skilled in asking questions and allowing the patients to speak what is on their minds. Not providing such an opportunity creates the possibility of failing to extract valuable information and thus prematurely arriving at a hypothesis as to the nature of the medical problem. Frequently the focus of the resident is on making sure to ask the right questions, rather than on listening to the patient. One can often get a more complete perception of the problem from patient comments than from the compact, dry notes of nurses, medical students, or residents. This is a result of the brevity of contact of medical personnel with the patient, which presents a challenge.

In evaluating a patient, it is critical to learn the essence of the manifestations of the illness through the patient's history and physical examinations. This information allows the doctor to see the reality behind the appearance. The use of technology, although a most valuable asset, should be controlled by the physician rather than their being a hostage to it by being overly dependent on its results. Lab tests, will tend to confirm what is suggested or is already known by the physician, whose diagnostic skills are high. Often, the tests may not add much to the moment of truth when you make decisions, but the supporting data can prove reassuring.

The emphasis of medical education is on facts, procedures, clinical pathways, and decision trees. Inadequate attention is oft times placed on perception and how to focus attention on events. This can be most illuminating in terms of strengthening one's diagnostic skills. The didactic training in physical diagnosis, although valuable, unfortunately usually does not get reinforced during the last two clinical years of medical school. This training gap should and can be compensated for during residency.

Along with the adverse medical impact of not adequately focusing on diagnosis by physical examination and observation, is the diminished quality of the doctor–patient relationship that is not uncommon. Patients want more time to ask questions and get answers, as well as gain reassurance about the condition of their health. They seek to feel that they are being adequately cared for. Similarly, doctors feel a loss of satisfaction from their deficient relationship with patients, which circumstances have forced on them due to lack of time. It has been estimated that their workload associated with reimbursement issues alone, depletes an hour a day from doctors' employment time.

One should be aware that patients are sensitive to the approach that their physicians use in their evaluation regimens. They seemingly are able to recognize qualitative differences in their physicians' professional routines as reflected in their physical examinations. Their reactions contribute to judgments made of their physicians' competence and dedication. Patients seek to be the center of their doctors' concerns and want to feel confident that they are in the hands of well-trained and caring practitioners.

In spite of the changed medical climate, the primary motivation to become a physician has remained essentially the same. It still is the desire to heal and help people in need. This is true for the majority of doctors, although for some it is to attain social status and wealth. There have been trends over the years in the career motivation aspects of medical students. In the 1960s monitory considerations ran high. In the 1980s technological interests were the vogue. Currently the majority of those entering medicine still do so for essentially altruistic reasons. Thus there is a significant level of frustration among physicians, generated by health care management changes that have strongly impacted medical practice. This situation can be partially offset and compensated for when physicians spend more time at the patient's bedside doing what they should do best, namely, making the critical observations that result in arriving at sound medical diagnoses. Residents who pursue such an approach may well enhance their chances of gaining career satisfaction by becoming more proficient in facing the intellectual challenges that medicine presents.

Using your heart

There is a paradox in practicing medicine. In order to serve as a devoted physician, you must be sympathetic and caring, but to function objectively, you must maintain an appropriate emotional distance from the patient. If you become too emotionally involved, it is difficult to be detached. Determining the proper balance in this context is one of the important skills required for the successful practice of medicine. This truism is rarely mentioned during the course of one's medical education.

The focus of training of physicians is usually directed at the head and hands but not the heart. Medical training encourages keeping a certain emotional distance from patients, which is understandable for a profession where pain and suffering are common. Moreover, you are also encouraged to put your own needs aside. Many physicians feel that this may not be the best strategy. They believe that overly detached and distant physicians do not fulfill their patients' needs, and that repressing emotions is emotionally not good for the physician.

The impact of emotional trauma on practicing physicians is not adequately recognized, nor do they usually have an acceptable mechanism for coping with their own inner turmoil. Some go so far as to weep privately at the loss of one of their patients. This response will arise as an expression of the deep empathy and sense of compassion for the patient and the disappointment of the failure of their best professional efforts to save their patients' life.

There is a strong need to find the proper emotional balance between you and your patient. This not only is essential to practice good medicine, but also is important for your own psychological well-being. There are those who believe that a suitable mentor can help a resident establish the appropriate emotional equilibrium when faced with delicate situations. Some have suggested that to ease the emotional pain of the loss of a patient, the resident should spend a little time at the bedside of the deceased, rather than making an abrupt exit after merely confirming the event. In addition, it is thought to be advisable to tactfully share one's feelings with family members, as well as with other physicians, concerning the loss of a fellow human being.

The stoic attitude of some physicians when making routine rounds can leave patients with the impression that they cannot wait to depart from the patients' rooms and that they are really not listening to what the patients are saying. This apparent lack of emotional involvement is not helpful to the patients' state of mind and unconsciously it may be damaging to the doctor's psyche as well. The deliberate emotional distancing of the physician from their patients can spill over into the physician's private life and can create all sorts of problems. These include difficulty in maintaining relationships, depression, and possibly even substance abuse.

One should not automatically assume that the medical profession is the essential source of the emotional problems that may arise among physicians. Some may arise from being raised in dysfunctional families that have left their impact upon them. The vigorous demands of practicing medicine and its intellectual essence tend to foster disregard or repression of inner emotional issues. Some doctors may subconsciously project their own needs onto their patients, thereby becoming either excessively involved or overly distant from them.

Some patients may inadvertently evoke emotional responses in their physicians. If the reaction is unjustified hostility, it is a signal that the physician needs to evaluate what personal issues are being stimulated within their psyche. For such individuals, the practice of medicine can consequently be a road to self-awareness.

The more recent direction of medical education facilitates students having contact with patients earlier, starting even in their freshman year. This can help further their adjustment to the emotional demands that arise when clinical contact becomes more intense during later phases of one's medical education and training.

Some physicians almost instinctively manage to strike a proper balance between too much and too little emotional involvement with their patients. Those gifted with unique personalities can establish a positive rapport with their patients in just moments. They have an inner charisma generated by their presence, which serves to establish bonding with the patient, while at the same time maintaining a balanced distance from them. For others, it takes considerable effort to learn how to connect and yet be disconnected, but it is very rewarding to able to do so and it is certainly worth mastering the art of doing so.

In responding to the complex issue of maintaining one's emotional balance, it is advisable to consider the following:

Utilize a personal physician. When emotionally distressing issues arise as a result of patient contact, it is wise to avoid self-diagnosis and self-prescribing, because of the obvious lack of objectivity. It advisable to seek the counsel initially of one's primary care physician and, if more help is necessary, consult a suitable psychiatrist.

Seek counsel. When stressful decision-making situations arise, obtain the counsel and help of a trusted colleague or a mentor. Gaining a different and fresh perspective on a situation, will provide a sense of reassurance or enlightenment. In either case, it may help ease any inner turmoil that may have arisen, which can be stilled by a supportive environment.

Secure a respite. Given the intense physical and emotional demands of serving as a resident, it is most beneficial for one's health to maximize the use of free time for relaxation and a change of environment. It is also of special importance that you engage in an appealing activity that you find enjoyable on a regular basis. This may be an exercise regime, phoning family, or attending a movie. This will add a dimension of personal purpose to your life and demonstrate the need for you to have consideration for and even compassion on yourself. Although establishing an emotional balance certainly is difficult, physicians-in-training have a unique opportunity to work at it so that they get it right at the onset of their professional careers. This serves to avoid difficulties later on, when the pressures of building and maintaining a successful practice arise.

In training, emphasis is placed by some educators on submerging one's feelings. Once in practice, physicians realize that being aware of one's feelings is important. Suffering patients and their families need the support of compassionate doctors who can be sympathetic to their pain, anxiety, and sense of concern. The sensitive physician can help such individuals work through the difficulties that they face because they have come to grasp its meaning internally. Thus the message is not to be overly concerned about showing your feelings. This should not be looked upon as a weakness and is likely to turn out to be a doctor's strength, if acted upon in a wholesome manner.

Thriving

The residency interval has many varied challenges. These involve working long hours, meeting both success and failure, and having periods of exhilaration and times of disappointments. In other words, you can expect to be on a physical and emotional roller coaster. This life-style certainly places enormous pressures on an individual's well-being. Facing such challenges generates a need to harness all of one's inner emotional resources to survive this lengthy demanding experience.

Beyond the goal of survival lies an inherently more meaningful achievement, namely that of thriving. This can be attained by recognizing that in spite of all the hardships, you are attaining and absorbing vital knowledge and essential skills that will bear fruit for many decades. In addition, you are able to do what you originally most likely intended, namely, genuinely helping people. This can provide you with a potential source of great satisfaction. When placed in its proper perspective, it should offer you a vision of a professional life filled with much gratification. If viewed accordingly, you should be emotionally thriving as you proceed through the varying experiences that you will be exposed to. Developing strong positive feelings about your work, will serve to ease your burden and enhance the training interlude, so that when you complete it, you will retain fond memories of this phase of your life.

PART FOUR

SUCCEEDING IN PRACTICE

MEDICINE AS A PROFESSION HAS BEEN CHANGING DRASTICALLY OVER THE PAST quarter century. Business concerns now dominate the delivery of health care services. Thus a resident nearing the end of their training and planning to enter practice needs to become familiar with the basic elements of the business of medicine in order to establish a successful practice. This is needed as an adjunct to mastering the clinical skills relevant to their specialty. Obtaining familiarity with the business side of medicine will enable the physician to advocate for patients with insurers, understand billing procedures in order to avoid government audits, be able to properly negotiate, if necessary, capitation and managed care contracts, and manage to decrease expenses while increasing productivity in the office. Being qualified to handle the business aspects of a practice not only will enhance the chances for financial success, but also will make your practice a more efficient, reliable, and worthwhile venture.

The revolution in medical practice has resulted from the evolution of managed health care and the consolidation of hospitals and clinics into vertical health delivery systems. By becoming adequately acquainted with the changes that have taken place in this area, you will find it easier to adjust and prosper in the new environment that you will be entering upon the completion of your postgraduate training. You will then be in a better position to make the critical decisions that can strongly impact your future success financial as a practitioner.

19 | Securing a Position

Overview

A common activity for a resident nearing completion of their postgraduate training is to seek a position with a group or managed care organization. Looking for an appointment is a challenging task. For what each individual seeks is not merely a position, but one that meets specific needs. This serious task has to be carried out at the same time one is fully preoccupied in meeting demanding professional and personal responsibilities.

A recent tactic employed by some hospital executives to secure attractive staff physicians is to recruit residents earlier in their postgraduate training. The information on the subject of securing a position found in this and subsequent chapters should prove quite useful in planning one's future.

Formulating an action plan

A key element in achieving success when starting to establish oneself in the practice of medicine is developing a well-thought-out action plan. In preparing such a plan, the type of practice setting being sought is a primary consideration. There are, however, many other issues that need to be considered, such as geographical location, salary considerations, and potential for professional growth. Each of these factors will now be discussed.

Practice setting. Thoughtful consideration needs to given to your work-style preference, at least in the initial phase of your career. This may be a solo or group practice, becoming a salaried hospital employee, or joining a physicians' organization (HMO, PPO).

Prior to the 1970s, physicians commonly maintained individual practices for the entire length of their careers. Economic changes over the past several decades, such as the increase in the popularity of managed care, dealing with reimbursement issues, and changing IRS regulations, decisively altered this pattern of solo practice. As a result, physicians gradually started group practices which offer significant benefits for their members. These include sharing of overhead costs, greater ability to provide full services, increased automation capability, more capital for start-up purposes, and the ready availability of associates to consult with and learn from. In considering joining a group, it is important to clarify the nature of your employment status. Options that exist include becoming an employee for a limited period of time, after which you assume a permanent status or serve as an independent contractor. In either of these arrangements you will have an opportunity to learn a great deal about the nature of the practice, without the need to invest a substantial amount of money as a partner would be required to do.

In considering a position, it is important to evaluate the level of financial security offered for any position you seek to acquire. Thus, when you consider a group practice, it is desirable to know about its efforts to maintain short-term and long-term viability with respect to marketing support, contracting opportunities relative to managed care organizations, potential referral sources, consultation opportunities, and accessibility to local hospitals for grand rounds, as well as responsibilities relative to committee assignments and other hospital meetings and educational programs.

When you are considering an opportunity that is part of a larger network, it will be important to know if you will have access to other medical services such as laboratory and radiology facilities.

Geographical location. This is a good starting point in formulating an action plan. At the outset you should evaluate all reasonably possible geographic options. Upon further thoughtful reflection, eliminate from consideration areas that you consider not suitable either to practice or to live in. You should then be able to focus your attention on areas that are more promising in terms of meeting your personal life needs. The more practical a plan you develop, the less of an interruption it will make in the ongoing aspects of your life. In making a geographic choice, bear in mind also that weather conditions throughout the year are a major consideration. They will determine much of the comfort level of daily life for you and your family.

Beyond the geographical location, there is a need to ascertain your preference for an urban, rural, or suburban location. Your clinical area of specialization will significantly influence your choice in this respect. For example, neurosurgeons are not in demand in rural areas but family physicians are. Other considerations have to be kept in mind to help narrow down your selection, once the area and type of location are established. These factors are residences of close family members and proximity to educational and cultural facilities.

Salary considerations. Salary is an essential element in any job search. This factor is influenced by geographical considerations, medical specialty, and the individual's background. Rural hospitals tend to be more generous, frequently offering attractive sign-up incentives. These are available because of inherent disadvantages in such areas resulting from professional isolation, heavy workloads, limited support services, and lack of backup from other physicians. Positions in federally designated Health Professions Shortage Areas, which may include many rural regions, offer physicians appealing opportunities for loan forgiveness. This is particularly relevant to primary care doctors and can be monetarily quite attractive. It should be noted that there has been a diminution in the isolation of rural practices as a result of the coalescing of free-standing rural hospitals into health care systems and of advances in telemedicine. This has facilitated closer relationships among physicians within such networks.

Applying for a position. Once you have made a decision regarding a geographical location and practice setting, you should prepare a suitable resume and cover letter. Actually you only need to update the resume you used at the time you applied for a residency appointment to make it applicable for use in your job search. Because these two documents are your initial introduction to a potential employer, you should make every effort to leave a favorable impression as you move forward. Thus, to help make your application stand out, you should devote attention to its appearance, so that it will be attractive (as described in Chapter 10).

The first paragraph of your cover letter should indicate how you heard about the position for which you are applying. Ideally you may have been referred to it by an acquaintance of the person to whom you are writing. This should obviously be noted. Otherwise, as is commonly the case, indicate the source, which could be a journal ad, a posting, a conference, or even the Internet.

In the subsequent paragraphs of your cover letter, briefly outline your qualifications for the position you seek and the specific reasons for your interest in it. Succinctly, indicate relevant clinical experience from your years of training that provides evidence of your special suitability for the position that is open. You may view your expression of interest in the position as being equivalent to a mission statement. By defining your interest in an attractive manner, your initial introductory step in securing the position will start things off on a positive note.

The closing paragraph of your cover letter should indicate the sincerity of your interest in the position and express your hope that the reader will pursue this matter further. Make sure to indicate how you can be contacted by giving your local and e-mail addresses and phone and fax numbers. Although presumably this information is on your resume, it should be repeated in the cover letter, because the two documents may become separated during the screening process. This precaution will facilitate your being able to be contacted when deemed necessary.

At times residents have an opportunity to leave their home base and attend a specialty meeting. This simultaneously may afford the opportunity to scout out a potential position in the city where the meeting is being held or in an adjacent community where a position may be available. If this proves to be the case, it is desirable to contact the appropriate individual program directors, advising them of the fortuitous circumstances, enclosing your cover letter and resume, and suggesting an interview while you are in the area. This direct approach should not be made at the last moment prior to a site visit. Rather, communicate several weeks in advance of any meeting. If no response is received you may wish to follow up with a phone call to the prospective employer. Pursuing reasonable opportunities can at times prove profitable in lining up a potential opportunity.

When calling a prospective employer, carefully consider what you plan to say before you place the call. Be prepared to respond to questions as to the reasons for your interest, your availability, and your clinical experiences and salary expectations. In turn you might ask important questions that are critical to your conceivably accepting such a position at a later date.

A dedicated effort to formulate a suitable action plan, supported by a well-prepared cover letter and resume, will set the basis for the next step in the process.

Searching for a position

There are two approaches to searching for a position, namely, finding the opening on your own and using physician recruitment firms. Both of these options will be discussed now.

Finding the opening. The basic approach is to employ multiple techniques on a simultaneous basis. This may involve networking, exploring leads suggested by your mentor, colleagues, or friends, and responding to advertisements (in journals or on the Internet).

Of the approaches mentioned, networking can be of special value in helping you achieve your goal. You should therefore consider this approach as a regular part of your day-to-day activities and certainly when attending specialty meetings. At such gatherings, carefully examine the program to see if it can clue you in to specific relevant individuals who can provide leads about appropriate positions.

As a resident, you may enhance your employment prospects by completing an elective at an institutional site that is relevant to your geographic region of interest. It may have potentially opportunities for a practice type that is closely compatible with your needs. This approach may put you in close proximity to an opening that is comparable to the position you are looking for.

It is important to be persistent in your search for leads in medical journals and on the Internet. Formal advertisements usually provide details about available positions that will help determine if they are worth pursuing. Many medical organizations, as well as journals, offer free online access to job opportunities. Some positions can be contacted initially online, prior to initiating phone, letter, and e-mail contact.

It is advantageous to try to secure a job description, which usually is available from the prospective employer. At the same time you can attempt to obtain literature that describes the organization offering the position. This will provide you with an initial assessment as to the possible potential of any such position.

It can prove quite helpful to develop and maintain a log relative to your job search. Keep accurate records of inquiries, contact persons, the dates and nature of communications, brief position descriptions, and the proposed salary scale (if known).

To succeed in a job search, it is important to (a) follow up all reasonable leads and (b) have an arrangement for keeping track of suitable openings. Be organized, thorough, and especially patient. This will serve your interests well during the search process, which can prove to be a challenging out ultimately experience.

Physician recruitment firms. Physician recruitment firms are another potentially useful source that you may wish to explore as part of your search for a position. Such firms may provide confidential access to openings that may or may not be publicized. Recruiters may develop a close relationship with clients and can provide them with detailed useful information about openings. In addition, a recruiter may promote your candidacy, contact sources and references, arrange for an interview, and even negotiate your contract. Because their goal is to maintain the employer as a long-term client, they will seek to provide an appropriate candidate to fill a vacancy. The remuneration for recruiter services rendered comes from the employer. Hospitals and large group practices (HMOs and PPOs) employ physician recruitment services to fill their professional manpower vacancies. Many professional societies also coordinate mailings to assist members in locating job opportunities.

Achieving a successful interview

After obtaining an invitation for an interview, the prospective new practitioner faces the challenge of leaving a favorable impression that will warrant their name being ranked close to the top of the list of applicants for a position. To help achieve this goal, this section will discuss a number of relevant topics, namely, your travel plan, your appearance, the nature of the interview, and questions to be asked.

Your travel plan. Once a positive contact has been made with a potential employer, your next major goal is to secure an invitation for an interview. When such an invitation is extended, inquire if you are responsible for financing the visit's costs. Feel free to request an itinerary of your interview schedule, which will help facilitate preparation for your visit. If relevant, inquire whether the invitation you received extends to your spouse and, if so, to what extent reimbursement may be available for them. Your spouse's input can be important in assessing the community you may settle in. Therefore you may wish to cover these expenses yourself, no matter what. In any case, do not bring an unexpected guest along, even if you are funding them. If you wish to do so, it is appropriate to notify your host in advance.

Your appearance. Appearance, as you well know, is an important factor, for it affords the interviewer an opportunity to form an initial impression of you. The clothes you wear should be fashionable as well as clean, should be pressed, and should serve to give you a professional look.

The issue of appropriate interview dress has been discussed in Chapter 11. A less formal outfit can also be taken along for use if participating in a social setting is called for.

Nature of the interview. It is common knowledge that the interview process is burdensome for both you and the prospective employer. This is because the outcome is uncertain and it is time-consuming and costly. Nevertheless, it is an essential component of the process of trying to ensure a successful match between a prospective employer and a resident completing postgraduate training.

General advice about interviews is outlined in Chapter 11, but the following basic suggestions deserve to be reemphasized at this point.

■ Bear in mind that you start to give an impression as soon as you walk into the prospective employer's outer office.

■ Come a little ahead of time, so that you can orient yourself to your surroundings.

■ Check your appearance in a rest room prior to entering the office.

■ Be courteous to everyone you come into contact with, including the receptionist.

■ Bring a copy of your resume with you as well as any other relevant papers (e.g., research articles or abstracts).

■ Demonstrate that you have good interpersonal communication skills.

■ Be especially effective in presenting your qualifications for and your special interest in the position you are being interviewed for.

■ Focus on leaving an impression of self-confidence and sincerity, while avoiding an attitude that implies arrogance.

■ Always provide a positive view of both your educational and training experiences as a medical student and resident.

■ Omit personal issues such as outstanding student loans or family matters.

■ Prepare in advance the message about yourself that you wish to convey and the questions you seek to have answered about the position (see below).

Questions to be asked. The interview for a position with a group affords your unique opportunity to secure important information about the position. You should consider asking the following questions:

■ Will I have any administrative responsibilities and, if so, what will they be?

■ What is the existing policy regarding physician on-call service availability?

■ Will my on-call responsibilities be the same as those of other members of the group?

■ What are the back-up support systems available (e.g., physicians, laboratory technicians, x-ray facility, secretarial help)?

■ Will my patients be covered when I am on vacation?

■ Do my responsibilities include supervising medical students and residents?

■ How would you describe the future direction of the department?

■ What is the current level of competition in this specialty within the marketplace?

■ What do you anticipate will be the demand for services from this organization?

■ Can I be provided with the fee schedule currently in use?

■ How will I be expected to contribute to the practice's business?

■ Who is responsible for billing and collections and how costly are these activities?

■ Are billing procedures automated, such as electronic filing of Medicare bills?

■ What can I anticipate will be my share of the office-usage costs?

■ What is the collection method utilized in the practice?

■ How long do you anticipate it will take to establish a full-time practice?

■ How are new patients assigned to physicians who belong to the group?

■ How much will my contribution be toward overhead expenses?

It is especially important that during the site visit, you tour the entire facility. Focus your attention on the manner and atmosphere in which routine activities are carried out (e.g., is it hectic or leisurely?). At the same time you should become cognizant of the equipment that is available and how up to date it is. Determine if it is adequate for your needs and if you will have enough access of time to it.

Although the main focus of your site visit is on exploring the nature of the practice, there are other important issues that you should bear in mind and look into. This is especially true regarding a possible future site of your residence. A source of good information regarding this matter is a competent and knowledgeable local realtor. They not only can provide useful information about available residences and their cost, but also may be knowledgeable about the cultural, educational, and other facilities that are available in the community.

After returning home from a site visit, it is appropriate and gracious that you send a note to your interviewer(s) expressing your appreciation for the hospitality extended and indicating your strong continued interest in the position (should that be the case). Should any additional information be requested at the interview, make sure to send it off as soon as possible. You now have done your part and need to patiently await a decision from the employer's side. You are now in a much more favorable position to know how to respond to a favorable offer.

Negotiating for a position

Once you receive an offer of a position, a number of important issues need to be discussed these include salary considerations and fringe benefits.

Salary considerations. Bear in mind that compensation for positions has markedly changed from a fee-for-service arrangement to a salaried appointment. Individuals are being offered one-year and sometimes two-year income guarantees. This issue should be raised during negotiations.

Attaining a mutually satisfactory salary arrangement is critical to formalizing a contractual agreement. By speaking to knowledgeable individuals you should become aware of the salary range at your level of experience in the geographical region in which the facility is located and for the specialty in question. You should thus be able to determine approximately what should be the appropriate level of the offer that you can anticipate. You may be able to obtain useful advice from your mentor or peers on the subject of salaried remuneration.

Being realistic about salary expectations is important. Although financial pressure may exist as a result of significant outstanding debts, if possible, this should not be the decisive factor in your formulating an acceptable salary level. That your personal needs should have a strong impact on your thinking is understandable. Nevertheless, it is essential to avoid exaggerated salary expectations at the time you are negotiating an agreement; otherwise difficulties in arriving at a contractual agreement may arise. You wish to start off by maintaining a favorable tone in the relationship with the department director. Thus having reasonable expectations is the best approach.

It is acceptable and frequently advisable to inquire as to the salary range of a position at the time of your initial contact with the prospective employer. This will enable you to eliminate from consideration positions that are significantly below what is financially appropriate, given your personal situation. Knowledge of the salary situation will serve to allow you to focus your time and efforts on positions that can meet your needs and expectations. Once an offer has been made and the salary finalized, a written contract or formal letter of understanding is needed to make it legally binding.

Fringe benefits. Fringe benefits, which include such items as health insurance, pension contributions, and reimbursement for travel to meetings, are a standard and essential component of a compensation package. The value of these benefits varies, but they can amount to as much as 25% above your annual salary. When negotiating your contract you should consider raising such issues as coverage of moving expenses, malpractice insurance, family health insurance, reimbursement for securing continuing medical education credits, sign-on bonus, coverage of practice management service expenses, and reimbursement for society membership fees and subscriptions to professional journals. Among incentives that some employers may offer are free office space and support staff and even loan forgiveness.

Another fringe benefit that is becoming increasingly popular is incentive rewards. This essentially involves providing bonuses to physicians for achieving enhanced patient volume of care above the standard level that is to be expected. Any such arrangement should be explicitly defined in your contract.

Contract considerations

Various additional components associated with a contract will now be briefly discussed.

Meaning of the contract. When you and your prospective employer have completed all your negotiations, the agreement reached needs to be formalized in the form of a written contract. This binds both parties to the terms stipulated in the document. A written contract ensures that both parties are fully and clearly aware of the obligations that each side assumes during its lifetime.

Given its binding nature, a businesslike contract is important to avoid possible misleading or ambiguous language that is subject to divergent interpretations. For the parties to rely on only a verbal understanding of the terms of an agreement, even with the best of goodwill, places the understanding in serious jeopardy. Securing a clear and precisely worded, written contract will help facilitate a good future working relationship between both parties. This is most desirable, especially when you are initiating work at a facility.

The standard contract that is relevant to a resident physician seeking to join a group or health care system is known as an *employment agreement*. Where an incentive payment is involved to induce the physician to sign up, a separate recruitment agreement needs to be drawn up. Other types of agreements are also possible (e.g., independent contractor, partnership, operating, practice management).

There is no set form or language style that is mandatory for use in a contract. There is, however, a general format to most professional service agreements. They usually consist of a sequence of standard sections, each of which may consist of several clauses.

Preamble. This section serves to identify the parties to the contract by stating their names, stipulating the residence or location, and identifying the license to practice of the physician-employee and the corporate status of the employer. The date when the agreement is signed or when it becomes effective later, is also noted.

Recitals. This section of background information serves to outline the purposes of the agreement. The location of the organization may be identified at this point. The specific nature of the relationship of the parties as employees or independent contractors should be stipulated.

Definitions. This section outlines the meaning of the terms used in the course of the agreement. This contributes very significantly to a clearer understanding of the document. Defined terms used in the contract are usually capitalized. Where there are few definitions this section may be omitted if they are incorporated into the text.

Major physician obligations. As outlined in the contract, these obligations usually consists of assurances that the physician is

■ Licensed to practice in the state where the organization is located;

■ Registered with the U. S. Drug Enforcement Administration and eligible to prescribe controlled substances;

■ Eligible to participate in treating patients enrolled in Medicare- and Medicaid-supported programs;

■ A staff member of a relevant hospital(s), with practice privileges;

■ Covered by adequate professional medical malpractice insurance;

■ Board certified or potentially eligible to obtain such recognition.

Additional physician obligations that may be included in a contract are

■ A requirement to perform services according to a given schedule. This may define the specific number of patient contact hours, on-call responsibilities, and attendance at medical staff meetings.

■ If specifically recruited, a requirement for relocation to a particular community to establish one's residency and practice there.

■ A requirement that the physician's residence be reasonably close to the hospital so that they can meet their on-call responsibilities.

■ A clause that prohibits competition with the organization while under contract.

■ A nondiscrimination clause stipulating that rejection of patient treatment on nonmedical grounds is barred.

■ A clause stipulating that in return for an agreed-upon salary, the physician in turn assigns payment for services rendered to the contracting organization, which will bill the appropriate agency.

■ A clause requiring that the physician provide continuity of care until the patient can be transferred to another party, irrespective of the ability to pay for services rendered.

■ A clause requiring that the physician be held responsible for acts or failings relative to provision of their medical services. This protects the organization from being a party in a medical malpractice lawsuit resulting from the physician's activities.

Major employer obligations. This segment of the contract identifies the responsibilities of the group or organization that has engaged the physician to perform medical services at its facilities.

COMPENSATION. The contract should stipulate the extent of compensation agreed upon by the parties for services that the physician will provide. The exact terms of compensation depend on the arrangements made. In an employment agreement, it can be as an annual amount (and a productivity bonus is also possible). Compensation can also be in the form of an hourly wage scale or some other time-related unit. In the latter situation, a guaranteed minimum amount of employment time will be stipulated, to ensure a minimum income.

BENEFITS. In an employment agreement, it is common to be provided with insurance coverage for health, disability, and malpractice. The extent to which the physician's family is covered by health insurance and the level of their participation in paying for it, if any, should be specified.

PURCHASING A PRACTICE SHARE. A clause may be included in an employee agreement with a group that after satisfactory employment over a stipulated time interval, the physician, upon an agreed payment, can secure a share in the group practice.

FACILITIES AND EQUIPMENT. An employee agreement will naturally stipulate that the employer will provide the physician with the necessary facilities, equipment, and supplies that will permit providing appropriate patient services that meet the physician's professional obligations.

PUBLICITY. A clause is usually present for those employed by managed care organizations, in which physicians agree to allow the listing of their name and relevant information in the employer's directory sent to member patients.

Joint obligations. Clauses in this section apply to both the physician and their employer.

MEDICAL RECORDS. This clause requires both sides to maintain appropriate medical records for a fixed period of time. Authorization is given to permit eligible governmental authorities to examine these records. Confidentiality of patient records also will have to be agreed to by both parties. This clause should indicate which side is responsible for keeping the records after the contract terminates and that it agrees to allow the other side to have access to them if and when necessary.

PROFESSIONAL RELATIONSHIP. The agreement should indicate whether the contract refers to an employment or contractual relationship.

SERVICES CONTROL. This provision is applicable to employees for managed care organizations. It mandates that the physician, under normal conditions, check the eligibility of patients to undergo certain procedures before ordering them. Securing precertification is the usual condition stipulated by many insurers.

LEGAL COMPLIANCE. A clause is frequently present that requires both parties to be committed to obey all federal, state, and local laws relevant to their professional activities. This serves to protect both parties if either one is prosecuted for some legal violation relative to their medical activities.

NOTICES. This clause defines the advance notice that must be given prior to formal notification of the termination of the agreement. Specific instructions are usually stipulated regarding how such notification should be provided.

TERM OF AGREEMENT. This defines the effective length of the agreement. The date when the physician will initiate their activities is commonly referred to as the commencement date. Some agreements are automatically renewed without the need to formally confirm them. Under such an "extended term" agreement, one or another party has to provide in advance a written notice of their unwillingness to renew.

TERMINATION. Termination clauses can be included in the contract for various reasons:

■ Agreements may contain provision for termination by mutual agreement prior to termination of the contract.

■ Some contracts may contain a clause that allows either party to terminate the agreement without specifying the reason for doing so, provided specific notice is given in advance (commonly 1–2 months). Including such a clause can have serious negative ramifications for both parties. Thus careful consideration should be given before agreeing to include such a clause in an agreement.

■ A provision can be included that allows termination by either party for cause, namely failure of one side to meet its obligations under the terms of the agreement. The term *cause* needs to be clearly defined and prior notice needs to be given and its nature stipulated.

■ A termination option may be incorporated for a breach of contract by either party. Notice is usually required to allow time for a claim of a breach to be rectified.

General conditions. Some general conditions are standard for most such contracts.

BINDING CHARACTER. The agreement may stipulate concerns relative to its binding nature, such as in the event of a physician's disability or demise, or dissolution or transfer of the organization to another entity.

GOVERNING LAW. This clause is inserted to identify which state's law is applicable to the terms of the contract in the event of a dispute.

BINDING ARBITRATION. This provision may be included in the agreement. It provides a means of using an outside party to mediate a dispute between the parties if they are unable to resolve the dispute themselves.

ASSIGNMENT. A clause may be inserted that allows the employer to transfer their rights and obligations to another organization, for example, a subsidiary. A physician is denied such a privilege, because their skills are considered personal and thus are not transferable.

AMENDMENTS. It is best to have a clause that does not allow amendments to the contract without the agreement of both parties. This ensures that the rights and obligations of both parties remain intact and cannot be altered by either one.

Signature page. This final page of the agreement, when signed, confirms that the document is legally binding on both sides. It thus behooves the physician to carefully read the entire document and, if necessary, have a knowledgeable attorney review its contents.

Getting ready to work

Once the contract has been signed, you can start formulating plans for initiating your activities. When you are employed by a group, this may involve sending out announcements, placing ads in local newspapers, and preparing informational mailings, brochures, and newsletters.

It is essential that you arrange to secure hospital privileges well in advance of your starting date by filing an application with the administration of each institution where you intend to admit patients.

Assuming a position as a staff member of a hospital will enable you to utilize the institution's public relations department. In addition, becoming linked to the hospital's physician referral service, where one exists, provides another avenue for securing referrals.

Determine who provides malpractice insurance for your employer's staff and obtain an application from them. This is a time-consuming process that requires a variety of documents. These includes documentation of your professional education and training, appropriate licenses, and registration.

20 | Practice Options

Overview

How times have changed! For a large part of the 20th century, most residents who completed their postgraduate training embarked upon careers as independent practitioners. Over the past several decades, however, the situation has drastically altered. As a result, a more complicated health care delivery system now exists. It consists of multiple practice options available to physicians completing their residency training. This change in the format of the provision of medical services is the result of dramatic changes in health care delivery.

The aim of this chapter is to provide some understanding of the forces that have driven this change and then offer an introductory discussion of the organizational options that are currently available to practicing physicians. These will be presented in four categories, namely, salaried, solo, group, and substitute (*locum tenens*) practitioners. An outline of the current approaches to preparation for business and management in medicine then follows.

Forces for change

The significant expansion of practice options is the result of a number of forces for change in the provision of health care. These are managed care, amalgamation, and market pressures. Each of these three elements will be discussed briefly.

Managed care. The standard form of physician compensation that was in effect for a very long time was indemnification on a fee-for-service basis. Individuals insured under this system have few prior limitations on obtaining medical services. Reimbursement of the physician for services rendered comes from the insurer and takes the form of all or a percentage of the health provider's fee. Reimbursement under managed care, however, is radically different and is known as *capitation*. This involves setting a cap for services rendered, based on their nature. As a result, fixed fees are paid to providers, irrespective of the specifics of the medical situation. The rapid growth of managed care plans in recent decades has been most impressive, so much so that it has assumed the dominant role in the delivery of health care and reimbursement for medical services rendered.

The stated goal of the managed care system is to reduce costs by providing incentives to physicians to practice more cost-efficiently. This is done by restricting the number of procedures that are performed to those that are considered unquestionably medically essential by the insurer, and restricting those they consider to be optional. This goal is achieved by the capitation approach, which involves transferring the insurance risk of obtaining reimbursement at a fixed rate to the health care provider, by mandating prior approval for procedures. This situation has thus imposed upon the health care provider the need to practice in what is considered a more financially cost-effective manner.

Amalgamation. A second trend that has impacted the provision of health care is the integration of hospitals, physicians, and other health care providers. The goal in providing a broader umbrella of services is to reduce costs and offer better quality services by greater coordination within the system. This change has had an obvious impact in generating new organizational options. Consequently, consolidation and integration have become the operational modalities in the new health care environment.

Market pressures. An additional factor that influences practice options is the law of supply and demand. Thus, an overabundance of vacant hospital beds can result in fiscal losses that can lead to closure or consolidation with another facility. Similarly, if there is an oversupply of physicians in some specialties, this will certainly influence the choice of medical students as to possible future career directions.

As a consequence of these three trends, a variety of practice options have come into being. These options essentially involve determining if you wish to work (a) for others as a salaried professional, (b) for yourself as a solo practitioner, including *locum tenens*, or (c) with others in one of a variety of group practices. The variety of opportunities available makes it necessary for residents, as they near completion of their training, to consider their choice of a practice option very thoughtfully.

Salaried practitioners

Salaried practitioners are physicians who work under contract for private hospitals, governmental institutions (hospitals, clinics, or agencies), commercial, industrial, or insurance companies, or HMOs and receive a fixed remuneration for their services, rendered over a given amount of time. This type of employment is especially appealing to those just beginning their practice. Over half of those completing residency training begin this way and then move on to enter solo or group practice. Employee physicians receive salary and benefits in the same manner as others, but obviously at a higher scale. They are also provided with office and support staff as well as appropriate medical facilities and malpractice insurance, where appropriate.

The advantages to those starting a medical practice as a salaried employee are clear. The principal reasons given by many for doing so are to avoid (a) the financial strain of having to cope with a relatively low income for many months after beginning a new solo practice, (b) taking the risk of not succeeding, and (c) being a new practitioner while still financially burdened by heavy student loans. It is extremely challenging under these conditions to sign an office lease, order furniture and equipment, engage a staff, and arrange for the many other requirements a new solo practice mandates. This explains the reluctance of many to enter directly into a solo, or even a group practice.

A further element influencing a physician's career planning at an early stage is the knowledge that national economic trends, such as inflation and depression, as well as such issues as personal and professional contacts, can markedly impact the success of a private practice. Achieving an active practice depends on more than one's technical skills as a physician; it also requires acumen as a businessman.

Being a salaried physician provides a means of avoiding the aforementioned challenges while at the same time usually realizing many benefits. These include (a) a secure position with reasonably good remuneration, (b) an attractive benefit package that includes health care coverage (medical and dental for both physicians and their families), (c) paid vacations, holidays, and sick leave, and (d) shorter, defined working hours. This tends to favor a less frantic and more easygoing lifestyle.

On the other hand, there are significant disadvantages to being a salaried practitioner, including a limit on one's income, which is generally less than that of successful solo practitioners (unless maintaining a limited outside practice is allowed). In addition, there is a loss of autonomy as a salaried practitioner. This includes having to respond to directives of the administration for which one works and having to satisfy one's immediate supervisor. As a result of these liabilities, there is a marked tendency for physicians to undertake salaried appointments initially and, after a few years, move on to solo or group practices. Within six to eight years of beginning practice, therefore, the number of initially salaried physicians diminishes from well above half to under a third. In addition, the decline in the number of salaried employees varies for different specialties. Naturally, pathologists are almost 100% salaried, with surgeons and psychiatrists being under 50%.

Solo practice

Solo practitioners have been the largest group of practicing physicians, but their numbers are diminishing as the health care system changes. These physicians have direct contact with each of their patients as providers of professional services. In exchange for remuneration provided, they are personally responsible for their patients' health. They operate out of their own office or time-share one with others.

A solo practice can best be considered from four perspectives: (a) advantages and liabilities, (b) properly managing patients, (c) managing the business aspects of the practice, and (d) increasing patient clientele. Each of these perspectives will be considered in detail.

Advantages and liabilities. There are several advantages to this traditional form of practice, particularly for primary care physicians, internists, pediatricians, and obstetricians/gynecologists. These include, in many cases, establishing long-term relationships. It should be recognized, however, that people do move out of the area or are dissatisfied and select someone else. Another beneficial consideration is the independence that solo practice permits. Solo practitioners determine the location of their practice, arrange their office to their liking, hire the type of personnel they think they need and whom they want to employ, select the laboratories that will perform their tests, and set their own office hours, fees, and all the many other elements associated with an effectively operating practice. To a large extent, therefore, the solo practitioner essentially determines the success of their own practice.

On the negative side, there is the factor of uncertainty in how rapidly their practice will grow and how frequently they will get referrals from other physicians and patients. Consequently, the rate of growth of income of a newly initiated practice is unpredictable. Initially their income may even be less than that of salaried practitioners, whose expenses are paid for by their employers. Another major considerations, is that solo practitioners assume full liability for the unavoidable overhead associated with such a practice.

With the marked increase in paperwork required for Medicare, Medicaid, and insurance reimbursement, an additional bureaucratic burden and expense has been placed on physicians. This issue adds to the already restricted autonomy of physicians due to federal, state, and insurance company regulations that evaluate the appropriateness of patient treatment and tests and set guidelines for the length of hospitalization.

(There are alternative practice options that reduce the negative aspects of a solo practice. These are discussed near the end of this segment.)

The health care marketplace is characterized by intense competition. Under such circumstances, a solo practice would not seem to be too appealing. Nevertheless, physicians do undertake such ventures, because they have the opportunity to design a practice that is conducive to their personal needs. They do so also due to the conviction that by this means, especially high-quality patient care can be provided. Moreover, many doctors enjoy the challenge of building up a successful independent practice from scratch and the genuine satisfaction that comes with it.

Establishing a successful solo practice. To achieve success, it is necessary to know how to market one's services in order to develop a growing practice over the course of time. The strategy for establishing a practice is challenging, but certainly achievable.

There are two key elements involved: (1) providing superior care and (2) capable business management. The two subjects will now be discussed.

(1) OFFER SUPERIOR PATIENT CARE. This is the key component in developing a successful practice. To achieve it involves a number of factors. Among these are keeping up-to-date with scientific knowledge in one's specialty. This is enhanced by regularly reading the most important journals in the field, as well as attending relevant major medical conferences annually. Such meetings may frequently provide the opportunity to meet recognized academic authorities who have special expertise with state-of-the art diagnostic procedures and treatment modalities. These contacts can prove helpful in your practice such circumstances as when

- You need advice regarding the management of complex cases.

- You seek information regarding sites where investigational medical protocols are being evaluated.

- By securing cutting-edge information, you may be able to offer patients a broader range of treatment options to help solve their medical problems.

(2) MANAGING BUSINESS ASPECTS. Whereas doctors receive professional education in patient care while in school and during postgraduate training, most lack knowledge or experience relative to the business aspects of medicine. This vital gap can to be overcome in different ways. The many strategies that can facilitate this goal are discussed below.

Secure qualified personnel. Obtaining a patient-friendly, knowledgeable, and efficient support staff is essential to operating a successful practice. The key person is the office manager. Characteristics for this position are loyalty, enthusiasm, good interpersonal and organizational skills, being self-motivated, and having an empathetic personality. It is also important to select personnel who can work compatibly with the office manager.

A wide variety of business functions need to be carried out by office staff, in order for operations to proceed smoothly. These include the following:

■ Selecting and maintaining office equipment. This includes timely purchasing of office supplies and contacting equipment repair sources for potential use as needed.

■ Purchasing routinely used medical supplies from appropriate vendors and maintaining an adequate stock at all times.

■ Keeping an up-to-date record of patient accounts, sending out bills regularly, recording all direct patient payments and third-party reimbursements, clarifying outstanding bills, and resolving payment issues with insurers.

■ Arranging that bills for business expenses are paid in a timely fashion and maintaining accurate business records to facilitate auditing.

■ Scheduling patient appointments, responding to patient inquiries, maintaining a suitable schedule in coordination with the physician's needs, and rearranging the schedule when called for.

■ Receiving patients courteously and arranging that they provide all appropriate information relative to insurance coverage.

■ Scheduling patients for hospital admissions and hospital tests and maintaining liaison with home care providers.

■ Keeping patient records in an organized fashion, so that they are readily accessible.

■ Arranging that the office facilities are maintained in a manner appropriate for a medical facility.

■ Arranging that all specimens are sent to the appropriate laboratories in a timely fashion and that their results are promptly brought to the physician's attention and properly filed.

Part-time employees. The use of part-time support staff in a solo office can frequently prove cost-effective. Many employees benefit by being able to meet their personal needs with a reduced work schedule, while at the same time being available to provide additional time when office demands call for it.

Maintain careful financial records. It is important to secure the services of a suitable accountant who is knowledgeable about operations of a medical office. The accountant should be given accurate records to work with and be a meticulous and reliable individual who meets deadlines. It is valuable to have access to a competent attorney as well as an insurance agent.

Specialized personnel. For some specialties, having an efficient office nurse or physician's assistant on a full- or part-time basis can prove highly desirable. This is especially true where the work of ancillary personnel can serve to generate extra time for the physician and thus allow an increase in their patient load. Under these conditions, such personnel will pay for themselves.

Another important factor is the quality of the personnel employed. One should aim to provide appropriate incentives for their services and thus secure the retention of those who merit it. This can be done by offering, if possible, bonuses and other appropriate benefits.

Stay on top of things. Although having reliable and knowledgeable employees and appropriately delegating responsibilities is absolutely essential, it is important for the physician to be cognizant about the business operations of their office. Patient billings, income accounts, and cash flow should be checked randomly and with regularity. Payments, at least above a significant level, should be authorized only by the physician. The physician should seek to keep expenses down and ensure that bills are paid accurately and promptly. In other words, there is a responsibility to maintain a proper ratio between accounts receivable and expenses and be fully aware of in which direction the financial aspects of the practice are proceeding.

Once the basic office overhead is established, largely by rent and salaries, adding new patients serves to increase receipts by reimbursement without incurring additional costs. This is true even though most health plans continue to lightly control reimbursement or hold down the rate of inflation of fees. Nevertheless, by increasing your patient pool, your reputation will become more widely known and your income can thereby be enhanced.

Business acumen in operating a practice may be strengthened by becoming active on hospital committees or being appointed to the board of directors of a foundation. Experience in such settings may provide a degree of sophistication and a more comprehensive view of the business of medicine.

Increasing patient clientele. Although operating an efficient office is an essential element in the growth of a practice, a more proactive stance needs to be taken. This should include enrolling in all appropriate health plans and payer networks. Physicians increasingly are grouping themselves into health care systems that contract directly with employers. Doctors with established referral bases and hospital associations will be able to operate effectively across a broader range of insurance plans.

To expand a practice, one should be cognizant that interactions with patients and their families, as well as contacts with other physicians and health plan administrators, should be viewed as opportunities for enhancing one's growth potential. This should be done by acting thoughtfully and competently in advancing quality care for one's patients. In addition, providing an appropriate professional appearance enhances a positive image, and helps promote a practice.

Maintaining communications, both orally and in writing, in a timely manner with both physicians and patients will serve to maintain important relationships.

Making oneself readily available to colleagues by phone or on the hospital floor will generate goodwill that can prove profitable over time. Extending goodwill usually generates grateful responses.

Support patients' rights. The managed care system may place limitations on the services that physicians may render to patients. When a rejection of a recommended service has been received and the physician feels that in this particular case the procedure or treatment is unquestionably medically justified, it is appropriate that the doctor serve as an advocate for the patient. This may involve contacting the HMO by phone or in writing and, when clearly essential, supporting legal action undertaken by a patient. This effort to secure what is deemed a *vital* service, in spite of bureaucratic obstacles, will certainly be favorably considered. It serves to enhance the physician–patient relationship and further one's professional standing and reputation.

Provide accessibility. Patients regard their ability to contact their physician when essential as a major priority in judging the quality of service that they provide. Technological advances in communications make accessibility relatively easy. Carrying a beeper or cell phone and having a car phone facilitate prompt and easy establishment of contact with a physician, when essential.

This applies to communication away from the office. In the office, it is very desirable for the staff to be trained in handling all patient calls in an appropriate manner. This means learning how to screen calls and differentiate between those that need prompt attention (e.g., patients exhibiting serious symptoms, such as chest pain) and those of lesser importance (e.g., those seeking results of lab tests or renewal of a prescription). All calls should be attended to on the same day to avoid a need for the patient to call again, which can induce a degree of frustration.

It is obvious that for a physician to be readily accessible to their patients presents a challenge. It certainly can impose some constraints on a physician's personal life. However, physicians should learn to juggle their schedules, when necessary, to meet both their personal and professional needs, without neglecting either.

Get to know your patients. A major asset in building a relationship is to know *by heart* the major highlights of your patient's personal life and medical problems and needs, as well as current treatment regimen. By this means, greater personalization of medical care can be provided. This is exemplified by

■ The physician who is discharging a hospitalized patient arranging for a post-discharge office or clinic visit when making the last inpatient visit.

■ Being able to respond promptly to inquires (e.g., from other specialists and pharmacists) because of familiarity with the patient's medical background.

■ Demonstrating an interest in the patient's overall well-being, even if it lies outside of your specialty. Thus, inquiring from seniors if they had a flu shot as winter approaches will be favorably received as an expression of personal interest.

■ Referring patients for a consultation after a meaningful discussion as an impression of personal concern.

Consultations should be viewed as opportunities for enhancing one's career growth potential.

Professional relationships. Maintaining professional communications, which is greatly facilitated by the use of e-mail, will serve to enhance important relationships. Making oneself readily available to colleagues by phone or in person on the hospital floor can generate goodwill that may prove profitable over time. Extending goodwill can generate professional friendships, which over time can help facilitate the growth of a practice.

Strengthening marketplace connections. Being a solo practitioner imposes a greater responsibility to remain closely linked to the marketplace. One can avoid being isolated in an office-based setting by gaining professional exposure and presenting challenging cases at affiliated hospital conferences, as well as discussing case management with other clinicians in your specialty. Attending national meetings on a regular basis contributes to broadening one's clinical perspective and professional connections.

Future prospects. For a variety of reasons, it is possible that the number of physicians in solo practice may slowly diminish over the next several decades. At the same time, the size of the population of senior citizens is increasing. If these assumptions are correct it can be anticipated that there will be an increased demand for medical services, potentially from a reduced pool of physicians. This scenario may particularly apply to primary care medicine and selected specialties.

It needs to be recognized that the average individual seeks options insofar as health care is concerned, especially relative to choosing his/her physician. Many patients are partial toward solo practitioners, and may be prepared to pay an additional cost for the opportunity for more personalized service that this option offers. This pressure may have stimulated managed care plans to generate enlarged physician pools, thereby offering patients greater choice of practitioners.

Undoubtedly managed care will retain its domination of the provision of health care services. Nevertheless, solo practitioners will likely continue to offer services and find it possible to conform to the clinical practice guidelines mandated by the managed care system. Independent practitioners will be able to work effectively within it to both their satisfaction and that of their patients.

Variations in solo practice. There are a number of variations of solo practice that seek to reduce its negative aspects. The following are four examples:

SOLO–HMO PRACTICE. Many established solo practitioners seek to maintain this form of patient care, which they have long been accustomed to. However, realizing the changing situation in health care economics, they have made a significant adjustment by deciding to keep their solo practice, but at the same time being linked to an HMO. Consequently, they are accepting lower levels of reimbursement and making up for it with a larger volume of patients, for each of whom they receive a monthly stipend, if in a capitated HMO, or a reduced fee-for-service payment, if in a noncapitated HMO.

ASSOCIATESHIP. For younger physicians, establishing an expense-sharing relationship with another physician in the same specialty can be mutually rewarding. In such an arrangement, both physicians agree to maintain their own solo practices and to share office expenses (i.e., rent, staff, etc.) in an agreed-upon proportionately acceptable manner. The details of this relationship do not necessarily require a formal legal contract, but a written outline in the form of a memorandum of understanding should be signed by both associates.

In the case of association with a senior physician, the benefits for the younger practitioner of being in practice with an established physician include an opportunity to more readily obtain community recognition, a chance to learn the management aspects of a medical practice, direct availability of a dependable consultant, and also a way to keep operating costs down at a time when one's income level is just building up. Very often, associateship can lead to a partnership; in such a case, a legally binding contract providing full details of the nature of the arrangement concerning the division of both income and expenses is essential.

ACQUIRING A PRACTICE. Another way to establish a solo practice is to purchase one from a retiring or relocating physician. One can seek to secure such a practice in which the financial potential can be roughly estimated based upon the practice's overall past performance. It is important to get an accurate assessment of the value of such a practice, which calls for a careful analysis of income, assets, liabilities, and opportunities for growth.

LOCUM TENENS. *Locum tenens* refers to being a substitute physician for an established doctor, who is on leave. This can prove to be a good transitional phase for some new practitioners. One needs to be fully aware of all of the ramifications of this type of position. An assignment may last for a few days or several months and may vary from steady work in one area to practicing in widely separated locations. In addition, practitioners are responsible for their own health insurance. A major consideration is the impact of relocating one's family, both in physical and psychological terms, and it can prove costly, in view of the need to store some belongings and ship others. Naturally, for single people, these problems are far less troublesome, but nevertheless, they are challenging.

There are currently about 25 agencies placing physicians in *locum tenens* positions, with Comp-Health-Kron being the largest. These practitioners, for whatever reason, have a preference for the freelance route. The key to financial success using this approach is the ability to arrange a steady flow of assignments using an organized marketing plan. In addition to this substantial challenge, freelancers must handle all the administrative details, such as obtaining and paying for medical licenses and malpractice insurance and making travel and housing arrangements. These chores can be taken care of by a booking agency for a fee, which may be up to 40% of the client's income.

Group practice

Group practice is the second most popular form of medical practice. It is defined as two or more physicians, who provide medical care, jointly using the same facility and personnel and dividing the income as agreed to by the group. A group practice may be a corporation, a partnership, or an association of solo practitioners, but the majority of group practices are professional corporations (PC's). This arrangement provides a legal mechanism to protect the assets of the corporation from being seized in the event that a member of the group is sued for malpractice, loses, and cannot make full restitution from personal assets.

The number of group practices is increasing because they provide several significant advantages. They allow pooling of expenses for facilities, technical support services, and equipment, all of which come from a common revenue base. In other words, where the purchase of a piece of expensive equipment, such as an MRI machine, by an individual radiologist may well be prohibitive, a group can more readily afford it. This is because groups have the financial resources and space, and can utilize expensive equipment more fully to make it pay off. In addition, patient loads can be juggled more easily so that, when one group member is occupied, another can be made available to see the patient. The group members can more conveniently schedule night coverage, vacation time, and emergency care, all of which facilitates a more amenable life-style.

Additionally, members of a group work shorter and more regular hours than solo practitioners. It has been found that when a group has five or more members, income is on a par with that of physicians who are self-employed. In a successful group, a business manager may be hired to handle the many time-consuming bureaucratic aspects of an active practice and also to supervise and coordinate personnel activities. Also, in a group practice, each physician has colleagues available to consult when necessary.

As is to be expected, there are some negative aspects to group practice, such as the loss of substantial independence. Also, major business decisions regarding purchasing equipment, hiring or firing personnel, and renovating, relocating, or expanding facilities require a consensus. For a group to practice successfully, compatibility of personalities and professional outlook is a necessity. Also, groups that are smaller than five, which are very common, have income levels that can be lower than those of solo practitioners. This may result from the fact that the number of patients seen may be restricted by space and personnel limitations.

As with most issues, there are both positive and negative sides to being a member of a group practice. If you are considering it, you need to be cautious, thoroughly evaluate the nature of the practice, and determine if you would be compatible with the group members. Naturally, you should be the type of person who is a dedicated team player before you enter any group practice. However, the rewards of being a member of a successful group practice can readily outweigh its disadvantages.

The changes in the health care system noted earlier in this chapter have resulted in the creation of a variety of group practices. The major ones will be outlined below.

Multispecialty group. Several of the major U.S. groups of this kind, such as the Mayo Clinic, were established decades ago. Such large groups are all-encompassing in the scope of the specialty services provided. There exist, however, numerous small multispecialty groups that offer a narrower range of services. The direction of developments in this area has been the consolidation of smaller groups into larger ones, for a number of economic reasons. One of the results of such amalgamation is greater stability. Most such groups are organized as professional corporations or partnerships.

Single-specialty group. This consists of from two to 100 physicians who are in the same specialty, working in a cooperative, unified fashion. Surprisingly, many such groups developed from solo practices wherein on-call coverage relationships blossomed into a closer association, ultimately resulting in the establishment of a permanent linkage as a merged unit. As a consequence of the complexity of operating the business aspects of medicine, increased numbers of single-specialty groups have been established over the past quarter of a century.

Physicians have come to recognize that group practices can serve to reduce overall operating costs and can perform more effectively under managed care. Consequently, such groups have become increasingly popular. Most single-specialty groups organize themselves in the form of partnerships or professional corporations.

Independent physician association. Some physicians are quite anxious to maintain their independence, but nevertheless seek to retain managed care contracts. To do this they may elect to join an independent physician association (IPA). This enables the practitioner to associate loosely with a physician's group in order to establish a favorable contractual mechanism for payer reimbursement.

Physicians joining such associations are not required to integrate their practices. Rather, they maintain their own independence while retaining a linkage insofar as payer contracts are concerned. This type of arrangement has become popular because, in an effort to achieve competitive reimbursement rates, there is a need to pool contract negotiation leverage. The desire to pursue such a course is the result of the current market climate. IPAs are organized as shareholder entities, governed by their members. These may consist of from a handful of physicians up to a thousand or more. Properly operated, IPAs have become reliable practice options.

Physician practice arrangements with IPAs depend on their by-laws. These can be of two types, exclusive and nonexclusive. In the former, the practitioner agrees to accept all payer contracts only through the association they joined. In a nonexclusive agreement, the physician has the option of becoming a member of other IPAs. IPAs are usually organized as professional corporations. This practice option can be attractive because it can combine small size and favorable business benefits.

Physician–hospital organization. This entity, commonly known as PHO, is usually a professional corporation. Such joint ventures maintain a distinction from both the hospital and its associated attending physicians, even though their makeup is derived from these two sources. PHOs are governed by representatives from both components, who appoint delegates to negotiate contracts on behalf of the PHO with insurers.

Hospitals are especially partial to PHOs, since they serve to strengthen bonds with their physicians. Many physicians also view such entities favorably. They see them as a means of being able to gain a favorable contractual agreement and influence hospital policy in a manner that is beneficial to them.

PHOs have also gained in popularity because they provide negotiating leverage with third-party payers. Such organizational options, however, do present problems due to the challenge of satisfactorily dividing capitation funds among participating members.

Modified group practice. This practice option, also known as a group practice without walls, represents a hybrid between a solo and group practice. Under such an arrangement, the solo practitioners retain their independence as service providers, but collectively share key fiscal operations, such as billing and accounts receivable, with their group. As a consequence, while retaining personal freedom of action, the physician nevertheless is able to reduce operating costs of maintaining information systems. Naturally this also means that business functions are no longer under direct control of the individual practitioner.

Management service organization. MSOs are relatively new entities that provide, as their name indicates, management expertise relative to general practice operations and managed care reimbursement. These outfits will contract to operate daily business operations of a practice by providing these essential services. Some of these organizations, which are hospital- or corporation-operated, offer physicians the opportunity to secure part-ownership rights. The legal structure of these organizations may vary, but their future is uncertain at this time.

Integrated service systems. Another recent development in the provision of health care is the establishment of networks that may consist of varying service provider models. These are linked together contractually to negotiate favorable payer agreements, because of the leverage they have as a consolidated unit. Such networks may be linked to hospital systems to form larger integrated units. The viability of such arrangements is still uncertain.

Business/management preparation

For the greater part of the 20th century, it was adequate for physicians to be compassionate, well-trained professionals and lack business/management skills. With the vast change in the delivery of health care, however, it has become necessary, if not essential, that doctors have knowledge of both the management and business aspects of medicine. Consequently, practicing physicians and those planning to enter into practice are seeking to become knowledgeable about relevant, nonmedical aspects of patient services. This should help enhance their professional chances for success, both clinically and financially.

Naturally, the extent of business acumen needed by physicians for their practice depends on the position held, their level of responsibility, and the size of the practice. Nevertheless, even those in a solo practice need to organize an office, meet mandated legal regulations, and deal with third-party payers. Consequently, it is advisable for independent practitioners to have some background in the business aspects of medicine.

During the last quarter of the 20th century, business, finance, and insurance specialists have played a prominent role in administering the health care establishment. This situation has created a challenge to the status and authority of physicians who are responding aggressively. This is reflected by doctors, with appropriate credentials, accepting positions as physician-managers or physician-executives. This changed climate is also reflected in the educational programs currently available in many medical schools. They provide opportunities to become knowledgeable in areas relevant to the business of medicine.

Training options. There are different levels of education that one can obtain insofar as business and management relative to medicine is concerned. The desirable option largely depends on an individual's current needs and future goals. The extent of interest on the physician's parts will also be influenced by the person's background, training, and prior experience.

Sources for the acquisition of knowledge in these areas are as follows:

■ *On-the-job training.* This traditional approach continues to be popular, because it does not excessively disrupt an individual's routine activities. However, it lacks structure and can be of limited benefit.

■ *Self-education.* This is possible by using textbooks discussing business and management in general, as well as those issues as they are related to health care. Computer-designed learning resources are available to facilitate strengthening one's background in the business aspects of medicine.

■ *Taking courses.* This can be done by distance learning, utilizing the Internet.

■ *In-house sources.* Group practices, managed care organizations, and insurance companies may offer management training programs for employees and affiliated physicians.

■ *Short-term programs.* Such opportunities deal with business/management issues and consist of workshops and seminars.

■ *Degree programs.* These formal, structured educational options can provide a master's degree in one of several areas.

The last two options merit being discussed in somewhat more detail.

Short-term programs. These programs fall into two time categories, brief (days) or medium-length (weeks). The former type will be discussed initially.

BRIEF PROGRAMS. If a physician, intuitively or as a result of exposure, finds administrative work appealing, enrolling in a short-term educational program can prove beneficial. Such exposure may be secured by attending a workshop or seminar. These programs may be offered by universities, professional associations, and private firms. Since they are usually limited to one or at most several days, the content is usually restricted to skills enhancement and problem-solving, rather than in-depth or complex topics. Programs such as these can be useful in providing an introduction to the fundamentals of business/management. Then, if desirable, the basic information acquired can be supplemented by further study at a more advanced level.

MEDIUM-LENGTH PROGRAMS. These extend over a few weeks or several months. Naturally, they do not offer an advanced degree, but they may provide a certificate upon completion. Such programs are rather costly and may require relocation during the educational interlude. These relatively short-term programs may possibly be taken as part of a fellowship, sabbatical, or vacation, when such opportunities are available and do not dislocate one's routine professional activities.

Degree programs. These opportunities are designed for those who actively seek advancement as physician-managers or physician-executives. Such career aspirations may come into consideration as a result of their positive experiences with short-term programs. They can have a significant impact on one's knowledge base and interest in this subject.

There are a number of issues associated with securing an advanced degree relevant to administrative activities in medicine. These include selecting the most appropriate degree and determining how best to attain it. The four generally relevant degree options for physician-administrators are as follows:

■ *Master of Science in Health Administration.* The program usually requires two years of study at a university campus. This degree program usually covers a wide range of subjects. These usually include the economic, legal, psychological, and social aspects of health care. Study involves becoming familiar with the organization, financing, managing, marketing, and delivery of medical services. Programs may require enrollees to participate in field work and submit a thesis in order to receive the MSHA degree. This degree is identified by some institutions as a Master's in Health Administration (MHA)

■ *Master of Business Administration.* The two-year MBA degree is offered by colleges of business at very many universities. Program content tends to vary depending on the institution. Completing basic prerequisite courses in economics, accounting, and statistics is recommended. Building on this background, one can proceed to take courses dealing with the marketing of goods and services, financing of businesses (both profit and nonprofit), managing information systems, interpersonal skills, and policy determination. The second year of such a program varies very widely, with the focus being on advanced business and analytical skills.

■ *Master of Public Health.* This degree program is usually offered at medical schools through their Schools of Public Health. Since they are offered at such institutions, the contents of these courses naturally has a distinct scientific orientation. One can secure an MPH degree after one year of study by attending on a full-time basis. Among commonly required courses are health services organization, epidimiology, statistics, social and behavioral sciences, and environmental health. There usually is a need to take electives to meet the degree credit requirement.

■ *Master of Science.* These programs very widely in content and usually extend for about two years. Courses may include those dealing with business and management fundamentals (e.g., health economics, information systems, capital budgeting) and those in medical management applications (e.g., health policy and law, technology assessment, quality measurement). Other programs focus their courses on the financial aspects (e.g., strategy formulation and implementation, payment systems, and risk management).

Insofar as choosing an option is concerned, it should be noted that the MSHA and MS are frequently sought-after degrees in the area of health care administration. This is because they are more suitable for physician-administrators by virtue of their subject balance. This is the result of a favorable ratio of business and health administration courses. When considering an MBA degree, it is important to select a program that is geared for health management and is not excessively focused toward business. MPH programs have less appeal because they tend to be one-sided in content and thus may be of lesser relevance for prospective physician-administrators.

How to attain one's degree depends on each individual's personal situation. Full-time studies are a major commitment, while part-time enrollment requires an extended period of time until completion.

21 | Marketing and Operating a Successful Practice

Overview

The preceding chapter outlined the various practice options available. For residents seriously considering entering private practice, the issues of properly marketing and efficiently operating an office are critical to the success of the undertaking. This is the result of the fact that the health care system is now widely regarded as an industry and medical practice is considered a competitive business. With this perspective in mind, physicians have to look upon their occupation as being professional entrepeneurs. A primer on the two aspects, marketing and operating a practice, will be presented in this chapter.

Keys to professional success

When one is involved in a residency there is a tendency to lose track of time, which passes all too quickly. Before you realize it, you will find yourself on the verge of thinking about your future professional life. As you approach your ultimate goal, you will be faced with many new challenges and decisions. To help lower your anxiety level and make you feel more confident, a summary of the main issues associated with getting a practice under way are outlined in this section.

When considering your future professional activities, remember that

■ Your residency is the best learning opportunity for preparing to go into practice.

■ It is advantageous initially in your career to work for someone else, in that you will have a regular salary, you will not have to be concerned about running an office, and you can learn on the job about operating an office if you later decide to do so.

■ Working for someone else, however, has some disadvantages in that you have less autonomy, you have less control over which patients you see and what procedures you perform, and in the long run you will earn less money.

■ Having your own practice will allow you establish it to your liking, to manage office operations, determine procedures you perform, have a greater income, and have transferable assets upon relocation.

■ Setting up and running your own office, however, requires knowledge and greater responsibility, a significant financial investment, and a possible significant delay until you recoup.

When working with a partner or group, remember to

■ Carefully examine your employment contract to determine if the salary is appropriate, whether there is incentive pay, and, if so, if it is based on gross collected income.

■ Determine if the agreement offers other benefits such as malpractice insurance and if there is a noncompetition clause.

When setting up your own practice, remember to

■ Develop a suitable business plan that can meet your needs.

■ Carefully manage the costs involved in setting up your office to avoid fiscal problems.

■ Consider electing to practice with a group that is distant from your own office where you can work part-time until your practice builds up.

■ Establish a comprehensive view of what is involved in opening an office.

■ See if a local community hospital offers loans or provides compensation guarantees to help a physician initiate a practice.

When opening your own office, remember to

■ Apply for a state license in order to be able to practice medicine.

■ Select the most appropriate site for your office relative to your specialty.

■ Develop relevant administrative forms needed to keep records for proper billing.

■ Carefully select suitable computer equipment and appropriate software.

■ Apply for hospital privileges at appropriate institutions in your area.

■ Apply to become a provider of services for various health plans.

■ Obtain phone service suitable for your operational needs.

- Apply to obtain a business license from the appropriate governmental agency.
- Apply to obtain a business loan from a suitable source at an attractive rate.
- Purchase suitable office furniture, or lease it, if circumstances warrant.
- Hire an experienced, competent office manager who will meet your needs.
- Develop a suitable filing system that will accurately keep your records.
- Establish a fee schedule relevant to your specialty and potential patients.
- Secure the services of a dependable answering service.
- Arrange for a reliable paging service to be sure you can be readily contacted.
- Establish an office schedule that allows you to meet all your commitments.
- Order essential equipment and supplies to prepare for prospective needs.
- Secure the services of a knowledgeable accountant with suitable expertise.
- Gain the potential to obtain additional full- or part-time office help as needed.
- Arrange your reception room in a manner that gives you a positive image.
- Announce the opening of your office in an appropriate fashion.
- Initiate seeing patients when arrangements are complete and ready.

With regard to insurance and billing remember to

- Maintain a credentials file in a secure place.
- Carefully examine managed care contracts with the assistance of your lawyer and accountant.
- Be aware that Medicare does not cover some health care services.
- Bill Medicare only for medically essential services to secure reimbursement.
- Realize that if you participate in Medicaid, you must accept what they pay.
- Remember that the determination of the appropriate management level in billing is based on the nature of the presenting problems, extent of history, review of systems, physical examination, and medical decision.
- Utilize current coding guidelines that are found at the AMA and HCTA Web sites.
- Remember that a call for consultation is valid if it is medically essential to evaluate the patient.

Regarding operating your office, remember that

- It is important to train your staff in the proper office protocol, in order to ensure patient satisfaction.
- The medical chart is a legal document and thus mandates a high degree of care.
- You should have a staff member with you in the examination room if you feel the patient will be uncomfortable being alone with you. This is especially essential if you have to examine the private parts.

■ You may want to use the early part of the hour for scheduled patients, leaving the later part free for late arrivals, walk-ins, and emergencies.

■ You must date all chart notes, so that you can accurately judge progress or lack thereof, as well as to be covered legally for the accuracy of the services rendered.

■ Physician calls are taken when possible or should be returned promptly if you are tied up.

■ It is important to be diligent in communicating with referring physicians and consultants.

■ Your staff needs to be trained in emergency procedures, should they have to be used in your office.

■ You must obtain a current DEA license.

■ You need to arrange to provide suitable access to your office for those with disabilities.

■ Your staff should be told to collect co-payments from patients at the time of their visit.

When dealing with patients, remember to

■ Caution them in a specific manner about possible side effects of medications.

■ Make yourself available to a reasonable extent to respond to patient needs outside of office hours.

■ Prepare your staff as how to tactfully deal with patients and respond to inquiries.

■ Caution staff about disclosing confidential information and providing medical advice to patients.

With regard to federal regulations, remember to

■ Be cognizant that billing for services not rendered, or billing for unnecessary services, is defined as fraud.

■ Be certain to correctly identify the level of services in the chart and make sure that it is consistent with your coding and billing statement.

■ Learn the art of billing during the course of your residency training.

■ Establish a protocol to ensure compliance with federal billing regulations.

■ Register and obtain a CLA certificate.

■ Make sure that when you advertise your services, the advertising is consistent with federal trade regulations.

Regarding legal liabilities, remember that

■ To prevail in a claim of negligence filed against you, the patient must demonstrate (a) that you had a duty to render nonnegligent care, (b) that you breached that duty, and (c) that the breach caused injury to the patient.

■ You should never terminate care to a patient without providing reasonable notice, preferably in writing.

■ When transferring a patient's records to another physician, you must secure the patient's written consent to do so.

■ You must clearly inform the patient of any proposed treatment protocol and/or procedure and the rationale behind your recommendation and obtain their written consent to do so. Inquire if they fully understand your proposal. This is especially essential in dealing with elderly patients and should involve a family member or friend if circumstances makes this necessary.

■ When in doubt about handling an issue, you should consult a knowledgeable attorney.

■ Your malpractice insurance coverage is initiated as of the first day you start to practice medicine.

■ If practicing in your own office, you will need liability insurance for office contents, as well as disability insurance, to best protect your interests.

Marketing your services

A student in the second half of medical school should seriously consider the choice of a specialty. So too does the resident, whose postgraduate training moves past the midpoint, need to give serious thought to their future professional plans. When contemplating going into practice, you are required to make a number of critical decisions. The first is deciding the type of practice you wishes to participate in. Should the choice be made to establish a solo practice or join others in a group practice? Establishing an entirely new practice requires determining the most appropriate location for doing so. Once this is achieved and a new medical facility is contemplated, it is necessary to plan its design and furnish it appropriately. It will then be essential for word to get out that your professional services are available to the public.

The traditional means of providing initial publicity is by sending out announcement cards to relatives, friends, colleagues, former classmates, and residents, as well as acquaintances. You may also place an ad in a community newspaper with a similar message. This should be only the initial step in promoting awareness of your professional presence.

Relative to building a practice, it needs to be recognized at the outset that

■ The medical profession has never been more competitive. Thus, being market-oriented is an important element in developing a patient clientele.

■ The traditional announcement of the opening of a practice, by itself, is no longer an adequate means of securing publicity.

■ It is essential to define the target audience you seek to influence in your favor.

■ It may prove useful to consult with a marketing expert, but check any data given to support the advice you receive.

■ The quality of your patient rapport can be the best advocate for selling your services to the public.

■ One of the cheapest sources for publicity is satisfied patients, since they will likely make favorable comments to others.

■ You need to distinguish your practice in some manner, for example, responding to patient concerns so that they are motivated to say, "My doctor really hears me out."

Strategy for success. It is advisable to use a multistep process to facilitate your marketing efforts. Elements of this concept will be identified and discussed briefly.

■ *Set specific targets.* To enhance the chances that your efforts will be productive, it is important to establish realistic goals. These should be communicated to your staff so that they actively cooperate in the effort and share in the sense of accomplishment. Before initiating a goal, secure staff input to determine the feasibility of the target set. Monitor the fulfillment of the goal as time progresses and allow a reasonable amount of time for it to be attained.

■ *Identify your market.* It is important to establish the geographic or demographic identity of your prospective patient base.

■ *Create a marketing program.* The best program is one that is straightforward, definitive, monitorable, practical, and appropriate.

■ *Activate your plan.* Before initiating your marketing program, be certain that all the essential elements are in place. Do not be impatient and act prematurely.

■ *Evaluate results.* When the marketing program has been completed, see if the results have achieved their set goal. If they have, all well and good. You may wish to build on your success based on your experience and undertake another campaign. If unsuccessful, you may consider using your experience to redesign your marketing program, so that it proves more effective the second time around.

Promotional tools. When you are considering the use of any of a wide range of possible media options, it is necessary to evaluate your writing capabilities and speaking effectiveness. Your abilities in this regard will impact the choice and extent of your usage of the various media outlets discussed below.

There are a wide variety of instruments that can be used to bring your services to the attention of your target market. Among these are the following:

■ *Publicity packet.* This is a professionally designed bundle of material that includes a well-written biography that identifies the highlights of your career and notes any special credentials that you may have. It should also provide a brief outline of the specialty as well as of its standard procedures that, if necessary, you can perform to diagnose and/or treat specific diseases. Relevant insurance issues of interest to prospective patients should also be mentioned, along with an offer to be of assistance in this regard. The members of your staff should be identified, and (preferably flexible) office hours noted. The physician's business card may be included in the packet.

■ *Open house.* This is a useful means to provide potentially interested patients exposure to facilities and staff. When you are ready to initiate your professional activities, arranging for an open house for several hours at a convenient time is seriously worth considering. This approach can also be used when a new physician joins a group practice or if the facilities are expanded.

■ *Bulletin board.* Placing a display unit in a prominent place in the office can be helpful. It can be used for posting announcements that enhance the physician's prestige, such as copies of any published papers and book title pages, lecture announcements, or appointments to prestigious positions.

■ *Local newspapers.* Many communities have their own neighborhood newspapers, which commonly are distributed free in banks, shopping centers, etc. Advertisements in such outlets can offer direct access to those in the vicinity of your office. Such papers may also be used as a vehicle to write an advice column in your specialty, which may then be cut out by an impressed reader and passed around among friends, as well as being posted on your office bulletin board.

Some areas may have weekly local newspapers that are sold at a modest cost to readers. You might wish, in addition to advertising in them, to offer to provide periodic interviews or write a column on topics of public interest on which you are knowledgeable. Arrange to identify the health section editor at the paper to secure his/her cooperation. Choose a topic for an interview that will be of widespread interest or is a hot topic of discussion in society. Think about your subject and the major points you wish to convey. Before contacting a reporter, realize that those people, by virtue of their profession, are very pressed for time. Thus you should make a quick but effective sales pitch for your proposed interview, highlighting the key elements you wish to get across to your audience, and hopefully get a positive response.

In the past, a medical advice column could prove to be beneficial to a physician's name recognition. Currently the situation has changed and this approach has been converted into "advertorials." These paid ads seemingly are messages aimed at enhancing public welfare, but also focus on promoting the sponsoring physician's practice.

■ *In-house publications.* There are medical centers and large health care facilities that develop and distribute their own publications. This can provide an institution's affiliated physician with an outlet to get to be known to the community. Such publications are usually mailed out to past patients listed in the institution's database, targeted families in the service area, and prominent members of the community.

The contact person who can facilitate your gaining exposure through in-house publishers is the director of public affairs at the institution. You can inquire as to the topics that are of interest to him/her and see if you would care to write on any of the subjects. Simultaneously, you can offer suggestions of your own and see if there is interest. In any case, try to establish good rapport with this person, so that they might think of tapping into your expertise at some time in the future.

■ *Newsletter*. Topic-specific newsletters can be a useful means of providing relevant current medical information in a format that is understandable to lay persons. This publicity medium can be utilized by both independent physicians and group practices. Thus a newsletter is a convenient way to convey information to the members of your community and influence their choice of a physician.

Developing a newsletter is a multistep process. At the outset it is useful if you establish a reasonable budget estimate as to what financial commitment should and can be made for such a project over its entire existence. This potential commitment should be put aside for a while, until you get one or more cost estimates as the project progresses. That will be the decisive time for making a judgment as to the project's feasibility. Of special import in this regard is the frequency of publication contemplated (monthly, quarterly, etc.). This obviously needs to be borne in mind before moving ahead with such a potentially costly undertaking.

The next step is to select the audience you seek to reach. This may be defined in demographic terms, facilitating forming an estimate of the prospective number of newsletters that will be needed for distribution. This will allow you to secure an estimate of production and mailing expenses. With the extent of the audience established, you should then proceed to determine the message or subject matter for your prospective newsletter. It is desirable to avoid being overly broad in the scope of the contents presented to your audience. This aspect of the project deserves to be especially carefully considered, to ensure that your readers will find your comments specifically interesting and useful, rather than being exposed to generalities.

Once the basic content of the newsletter has been established, you then need to carefully consider the amount of information you seek to present to your audience without overwhelming them with excessive detail. This will allow you to zero in on production specifications. You obviously need to consider the layout of your planned newsletter, because the format of presentation will strongly influence the extent of interest in its contents. The manner of presentation should be appropriate for a medical newsletter that is being presented to a lay audience, namely, not too lively nor too dull.

The format has a significant influence on the cost of production. Cost will be impacted by the number of pages, quality of paper used, and inclusion of color, photographs, and graphics. The outcome of your newsletter will ultimately depend upon the quality of the people who handle its production. It is important, therefore, to examine samples of the work that your prospective production people have done previously. You can also seek to find out from references how compatible and reliable your prospective printer is in meeting commitments, before engaging anyone for the job.

The last step in the process is distribution of the newsletter, and this is not a straightforward issue. A judgment has to be made, for example, about mailing it third class, which is cheaper but in which the material is subject to being damaged, or placing it in a first-class envelope, which is costlier, but more secure from being defaced. An even greater expense will be incurred by using a mailing company for distribution services. Sorting the mailing pieces by zip code is recommended to hold mailing costs down. Guidance on mailing might be obtained from your local post office manager.

The mailing list you use may come from your affiliated hospital database, focusing on those individuals who conceivably would be interested in your specialty. Marketing media consultants can assist you in securing target populations (e.g., senior citizens, prospective pregnant mothers).

In conclusion, a newsletter can prove to be a useful public relations modality, but it needs careful planning and proper execution. Speak with colleagues who have tried it and learn from their experience how appropriate it would be for you as a medium to gain exposure.

■ *Radio.* Newsletters are useful publicity outlets. Thus some physicians turn to local radio as a means to become better known. Radio is also preferred, because it requires far less complex technical arrangements when making a presentation than does television.

Your goal is to identify local radio listings that carry talk shows and utilize guest interviews in their format. This can be pinpointed by checking radio station listings in your local paper. Your yellow pages phone directory can get you the appropriate phone number that will enable you to contact the station's program director. Before doing so, you should become acquainted with the program's content and format and, if appropriate, make a sales pitch to try to obtain an invitation for guest appearances.

Should you secure an opportunity to be on the radio, make sure to prepare adequately for it. Practice what you plan to say until you can say it fluently. Time yourself so that you will be clear and concise and not overrun the time allotted to you. Radio has a good potential for physicians as a publicity outlet. Television, both local and network, while potentially more attractive, is not a realistic source to gain exposure, because of the intense difficulty of gaining access.

■ *Internet.* Web sites are very popular outlets to publicize one's medical services. However, the applicability of this medium in securing patients is not appealing. This is because the effort and time involved in establishing and maintaining a Web site, as compared to its potential rewards, are not compatible. Thus most independent practitioners will likely not use this resource. What can be done, however, is to ascertain if the institution that you become affiliated with has a Web site. If so, you can inquire from the Public Affairs director if you can gain exposure through this site. The use of a Web site by a multispecialty group may be more feasible and merits exploration, because it may have broader appeal to Web surfers.

Efficiently operating a practice

Many demands are currently placed on medical practitioners. Among others, these include pressures arising from the need to comply with all relevant regulations, efforts by insurers to lower reimbursement for medical services, the need for greater control over overhead expenses, and the desire to ensure patient satisfaction. All these pressures make it a challenge to run an office effectively. The best response is strategic business planning, which will be discussed below.

Strategic business planning. Having an action plan as how to operate your medical practice will smooth the road to success. This is especially critical when initiating or expending a practice. Before drawing up your plan bear in mind to

- Include all areas involved in executing your practice in the plan.
- Establish reasonable deadlines for achieving goals that are set.
- Assign specific responsibilities to appropriate and qualified personnel.
- Inform and involve the entire staff in both developing and executing the plan.
- Establish strategies that are few, realistic, and straightforward to execute.
- Develop the plan by a consensus of the members when dealing with a group practice.
- Allocate the necessary resources to achieve targeted tasks.

With the basic prerequisites established, we can turn to various issues regarding the strategic plan itself. This should consist of multiple components, each of which will be discussed separately.

Propose definitive goals. When establishing goals for staff, be certain that they are reasonably attainable. Put them down in writing in such a way that they are comprehensible and decisive, so that a positive outcome can be attained. Thus, for example, when seeking to enhance collection of accounts receivable, a number of options and different proposals can be offered, but their effectiveness varies widely. To achieve such a goal, the following possible objectives can be suggested:

- Focus attention on diminishing the outstanding accounts receivable.

This is a vague and quantitatively ill-defined aim that does not allow a determination of successful achievement of the set goal.

- Aim to diminish outstanding accounts receivable to a reasonable extent.

Although this goal is somewhat more meaningful than the previous one, it is still unacceptably ill-defined and indefinite and thus its effectiveness remains questionable.

■ Eliminate all accounts receivable by a specific date.

This may be setting an unattainable target, since monitoring implementation at any stage, to determine progress up to that point, is not indicated.

■ Seek to diminish accounts receivable by a fixed percentage within a fixed time period and then afterward do so again for a higher percentage after a second interlude.

This last strategy is thoughtfully developed and logically formulated. It allows for an initial collection phase and a follow-up effort to secure funds from more challenging accounts.

The above comments are relevant not only for a solo practice but also for a group practice. Moreover, all significant issues faced by the practice should be resolved in an amicable manner and by consensus of the participants, so that amicable relationships are retained.

Evaluate your practice. It is important to analyze the manner in which your practice operates in order to institute *corrective* improvements when necessary. Seek to determine the following:

■ If your decision-making process is proactive, as it should be, or is merely reactive.

■ If assignments are made randomly, or are delegated to appropriate personnel for effective action (except for training purposes).

■ Possible common demographic, geographic, and cultural characteristics of your patient population. You then can respond accordingly.

■ If there is an imbalance in the sources of reimbursement of the accounts of patients utilizing the practice. This enables you to avoid being overly dependent on one or a limited number of them for an adequate income.

■ If funds are being properly expended, so that your costs are being adequately monitored.

■ If specific managed care organization affiliations are profitable and if you also have suitably profitable financial arrangements with them.

■ If the medical services and procedures being offered in your specialty are generating appropriate income compared with others in your area.

■ If objectively you believe that you are obtaining the appropriate share of the patient market for your specialty. If not, consider ways to improve the situation.

Evaluate your plan. The basic goal of a plan is to facilitate a move from one level of operation to a more efficient and productive one. But before implementing any plan, it should be scrutinized carefully to determine its necessity and validity. To do so you should ask yourself the following questions:

- Is the plan comprehensive enough to meet foreseeable needs?

- Do all the elements of the plan need to be implemented simultaneously?

- Do you have adequate funds to invest to effectively implement your plan?

- Are your fiscal resources adequate in light of any prospective risks you will be undertaking?

- Do you have suitable credit resources to provide needed funds that would make the plan feasible?

- Is the implementation timeline for your plans realistic, relative to your goals?

As a consequence of your responses to these questions, you should modify your plans. Both drafts and finalized plans should be put into written form.

Implementing your plan. This step is predicated on the assumption that previous elements are effectively carried out. A business plan may involve making decisions on the following:

- Hiring new and various types of personnel to increase efficiency.

- Purchasing different types of equipment for various uses (both medical and clerical).

- Renovating and/or expanding facilities to enhance patient services offered.

- Changing schedules or office procedures to facilitate operations.

- Enlarging the scope of services offered to increase the patient population.

It should be noted that significant changes in office facilities may be planned over the course of a number of years. To accurately keep in mind the details of such plans and the scheduling of these changes, they should be carefully recorded in detail and kept available for ready reference.

Monitoring the plan. Once implementation of a plan is initiated, it is essential that its progress be monitored to determine if it is proceeding satisfactorily. Monitoring should be an ongoing process; this helps guarantee successful outcomes.

If your plan is working effectively, all well and good, but do not rest on your laurels; continue to maintain vigilance to ensure that things keep progressing satisfactorily. On the other hand, if things are not progressing satisfactorily, then

- Seek to determine the source of the problem, especially its root causes.

- See if any of the goals set are basically unreasonable and unjustifiable.

- Examine if any faulty assumptions were made when you established your plan.

- Evaluate the schedule to determine if their goals set are unachievable under normal conditions.

- Ascertain if circumstances have changed since implementation of the plan that may be impeding its success.

- Identify any areas that may be specifically objectively the goals you seek.

- Ascertain if the delay in attaining your goal is beyond your control.

- Find out if merely allowing more time will rectify the existing problem.

- Determine if the remedy for a problem is minor or major to see if it requires modest or drastic change.

- Consider if delaying some parts of your plan for a time or changing circumstances may facilitate your resolving current issues.

- Ascertain if you need outside help to advise you on how to solve your problem.

Focus attention on information systems. The driving force behind the way a practice is run is managed care. To avoid bureaucratic difficulties, it is best to process the required formalities in the manner mandated by managed care organizations, in order to facilitate prompt and proper reimbursement. This is an important consideration, because most patients belong to health insurance plans. It is vital that your computer system be kept upgraded to meet the demands of changes required by these organizations.

There are two major information source impacting a practice, namely, the computer and the telephone. Each will be discussed separately.

Computers. Computerization is the key to effectively interacting with the bulk of the business aspects of a practice, including managed care organizations (MCOs). It thus is worthwhile to invest in a good-quality system, whose reliability will pay off in the long run. As we know, this type of equipment rapidly tends to become obsolete and it also requires a support service. For commercially available systems, it is essential that the level of expertise of the office personnel using them be fully adequate. This is especially true where your system is linked to a network.

The computer system at your faculty will be the mechanism for billing for services rendered, submitting claims for reimbursement to insurance outlets, and collecting outstanding payments due, as well as keeping track of practice expenditures, accounts receivable, and revenue transactions. In addition, your system will be used to schedule patient appointments and provide a source for a wide range of significant information regarding patient treatment and outcomes. It is apparent that the computer, being a multipurpose instrument, will serve as the nerve center of business operations in a practice. It thus is a vital component in facilitating the success of a practice and should be utilized to the fullness of its potential.

Telephone. The phone system you install should have the option of expansion to accommodate foreseeable future needs. It is important that all personnel be fully trained to effectively use the system that is installed.

Having a voice-mail system for personal calls is extremely helpful. It is also useful to arrange multiple options on your phone system, with the emergency line being first. An operator option allowing direct voice contact can prove most helpful to properly route incoming calls. Your direct access to a cell phone is mandatory.

Another essential information system instrument is a fax machine. This is a most valuable piece of equipment. It is an essential asset to receive vital medical and business information (e.g., laboratory reports and authorizations).

It is also important that all incoming patient calls be properly handled so that most patients will obtain a favorable impression about the operation of your facility. Special care must to be taken with emergency calls and for this purpose a medically oriented individual, such as a nurse, if available, may be warranted. It should be established policy that nonmedical personnel *absolutely* refrain from giving any advice. They should not even suggest what is the physician's usual recommendation under the circumstances. Every effort should be made to facilitate that the patient (or caregiver) speaks with the physician directly to express their concerns.

Focus attention on personnel contacts. The initial impression given about the nature of your practice for anyone contacting your office, either by phone or in person, will be made by your office personnel. They interact intensively with patients and should handle all the business aspects of your operation. It is obvious that their activities can be decisive in enhancing your practice or vice versa. It it is essential that for office operations to function effectively, that

■ You secure the most personable, competent, and reliable office staff possible.

■ Personnel should be assigned the most appropriate tasks that they are qualified to do.

■ A positive and pleasant working environment is provided that will motivate personnel.

To achieve the above results one should focus on a variety of issues associated with operating a successful practice. These will be discussed below under a number of headings.

Develop job descriptions. Such documents are very useful in the employee recruitment and evaluation process. The details stipulated in a job description provide the prospective employee with a chance to determine if they are qualified and interested in the position and what will be expected from them. Over time it may be necessary to revise and update job descriptions to keep them relevant to the actual nature of the responsibilities they cover.

Secure suitable personnel. The guideline for filling a position should be its job description. Using current personnel to network for a new employee can be a valuable means of securing a competent staff. If an existing employee knows of a potential candidate, have them pass a job description on to the candidate. If it is necessary to place an ad in a help wanted column, word it precisely so that under- or overqualified people do not trouble your office by applying.

When applications and/or resumes for a position are received, compare the qualifications with the job descriptions. This screening method will help ensure that only essentially appropriate candidates will then be interviewed. For a group practice, have other physicians of the group also interview the most suitable candidates. The prospective immediate supervisor of the employee (e.g., Office manager), should also gain exposure to the candidate and provide input into the hiring process, so that they feel comfortable with the ultimate choice.

Carefully check the references given and verify educational credentials. If significant troubling questions remain, seek to reinterview a promising candidate to possibly give them the benefit of the doubt, before making a final determination.

Using part-time employees can possibly serve to cut your overhead costs. This arrangement can be made by incorporating two employees into a single job-sharing position, so that they complement their working hours.

Once you have identified the appropriate person for the position, you need to make it attractive to secure their services. To do this, the salary and benefit package (for full-time employees) needs to be competitive. This can be done by securing current information as to remuneration for office staff positions for similar situations. You should indicate what increases an employee can anticipate in due course. Advise employees that they will be evaluated annually. Any pay increase granted to employees should not be across the board, but rather a merit increase, as determined by the quality of performance. Explain to the employee the basis for the level of increase and, where appropriate, indicate what improvements in performance are desirable (or essential). Avoid recriminations and maintain an atmosphere of goodwill when dealing with this issue. When preparing an annual budget, allow an adequate sum to provide for appropriate salary increases for employees.

Create a command structure. To operate effectively, it is important to establish a chain of command so that individuals are given appropriate credit when warranted and are held accountable for their actions or omissions. Such an arrangement can also ensure that an individual carries out tasks delegated by *one* supervising individual rather than by a number of persons.

Create a stimulating environment. The efficiency of office personnel will depend in large measure on the working environment. To facilitate communication and minimize the need to look for personnel in a large facility, an intercom system is essential. Seek professional advice regarding lighting needs, which should be appropriate to the nature of the activity to be performed in the space utilized. Thus, patient waiting rooms may have soft light (and possibly pleasant music); lighting should be suitable for working with computers in the office area and for examination purposes in clinical rooms. The office manager should make sure that the facilities are maintained in a manner suitable for their function by being clean, neat, and pleasant to be in.

In dealing with personnel, it is important not to assign them tasks inappropriate to their positions, unless they receive special instructions for training or other purposes. Also, if you have a grievance against an employee, discuss it in private in a polite and respectful manner, so that your comments are taken as constructive criticism. Resolve any issue, amicably if at all possible, so that the professional relationship is not damaged and the continued employment of the person is not affected. In situations where a serious problem develops with an employee, keep accurate records of such incidents and of any and all your attempts to rectify the situation. If this proves to be unfeasible, then discharging the individual may be unavoidable. This should be done privately and with minimum rancor.

To maintain a favorable working atmosphere, it is important to recognize that for new employees, there is an adjustment period that understandably is initiated after employment begins. This should be followed by an interlude of growth on the job. To achieve these goals, it is important to recognize that the desirable progression that leads to a motivated and satisfied employee comes about in several stages, namely,

■ Developing a sense of becoming a member of a dedicated health care facility. This involves establishing positive interpersonal relations with the others on the team.

■ Securing satisfaction by being recognized for effectively performing one's duties.

■ Recognizing the challenging nature of the position and being motivated to achieve a high level of achievement by conscientious work.

■ Realizing that the larger the practice the greater the potential for advancement.

Physicians can contribute to creating a favorable working environment by strongly encouraging mutual cooperation among employees. This benefits all the members of the team. Harmonious interaction among personnel will inevitably lead to greater productivity, better staff efficiency, and a more satisfied patient clientele.

Focus attention on satisfaction. Aside from staff satisfaction, attention also needs to be focused on the staff generating goodwill of patients, referring physicians, and managed care organizations. Each of these constituencies will be considered separately.

Patient satisfaction. A successful practice depends on securing patient satisfaction. The efficiency of your office practice naturally will contribute to this goal. It is therefore important to focus specifically on maintaining a high level of patient approval that will encourage patients to become long-standing recipients of care and to refer others. A number of elements contribute to patient satisfaction:

■ *Provide Positive office experiences.* These involve being received politely and processed efficiently. The waiting room should have a professional appearance with current magazines and, preferably, free access to local phone service.

■ *Start your schedule on time.* To achieve this, arrange that the first patient of the day arrives somewhat prior to the onset of your initiating provision of services, so that he/she can be placed in an examination room awaiting you at the start of activities.

■ *Focus on your schedule.* Make every effort to keep your schedule of patient visits on time as much as possible. Patients are not surprised if emergencies occur or you have to stay longer at the hospital. However, they need to be advised if such an event occurs, and that a significant delay in seeing the doctor is likely. The staff should do so preferably by calling them at home or notifying them in the office waiting room. When excessive delay is inevitable, offer patients the option of staying for the doctor's arrival or being rescheduled to the next earliest time possible. Allow a reasonable standard amount of time for patient visits. A patient should not feel that he/she has been short-changed by not having been granted enough time to speak with the physician.

■ *Schedule appropriately.* Your office hours should not be focused on hours that are primarily convenient for you, but also seek to accommodate potential patients' availability. Thus, if feasible, you should include both day and evening hours, selecting those periods that you find most popular for your patients. Be prepared to make needed schedule adjustments as called for by the demand for your services.

■ *Facilitate walk-ins.* At times it proves difficult for patients to schedule an appointment because an emergency has arisen or their schedule does not allow for a delay. See if you can add to your regular schedule one or two slots for walk-ins. They should be advised that they will be seen, but there may likely be a delay. Inform them politely upon arrival that they are being accommodated this time because of special need, but in the future they will be expected to make a regular appointment. If increased patient volume occurs due to seasonal circumstances (e.g., a flu epidemic, a long weekend, many sick calls), adjust your walk-in schedule accordingly. Especially seek to accommodate long-standing patients.

■ *Delineate response time.* Arrange a fixed period of time to respond to routine patient calls that come in on a given day. Also, use any available time during this interlude to carefully check all lab and other reports that came in during that day. Note in some manner that you have checked them and make any necessary comments on the report. Promptly contact patients who demonstrate abnormalities that merit your or another specialist's medical attention. It is desirable, as a gesture of goodwill, to have your patients contacted and be advised of a favorable lab report.

■ *Meet special needs.* Thus, for example, if your practice serves a significant number of non-English-speaking persons, see if you can engage a person fluent in the appropriate foreign language (Spanish, Russian, etc.) to fill one of your office staff positions. This will allow such patients an opportunity to express themselves more fully and comfortably. For such patients, their exact problem can then be better understood and more successfully treated. This approach should also help obtain other patients from a similar cultural or regional background.

■ *Suggest related services.* If you have an interest in special areas where you recognize a need, insofar as your practice is concerned (e.g., nutrition counseling, alternative/complementary medical care, ultrasound, physical therapy), seek to gain the necessary information or contacts and then offer such services to your patients.

Maintain strong referral links. Many specialists and subspecialists are largely dependent on their professional colleagues for referrals. It is obviously essential to maintain their goodwill to secure patient referrals. This can readily be done by seeing referred patients for a consultation without any excessive delay and providing your evaluation to their physician in a prompt and thorough manner. In case of critical diagnostic findings, you should promptly communicate with the referring doctor by phone. If you assume responsibility for treating the referred patient, ascertain if the doctor wishes to be kept fully apprised as to his/her progress or simply wishes to be informed as to the outcome. If you are invited to be a member of a treatment team, recognize that the patient's primary physician has overall responsibility for the case and be ready to defer to his/her judgment. If you vigorously oppose the primary physician's approach, you have the option of withdrawing from the case. Clearly, developing good professional relationships will further your own practice. Thus make every effort to accommodate referring physicians whenever possible, and extend yourself to be of help to them. This will strengthen both your professional relationship and your practice.

Seek membership in appropriate MCOs. Determine the MCOs that serve your location and find out what they are looking for in terms of physician credentials. Become familiar as to how demanding they are regarding keeping costs down and high positive outcomes. Inquire as to the extent of services they cover, reimbursement rates, and utilization guidelines. See if your personality and standards for medical practice are compatible with theirs. See if it is possible to satisfy their needs by accommodating the health plan's standards, efficiently processing the essential paperwork, and establishing positive personal contacts with relevant MCO personnel. The goal should be to enhance their potential to gain enrollees to their health plans because you are on the list of physician providers.

22 | Monitoring Your Professional and Personal Finances

Overview

Just as the vital signs of an individual are an index of their health status, so too does monitoring the key financial components of a medical practice serve to provide insight into the state of its fiscal affairs. This information includes periodically elucidating patient volume, the number of procedures performed, billing practices, and collection results. These data should be available from the information stored in a suitable computer system and a condensed status report should be able to be capable of being generated regularly without excessive difficulty.

Maintaining fiscal oversight

To maintain careful oversight of your practice, it is advisable to print out a brief, basic monthly statement. It should outline the details of various essential parameters such as accounts receivable, fiscal operations, and procedural activities that have taken place during each cycle. By means of such regularly generated reports prepared by a suitable spreadsheet program, the direction of progress can be readily, accessed. This approach to the business aspects of your practice facilitates having the essential data readily available for your evaluation when needed.

Aside from getting an overview as to the current state of financial affairs, a specific insight can be secured from such a fiscal report into such issues as

■ What potential sources of fiscal weakness may exist.
■ How effective your business manager's performance is.

■ The desirability of pressing for the resolution of long-standing open accounts.

■ The advisability of considering the use of billing codes.

A major item under the financial parameters heading is *gross charges,* namely, basic fees prior to any adjustments. These adjustments may result from contractual discounts due to health plan affiliation or insurance write-offs. Consequently, you now have the adjusted or *collectable charges.* It is critical to be aware of the percentage of the charges being secured. The target should be more than 95%. The bottom line is that one needs to have a good grasp of the extent of revenue generation, insurance write-offs, and collections to appreciate in which direction the business is going.

It is vital to secure additional information regarding the status of your practice by being familiar with the following concepts.

Capitation revenue. In contrast to the fee-for-service approach, under capitation, a physician aligned with a managed health plan receives a monthly fee per patient regardless whether services are actually rendered. Health plans may withhold a portion of the capitation fee as a hedge against potential losses. If the financial outcome for the plan for the fiscal year is positive, the withheld funds may be returned, in part or in whole, to the health care provider. In addition, incentives for effective care management may be offered by plans. Some plans even provide bonuses for attaining cost savings. The three revenue sources, monthly capitation fees, incentives, and bonuses, make up the actual capitation revenue provided physicians under contract with health plans.

To appreciate the impact of capitation, you can compare its revenue with that which you would have accrued under a fee-for-service system. This will demonstrate the extent to which the practice's capitation revenue compares with that from the traditional reimbursement format.

Collection ratios. The comparison between capitation and fee-for-service is known as the *gross collection ratio* (or percentage). Should it be established that revenue realization from capitation is low (60% or less), then there may be a problem with the level of the capitation rate or the physician may be overutilizing managed care services. Should the revenue realization percentage fall far below that anticipated, this should suggest that you (a) review your efficiency in managing patient care, (b) possibly renegotiate a higher capitation rate, or (c) reconsider the advisability of remaining in the health plan.

The computer program used to print out the spreadsheet should be able to automatically generate the essential statistics that will allow you to monitor the fiscal data regarding both the gross and net collection ratios. Most specialties usually fall into the 60–80% range. What should arouse your interest and merit investigation is a marked change in this parameter, especially an unexplained substantial drop in the gross collection ratio.

The key statistic reflecting a practice's state of affairs is the *net collection ratio*. A ratio of 96% or higher indicates that practice is operating well. It means that bad debts are absorbing only a few percentage points of collectable charges. This situation reflects favorably on the efficiency of your business manager and billing service. Should this figure be in the low 90s or less, improvement is called for.

Managing accounts receivable. The data regarding this issue can also provide a measure of judging a practice's business effectiveness. Of special significance are the amount and percentage of overdue receivables that extend beyond 90 days. This deadline is selected because it has been shown that Medicare reimburses within 15–30 days and most other third-party payers within 30–60 days. Beyond this time, most reimbursements should have been received (including co-payments). The extent of outstanding receivables varies, depending on the specialty, but is commonly in the 20–35% range.

Pending insurance payments are another parameter that one should examine. However, an average acceptable range has not been established as yet, although a figure of about 65% is considered reasonable. It is important to make sure that all payments are posted regularly, thereby automatically updating the insurance pending category. This will facilitate the patient's receiving a statement for the balance due and thereby updating accounts and enhancing possible full payment.

Where a massive backlog of payments is found to be present, it is advisable to institute an intense collection campaign to secure payment from all seriously delinquent accounts. Appropriate personnel should be assigned to secure payments due. These could be resolved, if necessary, using the installment method. To achieve this important goal, overtime payments for personnel involved may be desirable. In the event that in some cases, you are not successful, using a collection agency should be considered. It may be necessary to institute a collection campaign periodically to avoid a backlog in reimbursement. In any case, one should not become alarmed if accounts receivable drop temporarily. However, it is important to keep your finger on the official fiscal pulse, to ensure that the decline is not excessively lengthy.

Another monitoring factor is the *accounts receivable ratio*. This is attained by dividing the total accounts receivable by the average month's gross charges. The latter will provide the amount of gross monthly charges held in accounts receivable. While this figure fluctuates with different specialties, a ratio of less than three months is acceptable. If it is greater, then a concerted effort should be made to remedy the situation.

Service utilization. It is beneficial to secure command of the numbers associated with various procedures performed routinely in the course of the practice. One should monitor new and established patient visits, as well as consultations, relevant to procedural activities. There are specific specialty-related data in the literature relevant to this issue that may also be desirable to track.

In dealing with reimbursement it is important to identify new visits, because the level of compensation is significantly higher for consultations than for new patient visits. Attention should be given to identifying patient referrals as consultations rather than as first encounters with new patients.

In 1992, codes were introduced to identify patient management and evaluation procedures. From that time on, there came into effect the concept of five levels and of numbers being assigned to services. The key services of a practice are new and established patient visits and office consultations.

One can identify office visits by various kinds of patients by the level of service provided. The care level can range from 1 to 5. The higher the level, the more comprehensive care is being provided and hence the higher the remuneration. It is obvious that it is essential not to understate the care level when submitting for reimbursement. Thus accurate coding of services is important for enhanced revenue return.

Regarding recording service levels on billing statements, it is important to recognize that level 2 is not applicable to physician services; rather it is the designation for care provided by paraprofessionals (e.g., physician's assistants or nurses). Designating this level or understanding your level of service will result in an unnecessarily diminished extent of reimbursement.

Cost control

After analysis of the business aspects of the practice, it, often proves desirable to institute cost controls. The question of cost control will focus on three areas; billing practices, personnel and savings mechanisms.

Billing practices. If a statistical summary of the use of the service codes is prepared periodically (e.g., every three to six months), a bell-shaped curve is a likely outcome. This provides useful data for a group practice to determine if it is on target. It also allows identification of which individual members fall outside of the mean distribution. Remedial action to improve code selection can then be instituted. Recognizing this solution can diminish "under-coding", indirectly enhancing remuneration and thus profitability.

You should identify the major procedures in the specialty that account for the bulk of your revenue. By doing so and determining how extensively they are employed in your practice, you can provide a good insight as to the professional activities in this important category. Stimulating activity in such procedures increases profitability.

Regarding inpatient services, there are five areas to keep track of, namely, hospital admissions, follow-up visits, consultations, procedures, and discharges. Knowledge of the direction of activities in these various categories will enable appropriate charges to be made.

In general, the lowest level of service a physician can provide is level 2, but this is not used for physician services. The most commonly used designation is level 3 (code 99213). This represents about 70% of the billings filled, with the balance covered by level 4 and 5 designations. Before assigning a customary level 3, one should review the billing chart to see if the services rendered would justify a higher level assignment. Service-level reports facilitate physicians mastering how to assign the proper level of care to their billing statements.

Personnel. One of the various areas where cost oversight deserves special consideration is personnel. This is a major item in any budget. When considering laying off or hiring personnel, recognize that this may significantly influence the operational budget of the practice and carefully evaluate the situation accordingly.

When considering terminating someone's employment, be sure that a vacuum is not created, and that key services are not significantly diminished. Be aware that such an action, if not fully justified, may introduce a sense of job insecurity among your employees. This inturn may affect the long-term commitment of others and consequently induce a high turnover rate. This type of environment can disrupt office efficiency and generate patient dissatisfaction. Thus layoffs should be carefully considered before being instituted, because they may have unwarranted and unforeseen repercussions.

It may be possible to control costs even when adding personnel, because they can contribute to more patients being seen over the course of the same time interval. The types of personnel who can improve professional efficiency are office nurses and medical assistants.

It is also possible to enhance practice income at a very active practice by employing *physician extenders (PEs)*. This term generally refers to physician assistants (PAs), or certified registered nurse practitioners (CRNPs). Such paraprofessionals can assume some of the more basic medical responsibilities and administrative duties from a physician. This approach leaves more time for the physician to perform essential medically sophisticated tasks. Physician extenders can perform such tasks as taking medical histories, assessing principal health concerns, conducting routine checkups, and ordering lab tests and/or x-rays. Both PAs and CRNPs usually perform their activities under the supervision of and in consultation with physicians, who bear ultimate responsibility for patient management. The salary level for such personnel is significantly lower than that of an associate physician, and thus physician extenders can prove to be a valuable addition to certain solo or group practices. It has been determined that such personnel as PEs can add to a practice's income significantly in excess of their salaries.

Medicare and other third-party reimbursers will cover the cost of services by physician extenders, if their services are provided under physician supervision.

For a very large group practice, employment of a *patient advocate* can be considered. The function of this employee is to familiarize patients with the essential parameters of their health plans in order to secure reimbursable medical services. They can also acquaint patients with the support resources that are available to them. Thus they will guide them on how and where to secure their medications, laboratory tests, and rehabilitation services. Such individualized services can help improve patient satisfaction and also reduce the potential for financial losses incurred by inefficient usage of services within patients' health plans.

There is a new type of employee that may be useful in some group practices, such as obstetrics gynecology, namely a *chaperoned scribe*. Functioning as a chaperone, the individual is present when the doctor is performing a physical exam. This will minimize any legal problems that can possibly arise. They can take notes as the examination proceeds and follow up on any postexamination needs (e.g., order medications, order follow-up tests, arrange for hospitalization). Such personnel, it has been reported, can result in increased processing of patients, thereby significantly improving physician efficiency and patient satisfaction. In a field such as ob-gyn, this can prove quite profitable over the long run.

Saving mechanisms. A variety of other measures that can impact the fiscal status of a practice should be considered. These are as follows:

■ *Physical plant*. Evaluate if you are maximally utilizing your facilities. If they are being underused, perhaps you can sublet some unused space, which will bring in income, without effecting the operations of the practice.

■ *Leasing*. The terms of your lease should be carefully examined at renewal time, to see if you have negotiated the best terms possible.

■ *Outsourcing*. For a large group practice, determine if it is more financially advantageous to have payroll services provided by an outside agency.

■ *Overtime*. If your overtime costs are significant, seek to keep your office hours on a tighter schedule so, that you do not incur such additional expenses.

■ *Fringe benefits*. These should be reviewed carefully to determine if you can provide essential benefits without excessive cost to the practice.

■ *Physician perks*. Review which of these are essential and if they can be reduced or consolidated. This applies to books or journal subscriptions, and travel to professional meetings.

■ *Supplies*. It is essential to avoid panic buying, for it is costly. An up-to-date, inventory should be kept of all standard supplies used in the practice. Supplies should be ordered in bulk amounts whenever possible. These should be secured by competitive bidding or by having your purchaser search the Internet for the most attractive prices.

Personal financial planning

The critical goal of employment efforts is usually personal financial security. This involves recognizing the basic elements associated with the key areas of financial management. These are insurance, investment, taxes, retirement, and estate planning. It is important, therefore, to take the time to be somewhat knowledgeable in these areas.

Getting started. To initiate strategic financial planning, it is essential to gather and organize your personal financial data. By this basis you will determine your assets and liabilities and thus establish your net worth as realistically as possible. To do this you need to focus on up-to-date information. Therefore you should secure copies of your most current bank statements, as well as investment accounts and retirement reports.

Your investments should be divided into liquid, marketable, and nonmarketable assets. These assets can be defined as follows:

■ *Liquid assets*. These are stable in price and refer to checking accounts and certificates of deposit.

■ *Marketable assets*. These can be converted readily into cash and are represented by stocks and bonds, but their value may be higher or lower than your initial purchase price and thus need to be evaluated to determine their current market worth.

■ *Nonmarketable assets*. These are difficult to evaluate. They are examplified by one's share of a medical practice, limited partnerships, real estate, investments, one's home, valuable jewelry, automobiles, and insurance policies (which possibly can be cashed in prior to maturity).

When determining your liabilities, be sure to include such items as auto loans and leases, student loans, credit card liabilities, and outstanding mortgages on your home(s) (and any other real estate that you own in part or in full).

Your financial statement should contain an outline of your income from all sources. Preparing a financial statement takes time, but it is a worthwhile effort.

Budgeting. To accumulate wealth, it is necessary to maintain careful control over your fiscal activities. The best way to do this is by means of proper management of expenditures in the context of a budget. This can be done by analyzing your expenditures under various headings, as outlined in Table 22.1. (Your income tax return can be a source of this information.)

One of the largest segments of income is commonly expended on your home mortgage. You should seek to keep your mortgage payments (including taxes and

Table 22.1 Income and liabilities

Income

Wages . . . .   _____
Taxable interest income . . . .   _____
Tax-exempt interest income . . . .   _____
Dividend income . . . .   _____
Tax refunds . . . .   _____
Business income (loss) . . . .   _____
Other income . . . .   _____
Total income . . . .   _____

Liabilities

Taxes

Savings and investments . . . .   _____
Federal income tax . . . .   _____
State and local income taxes . . . .   _____
Social security tax . . . .   _____
Medicare tax . . . .   _____
Personal property tax . . . .   _____
Other taxes . . . .   _____
Total taxes . . . .   _____

Insurance

Homeowners . . . .   _____
Automobile . . . .   _____
Life . . . .   _____
Medical . . . .   _____
Disability . . . .   _____
Malpractice . . . .   _____
Other . . . .   _____
Total insurance . . . .   _____

Standard of living

Mortgage/rent . . . .   _____
Utility bills . . . .   _____
Telephone, cell phone service . . . .   _____
Home maintenance costs . . . .   _____
Auto leasing or mortgage costs . . . .   _____
Auto maintenance costs . . . .   _____
Home heating costs . . . .   _____
Food expenditures . . . .   _____
Personal care costs . . . .   _____
Clothing costs . . . .   _____
Educational tuition costs . . . .   _____
Entertainment . . . .   _____
Vacation costs . . . .   _____
Groceries . . . .   _____
Charitable contributions . . . .   _____
Medical expenses . . . .   _____
Dental expenses . . . .   _____
Professional expenses . . . .   _____
Miscellaneous . . . .   _____
Total cost of living . . . .   _____
Total liabilities . . . .   _____

insurance) at 18–35% of your pretax income. Leasing an automobile may also prove to be financially more rewarding than purchasing one on installments. This is especially true if you trade in your car periodically.

Once you complete Table 22.1 you can focus on your personal financial aims. These should be definable and realistic. Possible goals include having adequate funds for purchasing a home/second home, educating your children, and having a comfortable retirement.

To achieve these goals, it is necessary to plan properly regarding

- Investing
- Insurance coverage
- Income tax management
- Educating your children
- Retirement planning
- Estate planning

Each of these money management areas will be considered separately.

Investment planning. Investing is a common activity among physicians, in an effort to accumulate wealth. This can be achieved if one's assets grow in value. Such growth permits planning for both short- and long-term projected expenses and anticipated needs.

To design a realistic investment portfolio, a variety of considerations needs to be taken into account. These include the time frame to achieve your goals, personal risk tolerance, tax bracket, income level, and your state of health.

The following primer can be given regarding investments.

- *Time horizon.* This factor will impact the extent of risks you may wish to take. It is essential to determine in advance when capital will be needed and weigh that against the risk of not having it available at that time. For a long-term investment (e.g., five years or more), volatility is less of a concern, but inflation is more of a consideration, and depending on its level, it can erode one's assets.

- *Diversification of assets.* Once your goals and time horizon are established, you can start considering asset class selection of investments between cash, stocks, and bonds. Diversification by itself is not enough to ensure investment success; rather it is the makeup of the allocation that counts. Bonds and stocks are usually both chosen for investment, because traditionally, but not always, a decline in one will be balanced by an advance in another. Thus, if the investments in a portfolio are properly proportioned, their combined value may be enhanced. This approach has been shown to improve chances of maintaining a stable and forward advancing fiscal equilibrium.

■ *Internationalization.* Diversification can also involve investing in international markets and not exclusively in the domestic one. It has been shown that such a mix can, under conditions of a declining domestic stock market, serve to reduce volatility. In any case, with asset allocation, you should view your performance by examining the return as a whole, rather than that of the individual components of the portfolio and then making a judgment.

■ *Anticipate market volatility.* It is generally accepted that stocks present a very volatile investment vehicle. It is also a long-standing premise that if one holds onto stocks long enough, they are bound to go up. There are those, however, who advocate altering allocation of assets in response to changes in existing economic conditions. However, it has been found that such portfolio changes generally do not have a higher probability of achieving success. This does not mean that one should follow a buy-and-hold strategy and feel restricted in regard to selling when prices are high and then relocating one's assets. However, don't be impelled to do so because of a rumor about an investment that sounds too good to pass over. It most likely should be passed over.

There are a wide variety of investment vehicles. Several of these will be discussed briefly.

■ *Stocks.* These offer the possibility of a significant increase in value, but simultaneously present a greater risk than bonds. Analysis of stock history has shown that generally one can secure a greater financial return from stocks than from other types of investments.

■ *Bonds.* These are loans to a corporation or the government. In payment, the investor receives usually regular fixed interest payments and return of principal. The fixed value of the bonds will fluctuate on the open market, depending on the credit rating and movement of interest rates. Bonds may be called for redemption prior to maturity.

■ *Cash or its equivalent.* These instruments, which include CDs, provide a haven from volatility, but are impacted by inflation and taxes. This can result in a significant loss of income when interest rates are low. This can occur even if inflation is low and taxes are not excessive.

■ *Mutual funds.* One of the easiest ways to invest is by purchasing shares in a mutual fund. Such a fund represents a pool of funds provided to professional money managers by many individuals who share a common investment objective. The difficulty for the investor arises in selecting which of the many thousands of funds to purchase shares in. The prospectus of a fund will indicate its objectives, which usually involve purchasing a portfolio of stocks, bonds, and money market instruments. When considering purchasing mutual funds one needs, before investing, to evaluate a fund's past performance, level of volatility (beta measure), rate of turnover, performance record, and operating expenses.

Insurance coverage. It is important to meet your insurance needs before you start investing. This includes life and disability insurance on the wage earner. The agent you use to obtain a life insurance policy should secure for you a cost-benefit analysis from various companies and an annual comparison. Additionally, health, automobile, and homeowner's insurance coverage are essential for your peace of mind. The extent of the deductible will determine the level of the premium in these types of policies.

Life insurance seeks to protect an individual's family in the event of premature death. The money awarded can serve to pay off a mortgage on a home, can fund children's education, and may be a source of income to meet cost-of-living obligations. There are two basic types of policies, *term* and *whole life*. The former is cheaper at first, but costs more in the long run. This is because you pay more as you get older, so much so that at some point it becomes prohibitive in cost. Whole life is permanent insurance, which has a fixed cost throughout the life of the insured. In addition, this type of insurance builds up cash value (equity). In any case, carefully determine your life insurance needs before purchasing a policy. Probably in the early stage of your medical career, you will elect to buy term insurance. You should monitor your future needs and revise the level of insurance accordingly.

Before you invest in insurance, it is important to maximize the value of your policy and secure its fiscal integrity. To do this, you should purchase a policy from a low-load company, rather than an agent, which will significantly reduce your acquisition costs. In addition, you should evaluate the status of any prospective insurance company by determining its standing using such rating agencies as Standard and Poor's or Moody's.

Another major issue in protecting your assets is having a scenario in place, in the event that a situation arises when a member of a group practice passes on. If prior arrangements do not exist, serious professional and financial disruption of the practice can take place. This issue is best resolved by means of a preexisting *buy–sell agreement* which defines each individual's status in the organization. The extent of an individual's business interest in the practice can serve as their will. The document should contain a statement of conditions for a buyout, the mechanism for determining the value of the practice, the method of funding the agreement, and the name of the trustee who will ensure that the agreement is properly executed should it prove necessary.

Although the death of a partner is clearly destabilizing, so too can be the impact of disability. Becoming disabled can limit or eliminate one's income potential. Although not a common occurrence, it is well within the realm of possibility, and thus one needs to be protected against such an eventuality by special insurance coverage. Policy coverage in this area can define disability in various ways. Some characterize it as being related to loss of income. Others, however, use loss of ability to practice in their specialty as the criterion.

Educating one's children. Three fiscal approaches can be used to facilitate educational planning for one's offspring.

■ *Establish a trust.* Parents and grandparents can create trusts to receive gifts for a child's benefit. Substantial sums can be set aside under IRS tax-exempt gift provisions. Thus contributions by both parents and grandparents, if made, can help secure the financial base for children. This is obviously predicated on all parties being willing to participate.

■ *Establish custodianship.* Gifts to minors given under such conditions qualify under the U.S. Treasury's gift tax exclusion provisions. However, they may lack the flexibility of a trust. This also presents the risk of the prospective student diverting the money to another purpose than college, when they reach maturity.

■ *Direct payment.* Grandparents can submit payments to the institution of higher learning that they anticipate the individual will ultimately attend. This method also avoids the annual gift tax exclusion rules. The amount that can be prepaid for tuition is unlimited. The funds, however, cannot be set aside to go directly to the school.

Income tax management. The foundation of the income tax system was set up when Congress adopted the 16th Amendment to the Constitution in 1913. Over the years the tax code has become a complex compendium of regulations.

The basic aim of any individual is to utilize legitimate ways of lowering their taxes. The following approaches may prove helpful in achieving this goal.

■ *Deferring taxes.* Postponing the time when taxes need to be paid to a more appropriate time is a favorable strategy for reducing your tax burden. This can be done by means of a supplementary pension plan or annuities, where pretax funds can be placed. When taxes become due, such as at age $70\frac{1}{2}$, you probably will be in a lower tax bracket.

■ *Reposition investments.* You should consider moving investments from taxable to tax-free entities. This approach is applicable to money market funds or bonds. However, it should be realized that transferring to tax-free vehicles does not automatically guarantee that you have fiscally improved your position. There is a formula that is available that can be used to test if this will likely be so. This involves taking the interest rate of the prospective tax-free investment and dividing it by one minus the percentage of your tax bracket. If your result is higher than your current tax-table rate, repositioning may be worthwhile.

■ *Shifting income.* If you have an income-producing entity, this can be transferred to the ownership of a family member (e.g., a child) who is in a lower tax bracket. Bear in mind that there may be a limit to the amount can be credited to a child by each parent or grandparent.

■ *Balancing of losses.* By reviewing one's portfolio, it should be readily possible to identify stock investments that will incur capital losses if sold. This can be done to balance profits from other stocks.

Retirement planning. Retirement is an event that most working individuals face sooner or later. All individuals have one goal in common, namely, having financial security when that time comes. For this to take place, appropriate planning is necessary early on in one's career. This involves several considerations that will briefly be discussed:

Basic planning. Aside from determining assets and liabilities, it is important to incorporate retirement capital projections into your financial planning. In addition, planning should start as early as possible. Also, periodic review of your retirement plan is essential to make sure that your fiscal strategy is achieving your goal. Finally, you should have the discipline to maintain your commitment to your financial plan to help ensure a comfortable retirement.

Retirement process. There are two phases to this process, the accumulation and distribution stages. As to the former, the amount of money you save to accumulate adequate capital to provide retirement income and the rate of return on your investment are the essential factors involved in establishing a basis for accumulating income. Saving can be achieved by two approaches, before and after tax. The pretax method, because of higher tax rates, is far superior, and can accumulate into a larger and more secure retirement account.

After-tax savings methods involve tax-free, tax-deferred, and taxable investments. These involve purchasing municipal, corporate, and government bonds and annuities. Utilizing the after-tax approach requires time, fiscal expertise, and money management skills and this approach is not encouraged.

The distribution phase of retirement requires more than noting if your retirement income is coming in on schedule. It necessitates monitoring the status of your retirement accounts, checking investment performance, and budgeting your spending. It is essential to secure competent advice regarding federal retirement distribution regulations. These determine how little or how much to take out to avoid penalties for not withdrawing the minimum distribution or excise tax liability for taking out too much.

Beneficiary designation. In making a determination of a beneficiary, careful thought needs to be given. This involves not only the financial needs of the retirement account holder and spouse but their present state of health.

■ *Estate planning.* Having just focused on retirement, it is now important to shift to estate planning. One's retirement account(s) are usually a major component of one's fiscal assets. The beneficiaries are usually designated on retirement allocation forms, which usually take into account favorable modes of distribution. But there are other components to estate planing, including property, investments, and savings. To this end, it is obviously important to arrange for appropriate decision-making regarding these matters, with a knowledgeable and trustworthy adviser.

There are several issues that you should be aware of when considering estate planning. These are outlined below.

■ *Tax-free inheritance.* For many decades the inheritance law was that once an estate reached $600,000 for an individual or $1,200,000 for a couple, the minimum federal estate tax became applicable at 37% and rose to 55%. The Taxpayers Relief Act of 1997 slowly increases the limit until it reaches $1,000,000 per individual by 2006.

■ *Tax-reducing gifts.* If an individual provides cash gifts to children or grandchildren during their lifetime their estate will be reduced and potential inheritance tax will consequently be lowered. Since one can allocate $11,000 to each individual and a spouse can do the same, if done annually, a very large sum can be taken out of an estate over the course of several years.

■ *Utilizing trusts.* Although a will is the most common document used in estate planning, other options exist, namely trusts. These can contribute to reducing estate tax. It is essential that the creator of a trust appoint a trustee who is responsible for all of the operations of the trust. When a trust is created during one's lifetime, it is called a *living trust.* This can be established so that the terms may be altered (revocable) or may not be changeable (irrevocable). Trusts are complex instruments, so competent legal advice should be sought if you are considering having one drafted as part of your estate plan.

In summary, the following brief guidelines regarding managing one's personal finances can prove helpful.

■ *Prepare a well-designed will.* Utilizing the services of an attorney who is also knowledgeable in estate planning, you should arrange for a will designed to minimize any future estate taxes. You should also arrange for a power of attorney and, if desired, a living will. Review and, if necessary, update beneficiary designates.

■ *Coordinate will and property.* To maximize benefits under the estate tax exemption act, it is important that the title to property held by a couple be appropriately designated. If it is jointly held with right of survivorship, you may not be able to benefit from estate tax savings. It is also important that your will be kept up to date and all relevant changes in personal circumstances be taken into account.

■ *Educate your spouse.* Both husband and wife should be aware of the locations of their respective wills. The same applies to documents granting power of attorney.

When these vital documents are kept in a bank vault, both sides should know how to have access to the vault.

■ *Simplify records*. To more easily maintain oversight over your fiscal assets, including retirement plans, investments, and saving accounts, consolidation of these assets will allow easier and more efficient monitoring of your portfolio. Facilitate record-keeping by making individual files for your investments. It is in these that you should keep all relevant information, reports, and literature.

■ *Review insurance needs*. An individual's insurance needs change over time. As noted earlier, it may be anticipated that the type of policy needed will change in the course of time and one should act upon changed circumstances appropriately.

23 | Responding to Complementary and Alternative Medicine (CAM)

Overview

A major study published in the *New England Journal of Medicine* (*NEJM*) reported that over the last decade, Americans were spending billions of dollars annually on alternative medical therapies. These expenditures occur as a consequence of more than half a million annual office visits to alternative health care providers. More than 40% of Americans utilized the services of an alternative or complementary medical practitioner over the course of a recent single year. The traditional medical establishment has for a long time been not fully aware of the extent to which people in need of medical assistance have been seeking help to treat their ailments elsewhere, such as from acupuncturists, herbalists, neuropaths, homeopaths, and many other healers.

The impact of the demand for nontraditional healing approaches is clearly evident in the mass marketing over the radio and other outlets of goods and services that claim to successfully treat a host of medical conditions, both minor and major. Some even strongly imply the potential of slowing down the aging process and thereby extending life. A disturbing consequence of this situation is reflected in the aphorism being popularized, "Take charge of your health," with its clear implication of calling for self-diagnosis and self-treatment. This approach emphasizes the need for the patient to be proactive rather than relying solely on their physician for maintaining good health.

The attraction of CAM is not primarily generated by the professionals in the field. Rather it is patient-driven by an intense desire for help, when traditional medicine fails to provide it. One consequence of the demand for CAM is that at least 30 insurance companies currently offer alternative medical coverage as part of their health plans. Moreover, the National Institutes of Health (NIH) have established an Office of Alternative Medicine (OAM). Undergraduates, graduates, and continuing medical education courses are being offered in this field. In addition, a two-year fellowship program at the University of Arizona is available for those interested in in-depth study.

It should be noted that in recent years peer-reviewed journals such as *Complementary Therapies in Medicine* and the *Scientific Review of Alternative Medicine*, as well as a host of books on the subject of CAM, have reflected the intensity of interest that has developed in this subject.

Finally, it should be pointed out that nontraditional therapeutic modalities are commonly placed under the heading of "alternative or complementary medicine." However, some will use only one of these two terms, because strictly speaking, each defines its own special approach. Complementary medicine can be applied to therapeutic approaches used in association with traditional ones. Alternative medicine, as its name implies, refers to a substitute for the traditional approach. Some others have a preference for the term "natural medicine" and more recently there are those who employ the term "integrative medicine."

Alternative option seekers

Most people who become seriously ill will usually arrange to utilize the services of a conventional physician. There are, however, a growing minority who are disenchanted with traditional approaches and motivated to look elsewhere. There are indications that people who choose alternative medical care may have certain personal characteristics, such as these:

■ Objecting to the need for invasive therapy to treat chronic, degenerative conditions (e.g., back pain, fatigue, cancer, arthritis).

■ Being frustrated or embittered due to their illnesses or the ineffectiveness of conventional treatment.

■ Desiring practitioners who provide them with more time to discuss their problems in depth than they have been able to obtain elsewhere.

■ Preferring a physician who is open-minded and will not only consider the use of traditional therapies, but also prescribe nonconventional ones such as herbal remedies (on their own or at the patient's request).

■ Suffering from anxiety, pains, headaches, and addiction, conditions not easily treated conventionally.

■ Wishing to obtain holistic therapy to gain healing of the body, mind, and spirit.

Nontraditional modalities

Because of the strong interest of many lay people in CAM, patients may raise the issue of alternative therapies with their allopathic physicians. It is therefore advisable that physicians should seek to become familiar with the most common nontraditional modalities currently being utilized. For this reason these will briefly be outlined below:

Acupuncture. This therapeutic approach is well known and extensively used. It involves insertion of steel needles into the skin at predetermined strategic points along 14 defined meridians of the body. This traditional Chinese approach was aimed at restoring the body's "life force." This is presumed to flow along the body's meridians. Reliable reports of the success of this approach are explained in modern medicine in terms of the release of endorphins and other neurochemicals in the brain. The potential therapeutic value of acupuncture for some specific clinical conditions has been endorsed by the National Institutes of Health.

From a historical perspective, we know that acupuncture has been a therapeutic modality in China for several millennia. It is based on a concept that the universe is composed of two opposing forces, *yin* and *yang*, with equal strengths. Internal factors operate to maintain an equivalent balance between them. If an imbalance occurs between these forces, the consequence is the development of disease. It is presumed that the application of acupuncture will serve to restore balance in the body.

Early healers sought to quantify medicine and developed formulas for diagnosis and selection, using logic to determine the appropriate acupuncture treatment. They aim to unlock the channels that transmit the life force. It is a challenge to understand this modality in modern scientific terms, but its usage is largely based on pragmatic experiences in patient care.

Chiropractic. Although classified among CAM professions, chiropractic has become so popular as to assume the status of a mainstream therapy. It was originated by D. D. Palmer, a self-educated healer who hypothesized that most illnesses, including serious ones, could be treated by adjusting the spine. Many current practicing chiropractors apply their skills to a narrower scope of problems, particularly those relevant to musculoskeletal disturbances, headaches, and tension, but some treat other conditions as well. There are chiropractors who incorporate other CAM modalities such as nutrition and herbal medications into their practice. It should be noted that some osteopathic physicians utilize spinal manipulation as a lower impact, more subtle form of chiropractic in their practice.

Herbal therapy. This approach is another contribution of the Chinese culture, called ethnobotany by some. For thousands of years, a wide variety of herbs were used for therapeutic purposes. Employing only small doses of medicinal plants is recommended, because they can act synergistically or adaptively and thus generate multiple effects. When they are taken properly, their side effects are minimal and, if present, are usually mild. The herb can be extracted from the entire plant, or only its flower, bark, twigs, leaves, roots, or seeds. The three most popular of the very large number of herbal medicines being marketed are *echinacea,* to enhance the immune system, *gingko biloba,* to stimulate blood circulation, and *St. John's wort,* which has an antidepressive effect.

Herbs have gained popularity because many cost much less than prescription drugs. Given the promise that some herbs have shown and the popularity of their use, there has been a concomitant increase in the number of studies of their pharmacology. While an intense efficacy debate regarding herbal medicine is ongoing, this approach has nevertheless been incorporated among many CAM options.

Homeopathy. This treatment modality was founded by a German physician and chemist, Samuel Hanneman, around the turn of the 19th century. It flourished in both Europe and the United States. In this country, at one time, about 22 homeopathic medical schools were established and more than 100 hospitals were devoted to treating patients using this approach. Over time there has been a dramatic decline in interest in this form of CAM. All the homeopathic medical schools and hospitals either closed or converted to allopathic institutions. Nevertheless, a revival of sorts is currently taking place as a result of a rise in ardent supporters (who are opposed by numerous fervent critics).

The homeopathic approach rests on the concept that a substance that causes the same symptoms as an illness in a healthy individual is the best treatment for that particular illness, because it stimulates the body to self-healing. Thus, the rationale behind the homeopathic approach was the belief that symptoms of an illness were natural, protective responses to a disease, rather than manifestations of a malfunction of the body systems caused by the disease. Moreover, it is believed that the more diluted the homeopathic medications, the more potent its therapeutic effect.

The initial favorable impact of this novel therapeutic approach may have been due to the fact that at the time homeopathy was promulgated (1796), drugs were being dispensed in large doses and their side effects undoubtedly were significant. Recognizing this problem has resulted in more careful prescribing of allopathic medications. As a historical footnote, it may be mentioned that because of opposition from fellow physicians and the apothecary lobby, Hahnemann was forced to close his practice in his hometown of Leipzig, Germany.

Massage. In early times, massage was included as a medical specialty, along with acupuncture and other modalities, among the treatments officially recognized by the Chinese Imperial establishment. Interestingly, among its many practitioners were numerous blind individuals.

Massage involves the application of firm pressure to specific areas of the body. The goal is to diminish muscle tension. There are various forms of massage. *Acupressure* involves the use of the fingers of the hand to massage acupoints, rather than inserting needles into them. Another massage modality is *shiatsu*. This is a Japanese form of massage, which literally means finger pressure. Conceptually, this approach may also involve meditation. *Reflexology*, a third form of massage, is based on mapping of organs or body systems to areas on the sole of the foot. It is hypothesized that massaging a particular area of the sole, can alleviate diseases that are in the corresponding body regions.

Biofeedback. This approach is based on the concept that an individual can intentionally affect their own health based on the mind–body connection. The biofeedback system involves monitoring an individual's blood pressure, skin temperature, pulse, brain activity, and other vital signs and converting them into signals. The patient uses thoughts and sensations to control these signals and thereby seeks to regulate the body processes they reflect. This is viewed as a training technique that is aimed at modifying one's autonomic responses. It is employed to alleviate stress, hypertension, migraine headaches, and arthritic pain. The efficacy of this modality has been documented.

Besides biofeedback, a number of other mind–body approaches fall into this category. These include *meditation*, *prayer*, *hypnosis*, and *guided imaging* (for the last, see below). Although not curing organic diseases, these approaches can diminish emotional concerns that the disease process may induce. Strong feelings of stress and anxiety can generate elevated blood pressure, sweating, a flushed sensation, and reduced immune response. These disturbances can be diminished by mind–body modalities.

Guided imaging. This mind–body approach is based on the assumption that the unconscious mind is somehow capable of reversing the disease process. Thus, interactive guided imaginary is utilized to encourage patients to visualize their immune systems engaged in fighting illness and thereby stimulating a patient's recovery.

Naturopathy. This approach emphasizes the natural healing capacity of the body and avoids any invasive procedures. Emphasis in naturopathic treatment is placed upon nutrition and herbalism. It should be noted that modalities used by these practitioners vary widely. Thus some may also include acupuncture, massage, and homeopathy in their practice.

Traditional Chinese medicine. This refers to a comprehensive medical system that involves diagnosis by palpation and pulse evaluation, as well as treatment involving acupuncture, herbalism, meditation, and moxibustion. The last involves burning of herbs on or near the skin. It is thought that the body will benefit from the effects of aromatic penetration of the aromas generated.

Ayurvedic medicine. This modality originated millennia ago in India. It has similarities to traditional Chinese medicine. The approach involves using a proper diet and life-style including meditation as preventive measures, as well as massage, detoxification, herbs, and breathing exercises as treatment modalities.

Electromagnetics. The healing power of this modality was hypothesized in 1990. The claim has not been scientifically verified, and thus this approach still remains a controversial issue. There are numerous supporters who vouch for its efficacy.

Chelation. This relatively commonly used CAM technique is the result of the finding that ethylenediaminetetraactic acid (EDTA) binds metal ions. Plaque in the blood vessels of experimental animals, such as rabbits, was found to be dissolved when this chemical was injected into them. Many CAM physicians have applied this technique to humans with claims of success. Nevertheless, it has not been adopted by traditional cardiologists, who remain skeptical of its efficacy.

CAM status report

Organized medicine has been antagonistic to its unconventional counterpart for decades. The AMA has at one time or another used its considerable political power against many groups of CAM practitioners, such as chiropractors and osteopaths. On occasion their lobbying impact on state legislators caused some nontraditional healers to be barred from practice.

In recent years there has been a marked deadline in the battle against CAM by the allopathic medical establishment. While there has been a significant increase in support for CAM from lay people and some professionals, a strong multitude of skeptics nevertheless remain. Traditionalists suggest that positive outcomes ascribed to CAM may be due to a placebo effect or that the disease may have run its course, rather than having been cured as a result of the modality itself. Claims of quackery still abound and charges are leveled that CAM may cause irreversible harm by deflecting people from electing conventional therapies or inducing them to withdraw from such treatments.

There clearly are major unresolved issues associated with CAM. These may be complicated by the fact that a diagnosis or a prognosis by an allopathic physician may have been in error and thus the CAM treatment that is thought to be curative may have been misapplied. At times sick individuals may distort the results they experience due to CAM treatment out of an intense desire to get better, and disregard an ineffective result. Given all the current uncertainties, what is essential are well-designed investigations and logical deductions from accumulated data. Indications are that both sides of the debate are calling for intensive clinical research involving double-blind, randomized studies. This would avoid the various sources of error that can mislead individuals formulating conclusions about complex events such as illness, disease, and recovery.

Reliable scientific studies on CAM are currently being funded by the NIH Office of Alternative Medicine (OAM). This respected federal agency is sponsoring over a dozen clinical trials at sites involved in research on cancer, AIDS, asthma, allergies, and aging. These research activities are taking place in medical centers and universities in various parts of the country. The budget for OAM has increased substantially and thus potential funding ability is much greater. The extent of research data on the many CAM modalities varies, being more prevalent in mind–body areas, herbalism, and acupuncture than in most others.

Of special interest is the fact that OAM is receiving inquiries from conventional professional medical organizations regarding how best to view CAM and integrate it into areas such as education, training, practice licensing, and reimbursement.

The OAM focuses on unconventional therapies that may have a public impact. It has access to professional advisory panels and other NIH institutes. When a promising area is identified, the OAM seeks appropriate researchers, who are able and willing to submit grant applications for support to execute projects and thus determine the validity of a proposed study.

Complicating the entire subject is the problem of the numerous contradictory CAM studies that have come forth, that reflect favorable, negative, and inconclusive judgments as to the efficacy this approach.

It needs to be recognized that much of CAM began as anecdotal evidence and remained underground until it gained strong grassroots support. Moreover, gathering evidence and expanding CAM research is only at its beginning and it is too early to arrive at definitive conclusions. Clearly each modality will have to be evaluated independently to determine its value as a therapeutic approach.

The increased popularity of CAM has resulted in more voices calling for regulation over usage. The call is especially loud because Congress in the mid-1990's exempted herbal remedies sold as diet supplements from oversight by the Food and Drug Administration. This was reflected in the report in the September 1998 issue of the *NEJM*, which raised serious questions about the effectiveness of several CAM therapies. The journal's management editorially expressed a strong call for applying the same standards of testing and regulation to CAM therapies, especially herbal remedies, as is done for conventional modalities.

There is increased recognition that nutrition, vitamins, and massage are not substitutes for mainstream medicines but only supplement them. They are certainly more acceptable to conventional practitioners than the more radical approaches that are available. It is hoped that the end result of the in-depth scientific investigation of CAM will elucidate and identify those modalities that have merit. This may result in a more respectful and perhaps collaborative relationship being established between practitioners from both worlds of medicine.

It might prove helpful if major medical educational organizations involved themselves in ascertaining how best to integrate CAM into medical education. Specifically, their contribution should aim at educating the generalist physician. Also, attention needs to be given to develop skills in gathering evidence. This will enable physicians to critically assess information and thus enable professionals to make more responsible decisions regarding the usage of CAM.

Getting exposed to CAM

The strong public demand for CAM services has impacted the medical education establishment. They are responding to the need to train medical students so that they are at least knowledgeable about the subject. Thus, a published study found that well over half of U.S. allopathic medical schools offer electives in CAM or include the subject in their required courses. The course titles vary from generalized ones, such as "Alternative Approaches to Medical Treatment," to more specific ones, such as "Chinese Acupuncture." Obviously those electing to take CAM courses do so because of their special interest, but their numbers are limited. It is not known how extensively CAM is discussed when it is incorporated into other courses, rather than being offered as specific electives.

Of special interest is the fact that several major medical institutions, such as Columbia and Harvard, have established CAM research centers. These and other institutions are sites for NIH grant-supported investigations in the field, originating from NIH's Office of Alternative Medicine.

The slow incorporation of CAM into the typical required medical curriculum stems from three sources. First, it has proven necessary to overcome the long-standing negative bias toward CAM in the medical establishment. Second, the medical curriculum is overcrowded as it is, and making room for a new subject means downsizing or eliminating a long-standing subject. Finally, there is a scarcity of qualified faculty available to teach CAM courses in medical schools.

It is not uncommon that CAM electives develop through the impetus of medical students who enlist an interested faculty member to undertake such a program. If success is achieved in such an undertaking, then over time such a course may become a regular component of the curriculum. Some medical students, not fully satisfied with their schools' offerings so far as CAM is concerned, have established interest groups in the subject that hold regular lectures and present hands-on demonstrations. The genesis of such a group or the stimulation of the formulation of a course as a result of student initiative is not surprising. Students tend to be fascinated by the ancient oriental origin of many of the CAM modalities. As a matter of fact, it has been suggested that when taught, CAM therapies should be placed in their proper historical and philosophical context to gain a genuine appreciation of their value.

Another appeal of CAM for medical students and physicians is that they may find the holistic healing approach to be appealing. Many of their modalities are usable within the context of holistic care. Medical students also favor active patient involvement in the entire healing process. Finally, medical students may be carrying over the interest in CAM from their youth. Being a more activist group, they have emerged as a force in urging the medical education establishment to become more cognizant of this long-standing conglomerate of unconventional healing modalities. They are anxious to ascertain if such approaches have significant merit and applicability to medicine in the 21st century.

An interesting initiative relative to CAM took place with the establishment by the University of Arizona School of Medicine of a two-year fellowship in the subject. The impetus for this came from Dr. Andrew Weil, widely known proponent of the virtues of CAM, which he calls integrative medicine. The goal of the program is to train physicians whose outlook favors

■ Encouraging practitioners to find the time to offer their patients an opportunity to adequately express their concerns.

■ An unprejudiced attitude to the concept of mind–body interaction.

■ Awareness of nutritional influences on health and the need to manage them properly.

■ The introduction of lifestyle changes as a mechanism of improving health.

■ Treating patients in a holistic manner by considering not only their physical ailments but also their emotional, mental, and spiritual problems.

■ Patients who seek a physician who is open to the utilization of some of the CAM therapies.

There are four other areas of emphasis in the Arizona program:

■ Physicians themselves being committed to a healthy lifestyle.

■ Research to establish the efficacy of CAM therapies.

■ A commitment to continuing education in the holistic approach to health care.

■ Being enthusiastic messengers of the concepts of CAM to the community, fellow physicians, and the medical establishment.

CAM in clinical practice

Guidelines have been developed and recommended to traditional physicians as to how to respond to patients seeking CAM care. They are as follows:

■ Clearly advise patients about their condition and be sure they understand its nature and the extent of its seriousness.

■ Clarify to the patient what standard medical treatments are available for their specific problems and the prognoses with such treatments.

■ Inquire as to the rationale behind the patient's desire for CAM care and react to their response with understanding.

■ Advise the patient that you are still available to provide them with traditional medical care, perhaps in a collaborative manner with an CAM healer, should you be comfortable doing so.

Where a practitioner is versed in some of the nontraditional therapies of CAM and wishes to apply one, as part of their treatment:

■ Have the patient sign a consent form that identifies the CAM therapy being used.

■ Incorporate the standard legal language that is commonly used in standard consent forms.

■ It is advisable to provide patients with a suitable brochure that provides a clear description of the proposed alternative modality and how it is applied in patient care.

■ The patient should be allowed to review the descriptive material before his/her consent is asked for.

■ Arrange that the patient receive an accurate itemized statement for services rendered. This should identify the cost for the alternative therapy in detail. This will facilitate suitable reimbursement to the physician for CAM services provided, whether coverage by the insurer is available or not.

■ It is essential to carefully document the procedure in detail in your notes, identifying the modality used, how and where it was applied, and any relevant responses to the treatment by the patient.

■ If the alternative therapy proves to be ineffective initially, repeat it, if warranted, but place a cap on the number of treatments to be given.

■ If multiple treatments do not provide relief, suggest other therapeutic advice.

■ Keep careful notes of patient comments regarding the procedure and your responses. This is especially true if there is a disagreement with the patient in the course of the therapy.

24 | The Art of Medicine

Overview

Practicing medicine involves more than acquiring an adequate fund of knowledge and securing the clinical skills essential to healing the infirm. It usually mandates an intense interaction between two human beings, the physician, a professional healer, and the patient, a lay-person. Success for both parties is in part determined by the nature of the interaction between them. Consequently, the healing process clearly extends well beyond the borders of science. Thus, having a solid grasp of the art of medicine can facilitate and at times be decisive in achieving a favorable outcome. This chapter will focus on the importance of the physician–patient interaction and desirable approaches to enhancing this relationship.

Experience has shown that the success of a treatment plan is significantly influenced by the nature and quality of the physician's interaction with their patient. Most of the intimate medical consequences of life are the result of the decisions and actions taken by patients. Making patients aware of this empowers them to recognize the possibility of achieving positive results based on clear and reliable therapeutic guidelines and their careful and consistent compliance. This is best carried out in the context of a favorable psychological ambience.

By having a favorable physician–patient relationship, treatment plans can be formulated that have an increased chance of being effective. This will facilitate the patient's desire to implement faithfully their responsibilities. In addition, a positive relationship reduces the risk of the practitioner being subjected to malpractice suits. Studies have shown that where patients feel that they were treated by their physician in a friendly and thoughtful manner, they are much less inclined to take legal action against them when something goes significantly wrong. The strong positive feelings that a patient may have toward their doctor tend, in many cases, to serve as an emotional barrier to undertaking legal action where the possibility of malpractice may exist. Patients tend not to be inclined to punish physicians they genuinely like.

Healing effectively

When a person becomes ill, it represents a status change in the entire balance of activities going on within his/her body. Symptoms of a disease or the disease itself will manifest the altered state of the body's condition. It may be perceived as a threat to the body's essential unity.

To reestablish physical and/or emotional integrity, the patient may seek his/her personal physician's advice, reassurance, and medical assistance. There is a desire to receive clarification as to the nature and seriousness of the problem. What patients generally seek from their physician is to be informed, enlightened, and educated about their state of health. Naturally, the uncertainty of the situation and its possible impact can be disturbing. This raises the question of whether there will be a loss of income and work time and disruption of life's routine activities. An illness will impact negatively all the components of an individual's life, namely, its physical, intellectual, and emotional aspects. As a consequence, patients will become dependent on their physician for their restoration to normalcy. The healing process should be applied to all three of these components of an individual's life.

The physician may have the ability to eliminate the "imbalance" that has emerged in the patient's body. In response to patients' needs, it is important to recognize their altered state of being and that they realize that you view them in this context. Moreover, it is imperative that through your behavior and actions, you confirm that your approach is not that of a mere repair technician, but rather that of an artist seeking to restore a damaged masterpiece – the human body – to its state of normality.

The healing process can be enhanced by the impact of practicing both the science and the art of medicine. The science of medicine is based on the use of distinct, measurable, and substantive diagnostic and therapeutic elements. This is in marked contrast to the application of the art of medicine, which involves approaches that are quantitatively impossible to measure, such as interpersonal bonding and expressions of empathy. Such intangible factors are activated on occasions when there is genuine interaction on a professional level between the physician and patient. The art of medicine transcends the diagnostic skills and technical abilities that doctors possess as a result of their education and training. It is reflected in the nature of their verbal and body language, the intensive quality of the verbal exchange, the tone of the relationship, the thoroughness of the diagnostic evaluation, and the level of cooperation that is established between the two parties.

Applying both aspects of medicine, science and art, mandates focusing one's full attention on the whole patient as the principal component in the proceedings, rather than exclusively on the technical or purely scientific elements, such as lab reports or x-rays. The effectiveness of the healer requires facing up to this challenge and seeking to have the practice of the art of medicine incorporated as an integral component of the mastery of medical care.

Physician–patient relations

The patient–physician relationship is an important component in formulating and successfully executing a treatment plan. This is due to the fact that the decisions made by the patient in response to the physician's input will likely have a decisive effect on the outcome. Regrettably, the state of the physician–patient relationship has dramatically declined over recent decades. This unfortunate situation is apparently rooted in multiple causes. These include the following:

- *Emphasis on specialization.* In most cases, this involves short-term professional relationships with patients and consequently there is insufficient time to establish meaningful bilateral rapport.

- *Technological advances.* The advent of sophisticated diagnostic and treatment equipment has generated a large pool of technicians who have become a new layer of personnel interposed between the patient and the attending physician.

- *Managed care.* This system has limited the physician's flexibility of practice and has reduced the time available for physician–patient interaction. This is due to the pressure to process an adequate patient volume within a fixed time frame.

- *Increased paperwork.* There have been greater demands on physicians' time to meet the requirements of complying with governmental and other third-party payer regulations. This has impacted the amount of time available to physicians that can be allotted to patient care.

Attitudes on the part of patients have also contributed to the deterioration in the physician–patient relationship. This has been made evident by patient apathy, as is manifested by

■ *Failure to communicate*. Patients frequently are reluctant to express their inner-most thoughts and concerns to their physicians. These may be underlying factors in their symptoms and thus they complicate the diagnostic process.

■ *Failure to inquire*. Patients commonly believe that their physicians are too busy to be troubled with what they feel are insignificant or time-consuming questions.

■ *Failure to discriminate*. Patients are not in a position to evaluate physicians. Hearsay is the major source of their information. The issues of affability and compatibility frequently do not rank high on the list of criteria used in judging a physician.

Given existing circumstances, it is important to focus attention on the bond between the healer and the patient. A special effort should be placed on intimately involving the patient in all aspects of the healing process. This can best be done by ensuring his/her participation in formulating and executing the treatment plan. This will strengthen the doctor–patient relationship, increase the potential for compliance, and consequently enhance the chances for therapeutic success.

Physician responsibilities

Physicians can serve a major role in the life of patients, utilizing their knowledge and talents to provide reassurance, help, and hope. To successfully achieve the goal of practicing the science and especially the art of medicine, a physician's performance should be based on the following criteria:

Practicing competently. Patients seeking medical assistance have every reason to assume that their physician is qualified in their specialty by virtue of their professional education and training. Moreover, they take for granted that their practitioner seeks to keep up to date with advances in his/her field. Patients also have the right to believe that the physician will, when appropriate, refer them to other specialists, if the ability to solve the patient's problem goes beyond the scope of their expertise.

For the most part, the various accrediting agencies and monitoring mechanisms serve to ensure that the physician's level of competence to practice the science of medicine is satisfactory. However, the level of competence to practice the art of medicine depends on the physician's ability and commitment to the goal of establishing meaningful interpersonal relationships with patients and applying humanistic skills in his/her practice. The satisfaction felt by the practitioner as a result of practicing the art of medicine will serve to enhance his/her commitment to this approach and will improve the quality of health care being provided to his/her patients.

Providing compassionate care. Although the practice of the science of medicine implies a need to provide care in a compassionate manner, the art of medicine conceives of this approach as being its cornerstone. This humanistic approach is predicated on the physician sensing their patients' disturbed physical and/or emotional state of being and consequently responding in an empathetic manner.

Assurance of confidentiality. The doctor–patient relationship demands that the infirm individual be as candid as possible in discussing their condition with their physician. They need to reveal their feelings and concerns frankly, openly, and completely. Adequate probing of these issues in the course of practicing the science of medicine is basic to the validity of the diagnostic and therapeutic processes. The search for relevant background information, however, is both deeper and broader in the course of practicing the art of medicine. In either case it is essential that the patient have the assurance that the doctor–patient relationship is highly confidential. This will strengthen the bond between them and encourage more open communication, which benefits both parties.

Providing encouragement. It is essential for the practitioner to be a source of inspiration to their patients. This is especially important in treating those with serious or chronic illnesses. They should provide encouragement even if prospects for full recovery are limited. You need to act as a military officer who is leading troops to battle against the enemy, the disease process. The patients should feel that they stand to be rewarded if they put up a valiant battle, whether victorious or not. Thus, by demonstrating a positive outlook, the physician will help dispel or keep in check the anxieties that are a component of all serious health situations.

Major components of the art

The practice of medicine has undergone drastic evolution over the course of time. Prior to modern medicine, physicians served as *sympathetic comforters,* merely easing pain and suffering, but unable to prospone negative outcomes. Starting in the 19th century their role began to change to that of *rational healers.* As a result of the remarkable scientific and technological advances that took place during the 20th century, physicians were able to provide genuine services as healers and to defeat many diseases. The latter part of the last century has produced many life-style enhancing changes, with an emphasis on preventive health care. This has resulted in altering the role of the physician once again, so that currently, in the 21st century, they need to relate to their patients not only as rational healers, but also as *health protectors.* Thus, the new role for physicians necessitates that they serve as patient educators in addition to being diagnosticians and clinicians. To facilitate serving in such a multiple capacity, gaining the skills associated with practicing the art of medicine can prove most beneficial for both the practitioner and their patients.

The skills associated with the art of medicine will be briefly outlined.

Visual interaction. One of the most important elements of communication with patients is maintaining eye contact as much as possible during the interview process. By coordinating both visual and verbal senses, one multiplies the impact of the message being conveyed, many times over. Moreover, eye contact serves as a favorable mechanism that facilitates bonding between doctor and patient, making each more responsive to the other. In this way the information or instructions that the patient wishes to transmit will likely come across more precisely and in greater detail. Similarly, the message that the physician wishes to relate to the patient will be more clearly understood and more amicably accepted.

Verbal communication. This is the prerequisite for practicing medicine that forms the fundamental basis for diagnosis and treatment. The extent of training of medical students and residents in communication skills unfortunately is limited in time and scope. The key to effective communication is being a genuine listener and compassionate inquirer. Given the pressures of the limited amount of time that can reasonably be allowed to each individual patient, it is essential to maximize the value of the information extracted during the course of a visit. This can best be accomplished by asking probing questions, which, for completeness, should also include an all-encompassing one, such as, "Is there anything else you would like to tell me?"

During the visit, the physician will apply the science of medicine while carrying out a symptomatic systemic evaluation. This is routinely performed as part of a standard physical examination. This should be done in conjunction with in-depth probing of humanistically relevant questions, depending on the patient's age, as part of practicing the art of medicine.

While recognizing the reality of the pressures of time, it is nevertheless important in order to maintain a positive rapport and secure critical information, during the interview, that you not interrupt the patient by anticipating their responses. Patients can readily sense when they are being hurried and naturally may become less responsive and cooperative. You may thereby jeopardize the accuracy of the diagnostic and therapeutic process.

During the course of an important verbal exchange, it is useful to employ the technique of repeating a patient's critical remarks. This will serve to reassure them that the physician is truly hearing what they have had to say. It also serves to suggest that the patient's comments are genuinely relevant to the medical evaluation process.

Body language. Contributing to establishing a meaningful rapport with the patient is this element, which is an integral component of practicing the art of medicine. Use of appropriate body language can help to generate a positive relationship between the parties. To this end, the physician's individual mannerisms can have an impact on the patient. Thus, placing oneself at the side of a patient's bed, rather than at the foot of the bed, may be taken be a more meaningful indication of personal concern.

Similarly, where one is certain that there are no religious taboos, shaking hands with a patient or patting them on the shoulder can for some prove to be a very reassuring gesture. It can also serve to reinforce the strength of the intangible bond between doctor and patient.

Patient inclusivity. In practicing the art of medicine, seeking genuine communication, establishing a bond, and exhibiting empathy all become standard operative procedures. The positive response that this approach elicits from patients, can help to generate in them a feeling of being included as a member of the treatment team. As a result of the physician's applying the humanistic aspect of the art of medicine, the patient will tend to be more compliant and thus the physician's efforts will potentially be of greater value. This is critical for the entire patient management process, because it is the patient who can best relay the core information about their illness and strongly influence the physician's therapeutic endeavors. By stimulating a sense of being a vital participant in the healing efforts, a more wholesome relationship will be established with the patient, leading to enhanced chances for a successful outcome.

Time management. This is one of the most challenging aspects of medicine. Except for emergency visits, patients traditionally are seen at scheduled intervals. It is during this time span that health status data are collected and evaluated. To accomplish this while practicing both the science and art of medicine means redefining your goals for patient visits. Thus your focus needs to go beyond the scientific aspects of clinical assessment, to establishing a meaningful personal rapport with the patient that will be beneficial to the totality of the medical process.

One should recognize that an element of flexibility is important in considering patient scheduling. The probing questions that form the essential part of the art of medicine may at times require extending the patient's visit when information being extracted seems crucial to achieving a proper diagnosis. Allowing more time in this regard is quite important, even if at times it may distort your patient schedule. Delayed patients will usually respond favorably to their physician's apology for lateness. Thus it is appropriate to express your genuine regrets to subsequent patients when a delay transpires.

Deliberate focusing. In the course of seeing a stream of patients in a clinic or office setting or during rounds, the physician is exposed to a multitude of experiences, all at the same time. Thus it is understandable that they become preoccupied with the plethora of events and activities that transpire as the day goes on. It is, however, very helpful for the doctor–patient dynamic to train yourself to be able to mentally disconnect from all preceding activities as you step in to meet a different patient. That individual needs and deserves to be the center of your full and undivided attention. The ability to give yourself completely over to a specific issue and disregard other extraneous influences is quite challenging, but it has been shown that with training it can be achieved. By detaching yourself so that you focus upon the patient at hand, you can concentrate more precisely and perceptively on their tone of voice, their body language, and what they say and also what they omit from their comments. This may well contribute to your ability to more effectively render medical services. Patient satisfaction undoubtedly will be enhanced, for they will realize that you are genuinely in tune with them and earnestly concerned with their well-being.

Clinical intuition. This concept is also a vital component of the art of medicine. It is by means of a thorough history and physical examination, supported by appropriate tests, that the physician obtains the vital data essential to develop a differential diagnosis. This is the rational approach of the science of medicine. In spite of highly impressive advances made in this realm, gaps still exist in our knowledge base and anomalous conditions frequently make it difficult, if not impossible, to formulate accurate diagnoses in some cases. Consequently, it is necessary, at times, to proceed with medical care despite considerable uncertainty as to the exact cause of a disease. Under these intellectually perplexing circumstances, clinical intuition can play a critical role. It can serve to fill the void created by the ambiguity of the situation at hand. The clinical intuitive ability stems from an inner sense or hunch that fits in well with the accumulated medical data and one's prior clinical experience.

The intuitive capability varies widely among physicians. It is to a considerable extent, but not entirely, based on one's exposure and expertise in the field. Over time, intuitive skills may be sharpened and they can be utilized effectively to provide more comprehensive health care.

Practicing the art

After recognizing the significance of the art of medicine as a practice modality, it is necessary to become familiar with its prerequisite skills and develop a commitment to applying it. To do so, there are implementation guidelines to incorporating this approach into one's practice. Practicing the art of medicine specifically involves

■ *Providing reassurance.* Infirm individuals not only suffer from discomfort as a result of their illness, but feel that they have lost control over their bodies. By providing reassurance, the physician, being an authoritative figure, can help establish a barrier to protect the patient from becoming emotionally overwhelmed. This process can be reinforced in the course of providing the patient with professional guidance and information as well as references to other relevant health care resources. The consequences of these efforts, are that the patient's reinforced psychological system will be able to better tolerate future medical consequences, whatever they may be.

■ *Strengthening the relationship.* Making a conscious effort to develop a positive rapport with the patient is an important part of the therapeutic process. This can best be accomplished by encouraging communication and achieving a mutually comfortable relationship. A patient frequently has a deeply personal story to relate and needs to be granted an adequate opportunity to do so. The mere ability to ventilate feelings can significantly enhance his/her well-being.

■ *Diminishing patient self-denigration.* Illness has many unwanted consequences beyond its unpleasant physical manifestations. On a physiological level, it may be reflected in a sense of guilt on the patient's part, because he/she became ill and dependent on the help of others. There is a sense of social disassociation generated by awareness of inadequacies in meeting his/her personal needs. To help ameliorate this situation, the physician can serve as a resource for empathetic support and encouragement. The positive approach can encourage a sense of self-worth during both the treatment and recovery phases of the illness.

■ *Being informative.* It is important to provide your patients in an *understandable* manner the essential information relevant to their problem. Even if the information is common knowledge, it is nevertheless worthwhile presenting it. This is because it demonstrates your concern for the patients' well-being and thus reinforces the strength of the relationship you have with them.

■ *Establishing a partnership.* To achieve the best chances for a successful outcome, the goal is to establish a treatment plan in collaboration with the patient. This involves outlining the options available, recommending the best choice (if there is more than one), explaining the details of the plan, and inviting and welcoming questions and suggestions. Seek to accommodate and incorporate into the plan all reasonable patient ideas. Assure patients, to the extent possible, that they will be provided with the essential resources and that you will help facilitate carrying out the treatment plan, which should enhance their chances for recovery.

■ *Securing support for the patient.* Where necessary and possible, arrange to enlist the help of family or even friends on behalf of the patient. Advise the patient that you will instruct the Social Services Department to actively participate in carrying out relevant parts of the treatment plan upon discharge from a health care facility.

The new frontier

There is a critical need to depart from the traditional physician "know it all" or "trust me" approaches common to the practice of medicine by some or even many physicians. The fact is that no one, including physicians, is infallible and that patients are being strongly encouraged by the media "take charge of their own health." All this proactive concern with well-being has generated the necessity for physicians and patients to establish a new relationship, based on mutual respect and active cooperation. An integral component of the new association is that the physician recognizes that his/she are linked to the patient by virtue of their shared humanity. The recognition of this commonality should generate a special sense of empathy by the physician toward his or her patients. This enhanced sensitivity should certainly be manifested by physicians undertaking to practice both the science and art of medicine.

The implications of sensing the impact of your patient's condition or disability, can be manifested by maximizing the help you can provide in the limited time available to care for each individual. This help can be physical or psychological or both. One way to do this is to have the office staff suggest that patients prepare a list of concerns and questions that they have *prior* to an office visit. By this means they are likely to be more fully satisfied with the visit after they depart.

It is also important to recognize the impact of the wellness movement that generated the concept of health promotion and disease prevention. This has made many patients more knowledgeable and informed (as well as misinformed). As a consequence, practicing medicine requires a more open approach and the need to recognize that healing should be viewed as a joint physician–patient venture. Moreover, the new health care climate can be supportive to efforts at stimulating improved self-help (e.g., eliminating smoking or losing weight). Patients being more knowledgeable allows the physician to speak more intelligently with them, which in turn generates a more satisfying and useful dialogue. The ultimate goal is to have patients recognize your genuine interest in their welfare.

To establish and maintain long-term relationships where appropriate, it is useful not only to initiate positive patient contact but to consistently strengthen it as time goes on. This can be done by applying the skills of the art of medicine as well as by small acts of thoughtfulness that leave a big positive impression. These, for example, can be

■ A personal phone call to a recently hospital-discharged patient to inquire as to his/her well-being.

■ Acknowledging a patient's success in achieving a medical milestone (e.g., recovery from an illness, resisting smoking for a fixed period, or the loss of a predetermined amount of weight).

■ Even when only limited progress has been achieved, using an office visit to acknowledge it and encourage continued effort to attain one's goals.

These are but illustrations of the application of the art of medicine. They are symbols of an approach to practicing medicine as a profession dedicated to service both by means of one's scientific expertise and by a deep sense of compassion for a fellow human being.

APPENDIX 1

Major Professional Organizations

Accreditation Council for Graduate Medical Education
515 North State Street
Chicago, IL 60610
www.acgme.org

Aerospace Medical Association
320 South Henry Street
Alexandria, VA 22314
www.acgme.org

AMCAS
2501 M Street NW
Washington, DC 20037
www.aamc.org

American Academy of Allergy, Asthma, and Immunology
611 East Wells Street
Milwaukee, WI 53202
www.aaaai.org

American Academy of Child and Adolescent Psychiatry
3615 Wisconsin Avenue, NW
Washington, DC 20016
www.aacap.org

American Academy of Dermatology
P.O. Box 4014
Schaumburg, IL 60173
www.aad.org

American Academy of Family Physicians
11400 Tomahawk Creek Parkway
Leewood, KS 66211
www.aapfp.org

American Academy of Neurology
1080 Montreal Avenue
St. Paul, MN 55116
www.aan.com/professionals

American Academy of Ophthalmology
655 Beach Street
San Francisco, CA 94109
www.aao.org

American Academy of Orthopedic Surgeons
6300 North River Road
Rosemont, IL 60018
www.aaos.org

American Academy of Otolaryngology
1 Prince Street
Alexandria, VA 22314
www.entnet.org

American Academy of Pediatrics
141 Northwest Point Boulevard
Elk Grove, IL 60007
www.aap.org

American Association of Colleges of Osteopathic Medicine
5550 Friendship Boulevard, Suite 310
Chevy Chase, MD 20815
www.aacom.org

American Association of Dental Schools
1625 Massachusetts Avenue, NW
Washington, DC 20036
www.ada.org

**American Association of
Neurological Surgeons**
22 South Washington Street
Park Ridge, IL 60068
www.neurosurgery.org

American Association of Orthodontists
401 North Lindbergh Boulevard
St. Louis, MO 63141
www.aaortho.org

**American Association of Public
Health Physicians**
c/o Armand Start, M.D.
1300 W Belmont Avenue
Chicago, IL 60657
www.aaphp.org

American Board of Medical Specialties
1007 Church Street, Suite 404
Evanston, IL 60201
www.abms.org

American College of Cardiology
9111 Old Georgetown Road
Bethesda, MD 20814
www.acc.org

American College of Chest Physicians
3300 Dundee Road
Northbrook, IL 60062
www.chestnet.org

**American College of Emergency
Physicians**
P.O. Box 61911
Dallas, TX 75261
www.acep.org

American College of Gastroenterology
4900B South 31st Street
Arlington, VA 22206
www.acg.gi.org

American College of Medical Genetics
9650 Rockville Pike
Bethesda, MD 20814
www.acmg.net

American College of Nuclear Medicine
P. O. Box 175
Landsville, PA 17538
www.rsha.org

**American College of Obstetricians
and Gynecologists**
409 12th Street SW
Washington, DC 20024
www.acog.org

**American College of Physicians–
American Society of Internal Medicine**
190 N Independence Mall West
Philadelphia, PA 19106
www.acponline.org

**American College of Preventive
Medicine**
1307 New York Avenue, NW
Washington, DC 20005
www.acpm.org

American College of Radiology
1891 Preston White Drive
Reston, VA 22091
www.acr.org

American College of Rheumatology
1800 Century Place NE
Atlanta, GA 30345
www.rheumatology.org

American College of Surgeons
633 North St. Clair Street
Chicago, IL 60611
www.facs.org

American Dental Association
211 East Chicago Avenue
Chicago, IL 60611
www.ada.org

**American Federation for Clinical
Research**
6900 Grove Road
Thorofare, NJ 08086
www.afmr.org

American Geriatric Society
770 Lexington Avenue
New York, NY 10021
www.americangeriatrics.org

American Hospital Association
1 North Franklin
Chicago, IL 60606
www.aha.org

American Medical Association
515 North Street
Chicago, IL 60610
www.ama.org

American Medical Student Association
1902 Association Drive
Reston, VA 22091
www.amsa.org

American Medical Women's Association
801 North Fairfax Street
Alexandria, VA 22314
www.amwa.org

American Ophthalmologic Society
c/o W. Banks Anderson, M.D.
Duke University Eye Center
Durham, NC 27710
www.aosonline.org

American Osteopathic Association
142 East Ontario Street
Chicago, IL 60611
www.aoa-net.org

**American Osteopathic College
of Rehabilitation Medicine**
2214 Elmira Avenue
Des Plaines, IL 60018
www.aoa-net.org

**American Osteopathic Healthcare
Association**
5550 Friendship Boulevard Suite 300
Chevy Chase, MD 20815
www.aoha.org

American Psychiatric Association
1400 K Street NW
Washington, DC 20005
www.psych.org

American Society of Anesthesiologists
520 Northwest Highway
Park Ridge, IL 60068
www.asahq.org

**American Society of Clinical
Oncology**
1900 Duke Street, Suite 200
Alexandria, VA 22314
www.ascp.org

**American Society for Colon and
Rectal Surgeons**
85 West Algonquin Road
Arlington Heights, IL 60005
www.fascrs.org

American Society of Hematology
1900 M Street NW
Washington, DC 20036
www.hematology.org

**American Society of Internal
Medicine**
2011 Pennsylvania Avenue NW
Washington, DC 20036
www.asim.org

American Society of Nephrology
1200 19th Street NW
Washington, DC 20036
www.asn.org

**American Society of Plastic and
Reconstructive Surgeons**
444 East Algonquin Road
Arlington Heights, IL 60005
www.plasticsurgery.org

American Thoracic Society
1740 Broadway, 14th Floor
New York, NY 10019
www.thoracic.org

American Urological Association
2425 W Loop South
Suite 300
Houston, TX 77027
www.auanet.org

**Association of American Medical
Colleges**
2450 N Street NW
Washington, DC 20037
www.aamc.org
www.aamc.orgstudents/eras/start.htm

**Canadian Resident Matching
Service**
151 Slater Street
802 Ottawa, Ontario K1P-5H3
Canada
www.carms.org

College of American Pathologists
325 Waukegan Road
Northfield, IL 60093
www.cap.org

Educational Commission for Foreign Medical Graduates
3624 Market Street
Philadelphia, PA 19104
www.edfmg.org

Federation of State Medical Boards of the U.S., Inc.
P.O. Box 19850
Dallas, TX 75261
www.fsmb.org

National Association of Advisors for the Health Professions
P.O. Box 1518
Champaign, IL 61824
www.naahp.org

National Board of Medical Examiners
3750 Market Street
Philadelphia, PA 19104
www.nbme.org

National Board of Osteopathic Medical Examiners
8765 West Higgins Road
Chicago, IL 60631
www.abome.org

National Dental Association
5506 Connecticut Avenue NW
Washington, DC 20015
www.nadonline.org

National Medical Association
1012 10th Street NW
Washington, DC 20001
www.nmanet.org

National Resident Matching Program
2501 M Street NW
Washington, DC 20037
www.nrmp.org

Rehabilitation Physicians Association
1101 Vermont Avenue NW
Washington, DC 20005
www.aapmr.org

Society of Critical Care Medicine
8101 East Kaiser Boulevard
Anaheim, CA 92808
www.sccm.org

Society of Thoracic Surgeons
401 North Michigan Avenue
Chicago, IL 60611
www.sts.org

The American Academy of Physical Medicine and Rehabilitation
One IBM Plaza, Suite 2500
Chicago, IL 60611
www.aapmr.org

The American College of Occupational and Environmental Medicine
1114 N. Arlington Hts. Road
Arlington Heights, IL 60005
www.acoem.org

The American Society of Addiction Medicine
4601 North Park Avenue
Upper Arcade
Chevy Chase, MD 20815
www.asam.org

The American Society for Therapeutic Radiology and Oncology
12055 Fair Lakes Circle
Fairfax, VA 22033
www.astro.org

The College of American Pathologists
325 Waukegan Road
Northfield, IL 60093
www.cap.org

The Endocrine Society
4350 East West Highway
Bethesda, MD 20814
www.endo-society.org

The Infectious Disease Society of America
99 Canal Center Plaza
Suite 600
Alexandria, VA 22314
www.idsociety.org

The Society of Nuclear Medicine
1850 Samuel Morse Drive
Reston, VA 20190
www.snm.org

APPENDIX 2

Sample Resumes

Resume

A resume is a formal structured itemization of one's accomplishments and experiences.

Purpose of a resume

A resume, also known as a curriculum vitae or C.V., seeks in a concise manner to summarize a person's career experience, personal qualifications, and accomplishments. The resume is the initial approach used to enhance one's chances to secure the position being sought. Its goal should be to

- Make an initial positive impression on prospective employers.
- Facilitate your chances of eventually securing an interview.
- Serve as a source of information in the preparatory material prior to an interview.
- Assist in selling yourself at interviews by highlighting major achievements.

Contents of a resume

A resume should contain accurate relevant information about your life. Its contents should include your

- Educational background starting at the college level and beyond.

- Rewards and honors received at college and/or during medical school.

- Research experience in the course of undergraduate and medical education.

- Clinical experience, especially if relevant to the residency area of interest.

- Organizational memberships, both in college and in medical school.

- Employment experience, at any level, relevant to the medical profession.

- Foreign language capabilities, both oral and written, and their depth.

- Computer skills and potential in terms of your training and experience.

When preparing your resume, be certain to avoid items that can leave a negative impression:

- Spelling or grammatical errors leave an especially poor opinion of the writer.

- Disorganization in presentation, so that the information is not logically arranged.

- Discussing your availability for the position, because it is premature.

- A gap in the sequence of activities, which can raise uncertainty about you.

- Indicating desired salary range, which is far too premature.

- Resumes are not the site to explain any unpleasant past events.

It should be noted that although applications for residency positions are usually made through the Electronic Residency Application Service (ERAS), nevertheless, both a resume and a personal statement are necessary to be sent (along with recommendations) to residency program directors.

Presentation format

Your resume, in terms of both its contents and appearance, should have a positive impact on those reviewing it. Thus, it obviously should be computer-generated, using a good quality printer and paper. Use of a laser printer and 25% cotton bond paper is preferable. Your resume should be sent off in an appropriate envelope, so that it is not bent during transit. Be sure to include a brief, appropriate cover letter to accompany the resume and personal statement.

Preparing your resume

There are a number of distinct steps involved in preparing a resume. The following suggestions should prove helpful:

- *Study resume formats.* Before deciding on the format of your own resume, familiarize yourself with different styles as shown in the samples at the end of this section. Then make your choice and follow through.

■ *Prepare an inventory of personal experience*. These data are needed to serve as a source of information and to ensure that your statements are accurate and complete. This inventory should be prepared using the basic categories listed above, where appropriate, namely, objective education, honors and awards, research experience and publications, extracurricular activities, and meeting presentations, as well as your clinical and personal interests.

■ *Prepare a first draft*. Using a computer, print the initial draft of your resume. Then review it carefully and set it aside for one or more days.

■ *Print a second draft*. After rereading your original text and making desirable changes, print a reviewed draft and check it over once again.

■ *Get feedback*. Show a revised draft to several knowledgeable individuals and secure their frank comments regarding your statements, style, and contents. Ask them for their candid opinion (and don't be offended by any negative criticism).

■ *Amend your resume*. Use your own judgment when revising your resume in light of the opinions given you by others. It is you who will benefit or lose out from any changes that will be made. Do not, however, feel that you need to accept all suggestions made. When the review process is complete, proceed to prepare a final draft.

■ *Print final draft*. Now that you have had your resume reviewed by others, and made changes that you feel are desirable, the final draft is not ready until its appearance satisfies you.

■ *Final draft*. Carefully review your final draft before you place it into an envelope (with adequate postage). Include your personal statement if called for.

■ *Update when appropriate*. Set aside a working final copy to update as any new relevant data regarding all aspects of your resume come into being.

Sample resumes

Two different formats using the same data are presented below.

FORMAT 1

Paul C. Rogers

739 West 94th Street
New York, NY 10016
212-571-3067
e-mail: crogers@yahoo.com

OBJECTIVE
To secure a superior residency training appointment in internal medicine, in order to become fully qualified to practice in an urban community.

EDUCATION
M. D., Columbia University, College of Physicians and Surgeons, New York, NY, September 2001–June 2005 (anticipated)

B. S., New York University, New York, NY, September 1997–June 2001, major in biology.

HONORS/AWARDS
Medical School:
    Noland Prize for outstanding achievement during the freshman year
    Class vice-president, sophomore year
    AMSA student representative 2002–2003
Undergraduate:
    Magna cum laude graduate
    Phi Beta Kappa for scholastic achievement
    Alpha Epsilon Delta – Premedical Honors Society

RESEARCH AND PUBLICATIONS
    Fellon, T. S. and P. C. Rogers, Electron microscope observations on annulate lamellae in Mice Ova. *J. Cell Biology* 114: 87–90, 2000.

PROFESSIONAL ORGANIZATIONS
    American Medical Student Association

FOREIGN LANGUAGES
    Spanish (written and spoken)

PERSONAL
    United States citizen
    Health status – excellent

REFERENCES
    Provided on request

FORMAT 2

Paul C. Rogers

Home: **School:**
1470 Westgate Ave.   **739 West 94th Street**
Teaneck, NJ 07666   **New York, NY 10016**
261-833-5876   **212-571-3067**

e-mail: crogers@yahoo.com

OBJECTIVES   To secure a superior residency training appointment in internal medicine, in order to become fully qualified to practice in an urban community.

EDUCATION   M. D., Columbia University, College of Physicians and Surgeons, New York, NY, September 2001–June 2005 (anticipated).
B. S., New York University, New York, NY, September 1997–June 2001, major in biology.

HONORS/AWARDS
   Medical school:
        Noland Prize for outstanding achievement in the freshmen year
        Class vice-president, sophomore year.
        AMSA student representative 2002–2003
   Undergraduate:
        Magna cum laude graduate
        Phi Beta Kappa for scholastic achievement
        Alpha Epsilon Delta – Premedical Honors Society

PUBLICATIONS
        Fellon, T. S. and P. C. Rogers, Electron microscope observation on annulate lamellae in mice ova. *J. Cell Biology*, 114: 87–90, 2000.

MEMBERSHIPS
        American Medical Student Association

FOREIGN LANGUAGES
        Spanish (written and spoken)

PERSONAL
        United States citizen
        Health status – excellent

REFERENCES
        Provided on request

Personal Statement

Personal statement

This is a written exposition of your background, abilities, experience, interests, and potential serving to significantly amplify the contents of your resume. The statement usually should be no longer than a single page.

Purpose

There are several reasons that mandate preparation of a personal statement:

■ It is a standard requirement for many positions, including applying for a residency appointment, as well as for a fellowship.

■ It allows you to elaborate beyond the concise factual information outlined in your resume.

■ It offers you the opportunity to emphasize in greater detail important special assets you may have, relative to the position that you seek.

■ It can make you stand out from other applicants competing for the appointment by making you especially appealing by virtue of your described assets and achievements.

Challenges

Preparing a personal statement can be a trying and time-consuming experience. Thus individuals may procrastinate before undertaking this important task. The reasons for this may be:

- *Innate modesty.* Many people take themselves for granted. They erroneously assume that others have talents greater than theirs. One should recognize that because all individuals come from different backgrounds and life experiences, each person becomes molded into a unique individual, with their own special talents and potential.

- *Self-praise difficulty.* Putting down on paper your own attributes, irrespective of the valid reason for doing so, may for some prove unappealing because it seems to be an exercise in egotism.

- *Comparison impeding.* There is a natural tendency to compare yourself to others in your situation who are also seeking a residency appointment. Those others tend to be individuals like yourself, and it is irrational to view them as being superior to yourself or think that you are not as appealing as a nonexistent idealized candidate.

- *Being deficient.* One may lack knowledge about preparing a personal statement, which impedes sitting down and beginning writing. It is a challenge to plan how best to organize and convey a considerable amount of information in a logical, organized, and prioritized manner about varied aspects of one's life.

- *Starting block.* Many individuals, when gathering information to be used in a statement, may become overwhelmed by how much they would like to include. They may not know where to begin their exposition or what can or should be omitted.

Goals

Several goals need to be set prior to preparing your draft personal statement. These include:

- *Identify needs.* Seek to determine what are the specific attributes that your specialty requires from all prospective candidates for an appointment in your field of choice, (see Part I the Book).

- *Establish an inventory.* It is essential to present assets that will enhance your stature and be especially appealing to program directors. For this reason it is necessary to develop a suitable personal inventory (or expand on the one you use for the resume).

■ *Utilize action words.* Words have an impact, some being more effective than others. Such words are called action words. Samples are:

analyzed	diagnosed	maximized
attained	enhanced	modernized
calculated	formulated	observed
communicated	implemented	prescribed
consulted	initiated	provided
coordinated	integrated	replaced
created	investigated	solved
designed	launched	strengthened

Preparation

The following stepwise guide to preparing a personal statement can facilitate this task for you.

■ *Read samples.* These are shown at the end of this section. They will demonstrate how others have prepared their statements. Consequently, you will gain better insight into how to do so.

After reading then see if

a. You gain a favorable impression about the individual after reading their statement.

b. You secure a mental picture of what type of person is writing the statement.

c. Any special feature of these statements especially caught your attention.

d. The opening paragraph was attractive enough to stimulate and maintain your interest.

e. The approach to presenting vital information had any special meaning for you.

• *Identify personal attributes.* From your reading, note the attributes that the writers are suggesting they have and see how they are presented. Determine if you have comparable attributes that may be relevant to the residency to which you are applying. Note any action words used in the statement that especially impressed you.

• *Traits and skills.* Identify those mentioned in the statements and determine their relevance to you and your personal statement.

• *Prepare first draft.* Prepare a preliminary draft of your personal statement in the form of a series of paragraphs which sequentially reveal your attributes, traits, and skills. Indicate how you are especially suited for the residency position you seek.

• *Draft lead sentences.* Carefully provide each paragraph with an introductory sentence from which the rest flows naturally. Set it aside for a day or so.

• *Develop a second draft.* Put the paragraphs together so that they present a coherent story. Check each sentence to make sure that it does not run on, is consistent with the paragraph's lead-off sentence, and is appropriately positioned.

• *Get feedback.* Have a knowledgeable person (e.g., mentor/advisor) critically review your draft text. Secure opinions as to whether the draft reflects you in the most effective manner. Inquire if you have made the best possible case for yourself in the light of the assets and strengths that you possess.

• *Final draft.* Revise the second draft based on the comments you receive. Incorporate those that you feel merit inclusion. Then carefully check your statement for clarity, accuracy, and completeness as well as for the absence of spelling and grammatical errors.

• *Send off.* Put your personal statement in the same envelope as your final resume copy and make sure that your name is placed at the top of the page (just in case it becomes separated from your resume).

Sample personal statements

SAMPLE 1

It did not come as a surprise to either my family or friends that I decided to become a pediatrician. My desire to work with children emerged even before I entered college, when I became involved in a baby-sitting and youth group working in my church. Further stimulus emerged when I participated in my high school's Special Arts Festival, which was geared to provide educational activities for physically and mentally challenged children. Working as a volunteer with a young Down's syndrome girl, I came to realize the need for patience, perseverance, and the appropriate acceptance of those with limited potential as individuals. The warm response from my client and her determination to achieve the limited goal set was a most inspirational experience for me and it left a profound impact upon me.

Early on as an undergraduate, I enjoyed the intellectual stimulation of my science courses and began seriously considering a career in medicine. I gained deeper insight into this subject by speaking to physicians practicing in different specialties about the nature of their work, problems, and rewards. After gaining direct exposure to some of their activities, as a volunteer at a local hospital, my enthusiasm for the field of medicine increased significantly. Consequently, I enrolled in additional college science courses. I also sought to strengthen my liberal arts background by graduating as a psychology major with a minor in Spanish. Knowledge in both of these fields can obviously prove beneficial in my future career activities.

I sought to extend my college career outside of the classroom through participation in a variety of extracurricular activities. I was elected as a class officer (vice-president) in my junior year and was an active participant in student council activities. Consequently, I became involved in working with school administrators and faculty on several programs. This activity proved very satisfying and made me aware of my responsibilities to further the well-being of the student body. All of these activities helped enhance my communication skills, which proved beneficial as a medical student insofar as establishing patient relationships is concerned.

During the course of my volunteer service at a local Indian reservation, I saw children being brought to the local clinic who were diagnosed as suffering from vitamin deficiencies and preventable infections. I was disturbed by the limited medical care available to these people and their poor standard of housing and of life in general. Nevertheless, the children were playful and happy, singing and dancing, although lacking the affluence of the general society. This experience reinforced my evolving decision to devote my career to improving children's health care.

My success in life thus far is due in large measure to the wholesome upbringing and unwavering support I have received from my parents. They have inculcated in me a strong work ethic and a sense of moral obligation to help those in need. Clearly work as a pediatrician will provide me with the opportunity to achieve these goals.

Currently I am engaged to a fine young man who is working for a master's in social work. We have much in common, with our mutual desires for service-oriented careers (among other things). He has been very understanding regarding my educational commitments and I believe he will prove to be a supportive husband in the years ahead. Our commonality of interests should be self-reinforcing and facilitate our achieving the career goals we set and our ambitions in a rewarding manner.

I believe pediatrics will provide me with fulfillment because it will enable me to heal sick children, educate parents in child care, and provide guidance to both developing youngsters and their caregivers. To work in an atmosphere where there are children has always been meaningful for me. Having to face the wide array of potential pediatric problems presents practitioners with a significant intellectual challenge. It is my sincere hope that my training and experience as a resident will facilitate my becoming fully qualified to meet my obligations, I hope that I will gain exposure to a broad range of patients during my residency. As I move up the ranks during my postgraduate experience,

I look forward to utilizing my teaching skills to assist junior physicians-in-training. I am hopeful that my residency experience will be stimulated by working in an atmosphere of collegiality that will further enhance my professional growth.

SAMPLE 2

I was the first member of my family to enter medical school. I was quite young when I exhibited an especially strong interest in science. Subsequently, this fascination became focused on medicine. Although my road through medical school has proven to be quite challenging, I am firmly convinced that I have made the correct career choice. I am now preparing to embark on a period of specialty training to prepare me to enter the field of family practice.

During college and medical school, I sought to maximize my personal growth and thus fully achieve my potential. My educational experiences contributed extensively to my personal maturation process. My participation in extracurricular and volunteer activities also had a very positive impact on my growth as an individual.

Already as a first-year medical student, I became a volunteer "big brother" to a chronically ill ten-year-old boy. I was matched to this patient suffering from sickle cell anemia by a local Cancer Outreach Society. I spent a considerable amount of my free time at the bedside of this youngster during his extended hospitalization. As I visited him almost daily, our relationship grew close. Developing a rapport with a youngster coming from a different cultural and economic background was quite a challenge, as well as an enlightening experience. My presence also served to help fill a gap in this boy's family life, because his parents were divorced. I came to realize at first hand that often a physician's role may extend beyond that of a healer-comforter to that of a healer-friend.

In my third year, I accepted responsibility for coordinating the work of fifteen volunteers at a very active pediatric clinic serving a local disadvantaged patient population. I developed activities and assigned them to first- and second-year medical students. My responsibilities demanded initiative and leadership skills, as well as a strong commitment to helping people in need.

I make sure to devote some of my limited free time to maintaining my relationships with family and friends, as well as with my girlfriend, who is studying for her MBA. Maintaining these relationships, in spite of my demanding educational commitments, is very important. To sustain family ties I travel, when time permits, to see my parents and siblings. Their emotional and material support and pride in my activities have helped to reinforce my determination to see things through, especially when the going gets tough.

For relaxation, I enjoy camping, as well as rafting and swimming at accessible lakes. I also have applied for an overseas clerkship for one month, to assist a physician practicing in Nigeria, which is dependent on securing the necessary foundation support. This should prove to be an enlightening experience.

My choice of a family practice residency stems from the fact that it is an area that will allow me to make full use of my talents and fulfill my career aspirations to treat the individual in a broader context. I elected to serve two clerkships in this field in order to secure an in-depth appreciation of its characteristics, challenges, and obligations.

In the course of my clerkships, I was engaged in treating both children and adults and frequently helping them solve their problems within a family context. I experienced the satisfaction that can come from building long-lasting personal relationships. This is what is especially appealing to me about the field of family practice.

To achieve my goal, I recognize the need for me to become competent in providing comprehensive health care, including preventive medicine and some psychiatric counseling. This care needs to be provided in a compassionate manner, on both an inpatient and outpatient basis. I also want to develop judgment as to when it is essential for me to call in specialty support in treating my patients.

I am looking forward to the completion of medical school, when I hope to initiate training that will ensure my gaining the exposure and expertise to competently enter private practice. I look forward to working as a resident in a stimulating environment that will further my growth as a person as well as a physician, in order to become fully qualified to practice 21st century medicine.

Glossary

Advanced Positions Residency positions obtained through a matching program at least 18 months before the slot opens.

American Hospital Association A professional organization of U.S. hospitals. It lobbies for and monitors hospitals and has significant input in the setting and enforcement of hospital standards.

American Medical Association An association of physician members that establishes standards of care, monitors legal issues, and lobbies members of Congress on issues of significance to physicians and patients.

American Medical Women's Association An independent organization representing the interests of women physicians and female medical students.

American Osteopathic Association An association of osteopathic physicians that establishes standards of care, monitors legal issues, and lobbies members of Congress on issues important to physicians and patients.

Association of American Medical Colleges An association of U.S. and Canadian medical schools that accredits schools in the United States, Canada, and Puerto Rico.

Audition Electives Senior clerkships taken to demonstrate your special interest and abilities to prospective residency programs.

Canadian Residency Matching Service The Canadian equivalent of the NRMP Match.

Categorical Intern A first-year residency position in internal medicine or general surgery designed for those who plan to complete a residency in either of these two fields.

Clerkship Structured clinical education provided to medical students, usually during their third and fourth years.

Clinical Research Fellow A medical school graduate engaged primarily in research associated with patient care.

Clinical Years This period, usually refers to the third or fourth year of medical school, when students rotate through the various clinical services.

Couples Match A method that allows couples to rank their residency choices in the NRMP Match so that they can ensure that they will match only with program pairs that allow them to remain in the same geographic area.

Educational Commission for Foreign Medical Graduates A nonprofit foundation sponsored by standard-setting associations and agencies to monitor competency of foreign medical graduates.

Electronic Residency Application Service A method used by prospective residents to submit their application. It is being introduced gradually, specialty by specialty.

Exchange-Visitor International Medical Graduates The largest subset of FNIMGs applying for residency slots.

Externship A clinical rotation taken at a different location than your primary training site.

Federation Licensing Examination A discontinued medical licensing examination.

Federation of State Medical Boards of the United States An organization that maintains addresses and telephone numbers of individual medical licensing authorities. It responds to inquiries regarding medical licensure.

Fellow An academic term referring to someone engaged in postgraduate training following completion of a residency program. It may be used for experienced scholars engaged in research, writing, or teaching.

Foreign Medical Graduate Examination An examination for certification that is no longer given.

Foreign-National International Medical Graduate A non-U.S. citizen whose medical degree was conferred by a medical school located outside the United States, Canada, or Puerto Rico.

Greenbook The AMA-produced *Graduate Medical Education Directory*. This book lists most residency and fellowship programs.

Health Maintenance Organization A managed care plan whose enrollees are eligible for medical treatment that is prepaid through monthly premiums. HMO physicians are paid set salaries rather than collecting patient fees.

Health Professions Scholarship Program Military-sponsored scholarships for medical students.

Independent Applicants Anyone enrolled in the NRMP Match who is neither a current student nor a graduate of an LCME-approved medical school.

Individual Provider Association The group contracting with independent physicians to provide services to an HMO's patients.

Intern The historical term for individuals in their first postgraduate year of training.

Intern Registration Program A matching program for obtaining AOA-approved internships.

International Medical Graduate A foreign national educated at a U.S., a Canadian, or an accredited Puerto Rican medical or school, a foreign national who trains outside the United States, Canada, or an accredited Puerto Rican medical school, or a U.S. or Canadian citizen who trains in a foreign medical school and then returns to the United States or Puerto Rico or Canada.

Liason Committee on Medical Education This organization accredits U.S., Canadian, and some Puerto Rican medical schools. (Foreign-national graduates of these schools do not have to obtain an ECFMG certificate to continue training in the United States.)

License A state's permission to practice medicine within its confines. Each state has its own licensure requirements.

Match Day The day on which residency applicants participating in the NRMP or AOA matches find out with which program they have matched.

Matching Programs One of the various methods by which medical students or physicians obtain a position for residency or fellowship training.

Mentor The faculty member who helps guide you through medical school and usually through the residency application process.

Moonlighting Supplementary clinical work done by residents for pay, usually away from the institution where they are affiliated. It is performed on off days or in off hours.

National Board of Medical Examiners The organization that develops national physician licensing examinations (including the USMLE).

National Board of Osteopathic Medical Examiners An organization that gives an alternative licensing examination for osteopathic physicians. (This examination is not widely accepted by licensing bodies.)

National Residency Matching Program A national program to match prospective residents with accredited U.S. postgraduate specialty training programs.

NBME Examination A licensing examination that is no longer given.

Objective Structured Clinical Examination A patient-simulation examination used to test medical students and international medical graduates.

Participating Institution One part of a multi-institutional graduate education program.

Postgraduate Year 1 The internship year, otherwise known as the first year of residency.

Preclinical Years The period of medical school preceding clinical rotations, which commonly occurs in the first two years of medical school.

Preferred Provider Organization A collection of hospitals or physicians that contract to provide comprehensive health coverage at a competitive rate.

Preliminary Intern First-year positions in internal medicine or general surgery designed for those who are not focused on completing a residency in that specialty. Such interns either are undecided about their career plans or are going into another field that requires prior clinical training.

Program The designation used for both a place and a curriculum to train residents.

Rank Order List The program rankings that each applicant submits and the applicant rankings each residency program submits to the matching program.

Rank Order List Input Code The code required for each applicant to enter a Rank Order List in the computer system for the NRPM Match.

Research Scholar A term used for an individual holding an M.D. degree who is in a research training program in which no patient contact is involved.

Resume Known also as a curriculum vitae or C.V., it briefly summarizes a person's accomplishments from various perspectives.

Shared-Schedule Position One residency position shared by two individuals for their mutual benefit.

Special Purpose Examination A one-day examination to test the knowledge base of physicians who seek licensure in a new state or relicensure in the same state at least five years after graduation from medical school.

Sponsoring Institution The main hospital or clinic responsible for a residency training program, which often is also the primary training site.

Subinternship A clinical rotation that gives a senior medical student added clinical responsibility when dealing with patients.

Transitional Internship Also called a "rotating internship," it allows interns to rotate through a variety of clinical services, usually in most of the same specialties they went through during their third-year clerkships. This facilitates their making a more realistic decision regarding their specialty choice.

Unmatched Day The day before Match Day when those who fail to match with a residency program begin an extremly intense effort to secure a position with a program that still has an opening.

Bibliography

Belkin, L. *First Do No Harm*, Simon & Schuster, New York, 1993.

Bing-You, R. *The Residency Survival Manual: Tools and Tips to Help You Make It through Residency*, Morgan Bay, Yarmouth, ME, 2004.

Bullimore, D. W. *Study Skills for Tomorrow's Doctors*, W. B. Saunders, London, 1998.

Cant, S., and Sharma, V. *Complementary and Alternative Medicine: Knowledge in Practice*, New York University Press, New York, 1997.

Cassell, E. *The Nature of Primary Care Medicine*, Oxford University Press, New York, 1998.

Castleman, M. *Nature's Cures*, Rodale Press, New York, 1996.

Chin, E. *This Side of Doctoring: Reflections from Women in Medicine*, Sage, Thousand Oaks, CA, 2003.

Coles, R. *The Call of Service*, Houghton Mifflin, New York, 1995.

Coombs, R. H. *Surviving Medical School*, Sage, Thousand Oaks, CA, 1998.

Dessi, S. P. *101 Biggest Mistakes 3rd Year Medical Students Make: And How to Avoid Them*, Mathew Medical Books, New York, 2002.

Duncan, D. *Residents: The Perils and Promise of Educating Young Doctors*, Scribners, New York, 1986.

English, D. C. *Bioethics: A Clinical Guide for Medical School*, Norton, New York, 1993.

Freeman, B. *The Ultimate Guide to Choosing a Medical Specialty*, McGraw–Hill, New York, 2004.

Garrison, H. *History of Medicine*, 4th ed., W. B. Saunders, Philadelphia, 2000.

Gawan, E. A. *Complications: A Surgeon's Notes on an Imperfect Science*, Metropolitan Books, New York, 2004.

Giza, E. *Hints for Success in Medical School and the Match*, J & S, Alexandria, VA, 2000.

Hammad, M. *Blackwell's Survival for Interns*, Blackwell Science, Malden, MA, 2002.

Heymann, J. *Equal Partners: A Physician's Call for a New Spirit of Medicine*, Little Brown, Boston, 1995.

Hilfiker, D. *Not All of Us Are Saints*, Hill and Wang, New York, 1995.

Hoffmeir, P., and Bonner, J. *From Residency to Reality*, McGraw–Hill, New York, 1990.

Kan, L. *A Medical Student's Guide to Strolling through the Match, or What, Where, When, Why & How of Residency Selection*, American Academy of Family Physicians, Lewood, KS, 2002.

Klein, K. *Getting Better: A Medical Student's Story*, Little Brown, Boston, 1980.

Ko, K. *Survival Bible for Women in Medicine*, Parthenon Publication Group, New York, 1998.

Kushner, T. R., and Thomsama, D. C. *Ward Ethics: Dilemmas for Medical Students and Doctors in Training*, Cambridge University Press, New York, 2001.

Lantos, J. *Do We Still Need Doctors?* Rutledge, New York, 1997.

Le, T., et al. *First Aid for the Wards*, 2nd ed., McGraw-Hill, New York, 1998.

Le, T., et al. *First Aid for the Match*, 2nd ed., McGraw-Hill, New York, 2000.

Marion, R. *Learning to Play God*, Fawcett, New York, 1993.

Marion, R. *Rotations: The Twelve Months of Intern Life*, HarperCollins, New York, 1997.

Marshall, S. A., and Ruedy, J. *On Call: Principles and Protocols*, 3rd ed., W. B. Saunders, Philadelphia, 2000.

Miller, L. T., and Donowitz, L. G. *Medical Students' Guide to Successful Residency Matching*, Lippincott, Williams & Wilkins, Philadelphia, 2001.

Peterkin, A. D. *Staying Human during Residency Training*, 2nd ed., Toronto University Press, Toronto, 1998.

Rafferty, F. W., and Mckinlay, J. B. (eds.). *The Changing Medical Profession*, Oxford University Press, New York, 1993.

Ramshell, M. (ed). *First Year as a Doctor: Real World Stories from America's M.D.s*, Walker, New York, 1995.

Retaguiz, A., et al. *Mastering the Objective Structural Clinical Examination (OSCE) and the Clinical Skills Assessment (CSA)*, McGraw-Hill, New York, 1999.

Rothman, E. *White Coat: Becoming a Doctor at Harvard Medical School*, Morrow, New York, 1999.

Seltzer, R. *Down from Troy: A Doctor Comes of Age*, Morrow, New York, 1993.

Silver, J. K. *The Business of Medicine*, Hanley & Belfus, Inc., and Elsevier, Philadelphia, 1998.

Smith, R. P. *From Medical School to Residency: How to Compete Successfully in the Residency Match Program* (with CD-ROM), Springer, New York, 2000.

Smith, R. P., and Edward, M. J. A. *The Internet for Physicians*, Springer, New York, 1997.

Tao L., et al., *First Aid for the Match: Insider Advice from Students and Residency Directors*, 3rd ed., McGraw-Hill, New York, 2004.

Transue, E. R. *On Call: A Doctor's Days and Nights in Residency*, St. Martin Press, New York, 2004.

Wischnitzer, S. *Survival Guide for Medical Students*, Hanley & Belfus, Elsevier, Philadelphia, 2001.

Index

Printed in the United States
By Bookmasters